Date Due

Home
Medical
Encyclopedia

BY PAUL KÜHNE, M.D.

Translated from the German
by JEAN CUNNINGHAM

Adapted for American Readers
from *Medicine for the Layman*
with an Introduction
by DONALD G. COOLEY

Newly revised

FAWCETT CREST • NEW YORK

A Fawcett Crest Book

Published by Ballantine Books

© 1960, 1976 CBS Publiactions, The Consumer Publishing Division of CBS, Inc. All Rights Reserved.

ISBN 0-449-20459-6

This edition published by arrangement with
Faber and Faber Limited

The English translation of HOME MEDICAL ENCYCLO-PEDIA was originally published by Faber and Faber Limited under the title MEDICINE FOR THE LAYMAN.

Printed in Canada

First Fawcett Crest Edition: April 1968
First Ballantine Books Edition: April 1983
Second Printing: April 1984

Contents

Introduction

Great advances in medicine make it more necessary than ever before for intelligent people to know something of how the marvelous mechanisms of the human body work in health and disease. The art and science of medicine has been almost unrecognizably transformed in the past quarter century by the advent of "wonder drugs" which control many hitherto uncontrollable diseases, by operations which no surgeon would have dreamed of attempting a decade ago, by better understanding of the hidden and omnipotent chemical processes of life, by ever-accelerating increase in research in universities, institutions and pharmaceutical laboratories at a cost of several hundred millions of dollars every year.

Almost daily our newspapers and journals report new advances in the form of drugs, techniques, and more exact understanding of factors which underlie heart disease, high blood-pressure, cancer, ulcers, the common cold and a host of other common and uncommon afflictions of mankind. Some understanding of the foundations of knowledge upon which such advances rest is more and more a requisite of healthful living in this modern world.

Such understanding does not lead intelligent persons to self-treatment of disease—rather the contrary. The very potency and effectiveness of modern treatments demands the utmost medical wisdom in administering them. Delay in seeking the help of a competent physician when symptoms present themselves may result in senseless tragedy, and the informed person does not wait until it is too late.

Such understanding is also of great value in helping your doctor to help you. It is difficult for a physician to give his best if his patient knows so little of the purposes of common medical procedures and tests that he harbors irrational fears and misconceptions, cannot cooperate to his own advantage, and perhaps is frightened by the mystery of the unknown.

7

Before medicine became a science in modern times, it was a form of magic involving strange—and generally useless—potions and mysterious "secrets" which the practitioner cannily kept to himself. There was a tradition that the public should be given as little information as possible about the practice of medicine—a tradition which had its roots in the unhappy fact that there was very little information to give.

That tradition has passed. Only quacks profess to have secret medicines today. There are no secrets in modern medicine and no magic beyond that worked by drugs or measures whose composition and action are well-known to all physicians. Responsible members of the medical profession today consider an alerted, informed and intelligent public to be an indispensable asset in the conquest of disease and in pushing forward the frontiers of medical knowledge.

In this book Dr. Paul Kühne succeeds admirably in communicating the basic knowledge which every physician would wish his patients to have. Dr. Kühne's style is not only lucid but delightfully informal; it is as if you were chatting at leisure with an authority who had all the time in the world to answer your questions and a warm desire to do so. The book does much more than answer questions which may be of concern to you. It gives a rich background of information about the workings of your body and mind, about the complexities of health and disease, which cannot help but be of long-lasting importance to you as you make the most of your life day by day. In addition to listing the most recent developments in medicine's fight against disease, this book in its American edition also presents the latest approved techniques for first aid, including artificial resuscitation.

DONALD G. COOLEY

1. The Human Being

THE RELATIONSHIP BETWEEN BODY AND SOUL

A body without a mind is a lifeless bit of flesh and quite dead. It is the thing that lives, the functioning of the body and not its mere existence that makes us differ so basically from the inanimate things around us, and therefore we cannot understand the human being until we have discovered first the meaning of the word "mind."

Perhaps the simplest description of the mind is to picture it as being built around a central core, the driving force. This driving force behind our whole being is, in fact, our instincts of hunger, love, and self-preservation, and our struggle against death. Around this central core we may draw—

The first circle which we call love in its basic sense. The urge to live on through one's children. It means protection, help and care for our blood relations whom we identify to a certain extent with ourselves. They are, as the saying goes, our own flesh and blood. They are nearer to us than—

The second circle, to which, however, we ourselves still belong. This group involves in its widest sense the people of our own country, but it also has a narrow sense meaning our colleagues at work with whom we feel a certain bond, and our friends. During the war everyone experienced this feeling of belonging to his company, his platoon or his particular group. In this way we give up part of ourselves to a greater entity, to a common cause and to a common enjoyment. But our energies reach out further than our own nation. We all feel within us as it were—

The third circle—membership of the whole human race. We are all proud of the achievements of our race and we are all troubled by any failing in the political organization of our society. We are all passionately interested in the fate

9

of mankind. We are all equally horrified by the tales which forecast the decline of the race or its ultimate extinction by a world catastrophe. We tremble at the thought as if it were a matter of life and death to us ourselves.

These feelings have inclined men towards religion and from this springs the feeling of morality of philosophical man. Out of this feeling we order our small inner world.

From this psychological picture it is easy to see that it is perfectly possible to consider men as children of nature without damaging the religious viewpoint. It is only necessary to remember that mind, as a technical term, is something quite different from the living soul of religious teaching. To make this clear: one would not credit the immortal soul with a feeling of hunger, and yet the hunger instinct is definitely an important mental factor. We must try to make this distinction clear so that everybody can understand it and talk about the mind rather than the soul as this might otherwise lead to a misunderstanding.

The controversies of our fathers and grandfathers have become outmoded and we should forget them. It is not a question of proving to the theologians and priests that their conception of the world is wrong. That has been attempted time after time by the materialistic scientists and the controversy has been violent. All this was a senseless waste of time and originated because they had false conceptions and tried to understand the religious conception of the word "soul" with the eyes of the scientist, which was impossible. In point of fact, both these sciences are dealing with two quite separate subjects. The priest is not concerned with medical aspects of the mind such as loss of appetite and hunger, and the scientist is not interested in the immortal part of the soul. The person who has really grasped this difference has won a great victory for his own mental well-being, and a conflict which has worried him incessantly will disappear. This is true also for people who do not consciously think about these things and have rejected them as being of no significance. These people too, in their youth, had once to think about such differences, but they came to no conclusion and the problem remained unsolved. They refused to resolve the conflict, and so it was gradually pushed into the background by the responsibilities of adult life. But we know today that such unresolved conflicts, even if we are unaware of them, can be detrimental to our whole well-being. They gnaw constantly at our innermost beings and they constitute a perpetual source of irritation, just as a foreign body or splinter does to the body.

We have lingered over the relationship between science and religion because it is important that the reader shall understand that the two are not in conflict. Unresolved conflict can disturb our mental health. We, like every modern doctor, shall soon discover that bodily health is greatly influenced by our mental health.

DEVELOPMENT

It is well known that we are made very like the higher animals. Everyone who eats a roast beef liver knows that he too has a liver in his abdomen. He usually knows as well that this liver can be very troublesome when he is ill. We also know, even if we do not like to admit it, that there is a great similarity in mental excitement, in the scientific sense, please note, between us and the higher animals. They too are hungry when they haven't eaten, and they also feel the same biological urge to mate which we in our complex human world call love. Animals too are drawn to their own kind.

In just the same way, everyone knows that there are animals which are like us physically and mentally and others which do not resemble us so closely. We also know that we of the human race belong to the most highly developed group, the mammals. In common with whales, elephants and mice, we differ from snakes, crocodiles, birds, fish, crabs and worms. This similarity in the mammal group goes so far that we can use important physical substances from the bodies of these other mammals as medicines for ourselves. For instance insulin is extracted from the pancreas of whales and used. This insulin is chemically identical with that which our own pancreas produces, and if our pancreas breaks down, as in the case of a diabetic person who cannot produce his own insulin, we can make good the deficiency by taking insulin from another mammal.

This is not all, however. Our membership of this animal world is even more closely knit. For instance, if we observe the development of a living creature in its mother's womb we can watch the stages of development of this growing embryo. In their early stages of development the organs are just the same as those found in the most primitive animals. We have this in common with all other mammals.

In this connection it would not be wrong to assume that we, in common with this large group of higher animals, have evolved in the course of millions of years from more primitive forms of life. There is no doubt that our forebears at one time lived in water because all mammals bear the trace in their embryonic development of gills. In an even earlier embryo stage we find other forms of primitive life; for instance, there is a stage when the embryo is like a stomach tube, a primitive creature which only consists of a tube with two openings, something like a worm. Before that, in another stage, the embryo is only like a bag with a mouth. Now it corresponds to the sea anemone that takes in nourishment through the opening and then ejects the residue through the same hole. Both masculine and feminine forms occur in what are quite primitive forms of animal life.

It Was Not the Monkey

As you can see, we are not alone. Our human race evolved from primitive beginnings which we certainly shared with the whale, ox and monkey. I might add at once that the controversial subject as to whether man was descended from the ape, which has been the cause of many coarse jokes, has been as completely forgotten as the controversy about the soul of the rainworm. Man is not descended from the ape, but both man and ape are descended from a more primitive form of life, from a creature which was much more stupid than man and monkey put together. The higher apes are far more akin to us in intelligence than are other animals. The build of their bodies too is much more like ours than an ox; but no one can maintain that man descends from chimpanzees or gorillas. As far as anything is certain, we can say with confidence that the gorillas of today and we human beings of all types have evolved in our various ways from one common four-legged mammal form. As we know, the monkeys have come off worse, at least so we think. We have asserted ourselves to rule the world, while they are still shy, timid things that live in the jungle.

This opinion has been confirmed by the skulls which have been found in all parts of the world. Remains of living creatures have been found which were doubtless man in his primitive form because the brain was far less developed than ours is today. We can say with some certainty that these primitive people—we don't know when the higher apes broke away from this line of descent—were able to walk upright. By and large they must have been ape-like people.

Being able to walk upright may be a fairly recent achievement, for our human vertebral column is not well adapted to carrying heavy loads in the upright position. Only humans suffer from that very trying and prevalent complaint—a misplaced vertebral disc. The vertebral column is so constructed that it makes an ideal peg for the soft parts and limbs of four-legged animals. Since man insists on walking on his hind legs his vertebral column has to bear the burden of the body vertically, although it was not designed for this. It is therefore understandable that the soft cartilaginous discs between the joints of the vertebrae become painful if they are repeatedly jarred.

REASONING MAN

Any attempt to pursue the interesting subject of the development of reason in man must prove abortive since nothing is really known about it. In any case it does not concern us because we are supposed to be dealing with present-day man in health and sickness. At any rate we can definitely assume that man has not existed since the beginning of the world in his present form. He has, in common with the higher animals, evolved from a primitive form of life. Our forbears, after a series of physical and mental changes, gave up living in water and went on land, where they developed from a four-legged running animal into ape-like primitive man able to walk upright. Then they discovered how to speak and after a final stage of development eventually became man as we know him today.

This human species, called *homo sapiens* by the zoologists, has definitely been in existence in his present form for one to two hundred thousand years. Any evolution which has taken place since then is just mental development. There appear to have been no vital changes in the body or in our basic instincts during this time. The whole difference between a primitive savage and a modern man is purely cultural: the modern man is considered more educated. The size of their brains is the same. The brain is the central organ guiding all mental and physical functions and one can assess the relative intelligence of the various species from the size of the brain in proportion to the whole body, at any rate among different animal species.

So we are confronted with the surprising fact that the mind has had a decisive influence on human development. Between the primitive man and people of today there is, in all probability, no further structural development of either the body or the brain. Right down in the depths of our innermost being there is probably no difference. The proof of this today is the fact that so many aborigines have been Europeanized after being sent to America as slaves and they are now just as civilized as white Americans who emigrated from Europe with a much higher standard of culture. All that was needed was adaptation to the prevailing conditions of life. The step from the African jungle to a European or American city can be completed in a generation.

The development of humanity as a whole, which had to civilize itself as it were, was much more laborious. Unlike the aborigines of today, it had no example to follow. It had to create better conditions of living and adapt itself to them by trial and error. By conditions of living we mean housing, building of streets, organization of states and towns and, above all, high moral values.

EARLY LIFE

There is a mysterious group of living creatures which it goes against the grain to have to call a being at all. This is the most primitive form of life. The whole body of these beings is composed of a single large molecule of protein. A molecule is the elementary part of every stone, every substance, every tree and every bit of matter. There are living creatures which can be isolated chemically and preserved as powder in bottles. If one dissolves them again and gives them the necessary foodstuffs and living conditions, they multiply—that is to say, these chemical molecules live and create out of themselves new and similar molecules. At one stage they are living beings, and at another, dead pieces of matter which the chemists work on. As I have said, one is reluctant to use the words living being for this chemical substance. One would feel more inclined to describe it as a substance capable of multiplying.

We shall encounter living substances of this kind when we deal with human infectious diseases. We know of such molecules which have an individual life as invisible parasites on plants, animals or people. They are known as viruses and the diseases which they cause are known as virus diseases. We know hardly anything about their life force, but we may assume that it is confined to chemical stimuli for which there is only one answer by the virus, that is seizing groups of atoms and bits of other molecules to collect them round themselves, thus forming a new and similar molecule. The substance has enlarged itself only to divide itself again. A primitive form of birth has taken place, for there is only one sex among virus bodies. They grow and divide until all foodstuffs for this multiplying process have been exhausted and the living molecules revert to their condition of lifeless matter. To put it in human terms, with a virus, hunger and love are synonymous.

If anyone wants to be really bemused, he can interest himself in the size of such a living being. The millionth part of a gram of the virus substance which, for instance, causes the "mosaic disease" of tobacco plants, contains approximately 100 billion virus molecules. That is to say, in a millionth part of a gram of this substance are contained twenty-five times as many virus creatures or living beings as there are human beings on the earth. If one wants to write down the number of viruses which altogether weigh a gram, it looks like this:—

$$100\ 000\ 000\ 000\ 000\ 000\ 000$$

This so-called living creature is about a forty-thousandth of a millimeter long. It cannot move independently and exists in a world which we cannot visualize—that is to say, in the gaps of firm matter. It is pushed hither and thither by the molecules of other substances which penetrate every space and which are in a constant state of agitation. When we diagnose a virus disease, we mean that these viruses are multiplying in the human body. The virus molecules form out of themselves new molecules and this happens most quickly whereever food conditions are most favourable. For instance, the virus substance might wander along a definite nerve route in the body, just because food conditions were best for that particular virus in nerve tissue.

THE FIRST ONE-CELLED CREATURES

There are virus bodies of sizes which extend upward in an unbroken sequence which merges imperceptibly into that of the smallest one-celled living creatures which we call bacteria. We all know something about bacteria, which we often call "germs." Not all bacteria are harmful. Most of them are harmless, and exist outside animal bodies; some of them are very useful to us. There are, for instance, numerous kinds of bacteria which do nothing but transform milk into a variety of delicious cheeses. There are also one-celled yeast species which make most delectable wines out of simple grape juice.

While considering the size of these things, let the tubercle bacillus serve as an example. This dangerous beast is thirty thousand times as heavy as a small virus, and is rod-shaped. Even then, it is not much more than a thousandth part of a millimeter long. One gram of bacteria would consist of more than three million of these living things, which are, as you see, extremely small.

Virus bodies are not visible under the high powers of ordinary microscopes, but bacteria are. We can therefore actually see the cell body of a bacillus, and so do not fear to use the term living creature in relation to it. The body of a single bacillus is made up of countless molecules bound together into the visible structure of the cell body. Some bacteria have little whip-like tails with which they propel themselves forwards, but others have no means of locomotion.

We know very little about the moving force behind bacterial life—that thing which makes them different from dead matter. We do know that they have a complicated metabolism, and that they absorb food fast and grow very quickly, and multiply at the same time. They multiply by splitting into two: so do virus molecules. Bacteria are not divided into two sexes as are higher plants and animals. Bacteria seem to have only one urge or instinct, and this is a blind desire to take in the necessary foodstuffs from the liquid world in which they exist, and build them into their own bodies. Then, when they have grown sufficiently large, they divide into two halves. The process goes on continually until all available foodstuffs have been used up; at that point, the life of the bacterial colony in that place is at an end.

It is difficult to say how long any bacillus lives. The better the life of the organism, the faster it grows, and the sooner it divides into two or more parts. Simple chemical stimuli are probably responsible for virus multiplication, but the process is more complicated in the case of bacteria. First, foodstuffs entering the cell have to be passed on in the interior of the cell body until they reach the appropriate centres of growth. Later, when division begins, commands must travel from one part of the cell to another, organizing this. This is particularly apparent in those species of bacteria which divide, not into two, but into four parts. Some primitive form of signalling must pass through the vast numbers of chemical molecules which make up the bacterial cell. In a sense, this primitive form of signalling which we believe to exist inside the bacterial cell, corresponds to the much more elaborate nervous and chemical methods of signalling so well developed in our own bodies.

ONE-CELLED ANIMALS

Bacteria are not the only one-celled living creatures. There are minute little animals which consist of a single cell. Incidentally these were the first microscopic living creatures which Leeuwenhoek discovered when he invented the microscope three hundred years ago. They are called infusoria, because they are always to be found when one makes an infusion by pouring water on grasses or hay. In their dry form the infusoria cling to the stalks of plants, but they cannot survive long in dry air. These infusoria—some of you may have heard of the name *slipper-animalcule*—are proper animals even though they only consist of a single cell. Our body is built up of countless millions of rather similar cells. In a single drop of human blood, in one cubic millimeter, there are five million cells. The infusoria, unlike blood cells, have orifices in their cell wall through which they take in food and pass out undigested remains, and, moreover, they can move. They can flee and escape from excessive heat, from chemicals which get into the water, and from light. We are already well acquainted with the driving force in these infusoria. We can use our own expression "flee" when describing their actions.

Of course these animals cannot think. They have no consciousness with which to feel pain, but they do react to harmful stimuli, as, for instance, to a light that is too bright; they instinctively run away into the dark. There is no doubt that they can see. It is true that they cannot recognize definite objects, but they can distinguish between light and dark, and all this is done, one must not forget it, by a single minute solitary cell. But light is not the only thing to which the one-celled creatures are sensitive. They are also sensitive to smell and taste. They can distinguish between heat and cold and they react to pressure. This feeling for pressure is the first step towards hearing, for sound waves are waves of pressure.

But there is an important new phenomenon found among these one-celled creatures, protozoa (the infusoria are only a sub-species of this whole group of creatures). They usually multiply by fission, or dividing as it is called, but some of the protozoa show the beginnings of sex development. In some cases two individuals completely similar in appearance fuse, and then divide into four or more progeny. In other cases there is an obvious difference between the male and female cells. So these one-celled creatures must already have a sexual power of attraction which probably makes itself effective through a chemical sense. The partners wanting to mate recognize each other with the precursor of what we describe as smell and taste.

The mental aspect of these one-celled animals is quite simple. Their reaction, for instance, to light of a certain brightness is immediate flight, but they are immediately attracted to a pleasantly warm temperature. One can see that these two stimuli might cause conflict of feelings, but the creature always takes the line of least resistance. Driven away from the bright light although attracted by its heat, it will move about in a place which is neither too cold nor too bright.

So, it is completely dominated by the world in which it lives, but its simple automatic reactions to stimuli are such that it always finds for itself the best possible living conditions.

If it has a mind, then that mind deals solely with the problem of self-adaptation to its surroundings. This is a formula which we should bear in mind, if we are to understand life.

MANY-CELLED ANIMALS

The relationship between all living creatures is so close that despite this excursion into ancient evolutionary history, we have not lost sight of our prime objective, which is the understanding of ourselves. On the contrary, that which we have in common with primitive animals will help us later to recognize and understand clearly what is really human and exceptional in us.

The road from the one-celled animal to man is not as long drawn out as one might imagine. Almost all our mental abilities were in evidence in embryonic form in the unicellular organisms. It is perhaps sufficient to say that the simple reactions to stimuli like light, heat, pressure and sound are described as reflexes in many-celled animals.

We humans, too, have automatic reflexes. We know that when we go to the doctor and he hits us with his little hammer on the tendon below the kneecap, the leg shoots forward. No thought or consciousness is involved. The leg just does it automatically. That is a reflex. A stimulus is transmitted to the muscles (or another organ) via the nerves and so it happens. The leg shoots forward in this case, or in other examples, there is a flow of saliva, the stomach is excited, etc.

The ability to smell, to taste, to see, to feel heat, to hear and to feel pressure which are all combined in the minute cell body of the one-celled creature have each distributed themselves to specialized cells in the case of the many-celled animal. Originally there was a spout which was sensitive to light in the skin of the body. That then became an eye which was able to distinguish light more clearly and then one could actually see objects.

With the development of the senses the number of stimuli to be taken into account grew beyond all proportion. The many-celled creature had to find in its central organ—later called the brain—the line of least resistance between the many kinds of reflexes. All bodily and organic activity of the many-celled body had to be co-ordinated and adapted to the influences of the outside world.

A first attempt to evade the "torture" of this choice is shown in the instincts of primitive animals—for instance, ants, bees and species of wasps. They developed linked reflex movements. If, for example, a mated wasp catches sight of a particular kind of caterpillar it pounces on it, stings it in a certain place and lays its eggs there (the young are hatched in the dying body of the caterpillar). Nothing can stop this happening, for it is an instinct.

The whole scheme of behavior is unchangeable and innate. It takes place in the animal like a film-strip which has been made by its forbears and shows the same series of pictures generation after generation.

Unchangeable instincts are no longer found among the most highly developed animals. In all youthful mammals we find a time or a period in which they work out through play some of their later activities. So their instincts lose their fixed patterns, and are cut short so that the driving force may be more easily adapted to a suitable channel.

It is the same with human beings. We, however, can be trained to act by reflexes. For instance, we react promptly and instinctively to certain words of command just as our knee shoots out when it is hit with the doctor's hammer. But there is one great difference. There is something which only we human beings possess. It has never been achieved by any animal and it is something which makes our own mental achievements far more complex and more complete. This is our human language. The animal answers to definite sensory stimulus unconsciously. For instance, the furious barking of another dog causes the dog who is barked at to respond automatically with equally furious barking.

Our language and all it involves makes our reactions much more varied and complex. We can react to a letter or communication or a story just as we do to a sensory stimulus. We can fly into a rage about a letter just as a dog might should you pinch his tail. We react to words and their meaning just as an animal reacts to sensory stimuli. We possess a second system of signals and one connected with the meaning of things with which we can adapt ourselves most completely to the demands of our environment.

That is briefly the history of the mind among the creatures of the earth. We have seen that both the innermost circles, shown in the first picture of the mind, were already in existence in embryonic forms in the one-celled creature hundreds of millions of years ago. We must add that with animals living in herds, the instincts of the third circle, that is the herd instinct and the feeling of belonging together, developed with the fighting or the fleeing group.

REVOLT AGAINST THE LAWS OF NATURE

The development of the mind is a story of revolt against the laws of lifeless nature. The law says, for example, that bodies take on the temperature of whatever surrounds them. But the higher living creatures refute the law. A temperature of 98.6 degrees Fahrenheit suits them better as a constant temperature for their bodies and they maintain this temperature independently of the fluctuations in temperature of the earth and air. This has great advantages as chemical and physical processes take place more rapidly in a high temperature. All life processes behave in the same way as chemical processes, which means that when the temperature goes up 50 degrees Fahrenheit they take place two or three times as quickly. Species with a constant body temperature have made themselves independent of the outside temperature and are therefore in a position to dictate the speed and tempo of their own life. By contrast, the temperature of lower animals is governed by their surroundings. They move more quickly in the warm sunshine than in the shade, and when there is a frost they cannot move at all.

These attempts at independence have their own revolutionary history. Our first example, one's own body temperature, is a very late acquisition and the birds and the mammals were the first to achieve it.

A much earlier bid for independence was that of self-government over the salt content of the animal body. The earliest creatures used to bathe their cells with a liquid which was very similar to blood and the salt content of this liquid was equivalent to that of the sea. Their blood was just as salty as the seawater in which they swam. This was inconvenient for the development of more sensitive and delicately functioning cells but it was difficult to do anything about it. If one has a skin consisting of a thin membrane and there is a greater concentration of salt inside than outside, an enormous difference in osmotic pressure results, and one swells up.

For example, if one throws human blood corpuscles into a solution which contains only half the amount of salt as that in the blood, they burst. The higher quantity of salt attracts water through the partition wall and the result is that the cells are exploded by the water pressure from inside. So at one time living creatures were not only a prey to environmental temperatures but also to the environmental amounts of salt.

Now with the help of a more perfectly functioning kidney and an impermeable skin it has become possible to escape from this great physical inconvenience of the laws of nature. The flowing blood is constantly filtered in the most careful way in the kidney, so that it always contains the correct and same concentration of salt. With the higher living creatures these inner physical processes are regulated with the utmost precision. Our blood is practically independent of the kind and quantity of salts which are taken in with food. Anyone who eats a lot of table-salt knows that he will get thirsty, and that his kidney alone cannot correct for it. His thirst compels him to dilute the salt in the way demanded by his body.

And so in the course of their development living creatures have made themselves more and more independent of surrounding nature. They have learned to regulate the salt content of their body. They have learned to live in the dry air and to protect themselves from death by "drying up." They have learned to make themselves independent of the surrounding temperature. All this has necessitated an increasing number of new and more complex mechanisms in their body which help them in their struggle for independence of their environment.

MIND AND BODY

Our body emerged from its earliest form and finally became as it is today. Its development we have described in the previous pages. We have inherited from our earliest ancestors the constantly developing driving forces of the mind. This forms the foundation of our higher human existence. Superimposed on this foundation of instincts we have developed human language, which is the basis of our thought, our consciousness, and the alertness of our mind; through it we have learned to recognize and understand the highest values. Good health, as the ancients knew, is a necessary foundation for a well-functioning mind. The Romans used to say "Mens sana in corpore sano." We could translate it thus: Only in a healthy body can a completely healthy mind live. But one can also interpret the saying this way: that a healthy mind can itself compel a healthy physical foundation. Probably both interpretations of the proverb are equally correct, and both together make the truth.

Some readers may deny this. They will maintain that there have been geniuses who had a weak constitution and who were always ill. If, however, one regards the matter more closely, one will find that the majority of these people had an extraordinarily tough will to live and by sheer determination overcame their physical weaknesses. Of course it is a different matter with geniuses who failed because of the backwardness of their times and whose achievements were not recognized until many centuries later. With such people, there is a sudden collapse or breakdown which leads to illness or general ill health. They have failed in their struggle. The backwardness of their times has got the better of them. The contradiction between their conviction that they are right and the lack of outward success undermines their mental health and thus paves the way for a physical breakdown.

Only a few of us have to bear the hard fate of a genius. Our mental health does not depend upon gigantic conflicts with the spirit of the time but on our adapting ourselves feelingly to our own small circle. For all of us there is the possibility that conflicting emotions may paralyze or impede either the development or the use of a healthy mind. The latter may result from continual failure in our profession, or in our claims for recognition; or it may be due to lack of loving care which has been denied us, or to the unfulfilled desire to have children, or to a thousand other worries and cares which continually gnaw at us.

We must avoid misunderstanding. When we wrote of "a healthy mind in a healthy body" we did not, of course, mean that when our mind makes a mistake we necessarily become ill. We often feel that our political opponents are somewhat mad, but they are not going to become physically ill as a result of their "madness." It is not the outright errors of one's mind, the wrong opinions, which endanger one's health, but it is the conflict among our own ideas which can make us ill. Such conflicts make our hearts beat more quickly, embitter our lives, break our hearts. These are the problems which are apt to bring need for medical attention. They are problems peculiar to human beings, and are the price we may have to pay for the development of independent thought. It is this which distinguishes us from animals. You cannot have a flower without a plant and a root. A dead man cannot think. It is possible that when a man is sick his thoughts become sick too; just as a stunted plant brings forth a stunted flower, or does not flower at all.

THE IMMORTAL CELLS

All the smallest forms of life, those which consist of single cells, and which multiply by division, may seem to us to be immortal, because their bodies never die. Bacterial races maintain themselves over the years by endless rapid division. A single bacterium lives as such only for a few hours before it divides and becomes two individuals. Even our own cells, if isolated from the body in suitable vessels and in an appropriate food-containing medium, divide, just as bacteria divide, without death, to form new individuals. Cells from a chicken's heart have been kept alive in this way for fifteen years, which is three times the life-span of an average chicken. But when these cells, each capable of outliving the whole animal in a separate existence, are built together into the complex body of the chicken, their natural tendency to endless multiplication is checked. They grow and multiply in ordered fashion, making one perfect chicken heart: then they stop: the perfected heart remains and functions in the ordered body of the chicken, for about five years. The chicken will die, but her chickens, each as complex as she, outlive her, and have chickens in their turn.

LIVING ENEMIES OF MAN

Cave-men survived the terrors of the greater beasts of prey because they were the more intelligent, though less powerful than the wild animals. Man made weapons which were more effective than tigers' claws. Soon the world belonged to man, and man's remaining enemies were, sometimes other men, but always those viruses and bacteria which can cause disease. Men decide whether or not they will fight each other, but man must fight germs. Daily and hourly the cells of our bodies kill off invading germs. Daily and hourly countless research workers in every part of the world are seeking by experiment to make new weapons of defense against these microscopic and submicroscopic enemies.

Not very many years ago plague, cholera, and smallpox spread in wave-like epidemics across Europe, and killed many, many times the number of people killed in a world war. Plague, cholera, and smallpox have now been conquered in the laboratories. Some enemies, especially the viruses capable of causing disease to man or to his crops, remain as the great targets of medical research.

THE CHEMICAL FIGHT AGAINST BACTERIA

We have seen that two things are characteristic of the human species. The first of these is man's physical independence of his environment; the second is man's ability to think and act freely. Both these characteristics aid man in survival. One of the triumphs of man's reasoning has been the manufacture of drugs which he can use to fight bacteria which have invaded his body and are causing disease. Year by year, this work, which was begun in the 1870s by the Frenchman Louis Pasteur, and the German, Robert Koch, is becoming more and more successful. New drugs appear and soar like rockets into the sky of the medical world. The first really successful drug of this type was Ehrlich's salvarsan: he produced it in 1905 for the treatment of syphilis. The sulfonamides entered therapeutics in 1935. Penicillin (English) 1943, streptomycin (American) 1945, Aureomycin, chloramphenicol, and Terramycin (all American) in a stream thereafter. Now every year, or half-year, a new drug comes, and another group of bacteria is conquered. Day by day human life becomes more secure from bacterial invasion.

We are still faced by a host of dangerous viruses against which we still have no really effective weapons. These minute uncanny creatures, which are not creatures, but large chemical molecules capable of multiplying, are the tigers, lions, bears, crocodiles or dragons of modern life. Diseases caused by viruses include smallpox, "flu," poliomyelitis, mononucleosis, measles, colds, and some forms of jaundice. We have no effective drugs with which to exterminate these pests. Viruses do not live between the cells of our bodies, but in them. Unlike bacteria, the viruses do not have a metabolism of their own, different from that of our body cells. Instead, the virus gets inside a cell of our bodies, and supports itself by means of participating in the life activities of that cell. Our drugs do not yet differentiate between the virus and our own body cell. We cannot yet kill one without killing the other.

Fortunately for us, our body cells do slowly, in the majority of cases, manage to fight and kill these virus parasites. Our cells produce proteins which make us immune to attacks from such viruses. Once a person is immune to a particular virus his blood serum contains these defenses against this particular virus, and his serum can be used to help another sufferer fight his virus infection. This is the basis of serum treatment. Alternatively, we can grow and kill or make a particular species of virus very weak, and then give minute amounts of it to a human being (with or without protective serum) and so entice the human being to make defensive substances in his body which will protect him from attack by the strong live strains of virus that cause the particular disease we are trying to prevent. This is the basis of active immunization.

When we vaccinate a baby, we are actively immunizing it against smallpox. The first attempts at inoculation against this disease date from the eighteenth century. Smallpox used to be a devastating plague in Europe. During the eighteenth century it was noticed that cowhands who had previously contracted cowpox from cattle never, or hardly ever, died from smallpox in these frightful epidemics. Experimentally therefore, humans were given cowpox deliberately, because that was a mild disease, and this procedure was found to protect them from the ravages of smallpox when next it broke out. When we vaccinate nowadays, we do not induce generalized cowpox. We use instead a harmless version of virus which will produce only a localized pox, and yet will stimulate our bodies to set up defenses against the fierce strong virus which causes the disease of smallpox.

We are still dependent on the chemical factories of our own cells for the prevention of virus diseases by immunization. We know how to make a human body immune to attack from large viruses, but the process takes time (weeks). That is why it is so important to protect the population by immunization before they become infected—i.e. before, and not during, an epidemic.

Man as the Enemy of Man

One must admit that nowadays we are pretty well equipped in our struggle for existence. We have virtually removed all competition and threats from other living creatures on this earth. Savage wolves and man-eating animals only appear in our fairy-tales and dreams and are no longer a significant part of our daily life. We have even created animal preserves for the purpose of preventing the complete extermination of these beasts and to keep our old enemies on view.

Neither need we fear plague today. People prayed for protection from war, pestilence and drought a few hundred years ago; today we have practically forgotten about the "plague." We are, of course, afraid of war, of starvation and, quite remotely, of natural catastrophes such as earthquakes, floods and hurricanes against which we are powerless.

But with regard to starvation and war we know only too well that both these dangers rest in our hands and that we, the human race, are alone responsible to ourselves for them. This may not sound very comforting, but it means that such dangers should now be easier to banish than pestilence and the plagues of locusts in ancient times. One can imagine the impact and effect of such plagues on humanity in former days. No one knew whence they came. They swept uncannily over villages and towns.

In those days one dared to think that if kings and princes really saw sense and sat down and made peace, then war would be at an end. But nobody could visualize the advent of people who would be able to check the plague. No one suspected that it would be easier for mankind to destroy the invisible and uncanny and at that time still unknown enemies which took their toll of human life in ever recurring waves of pestilence, than to avert repeated warfare.

The Inner Enemy

Man, by the invention of gunpowder, freed himself from the danger of wild beasts. Then, by the building of dams and dikes, and the whole structure of civilization, protected himself from all but catastrophic events in his external environment. Then, by medical science, he has come near to complete success in the control of bacterial diseases, and has made some progress in the prevention of virus infections.

His greatest dangers now are international, those of man against man, and internal. A man can still be his own worst enemy.

We are all well aware that we are living creatures—human beings, each with our own gifts and abilities—but none the less, living creatures like all others. Like all living organisms, man feels the urge to reproduce, and has exerted all his powers in the struggle for survival. Superficially it seems absurd to impute desire for self-destruction to man. We immediately reject the idea that man desires to hurt or destroy himself. Yet, we know that man can become the victim of mental disease, or of deep anxieties, which cause wasting and chronic illnesses in which bacteria and viruses play no part, or of cancer. None of these things could happen to a primitive organism like a bacterium.

The cause of man's ability to destroy himself from within lies in his complexity. Primitive human races have tried to explain the mental and some of the physical troubles which may arise in and even destroy a human being in terms of possession by evil or sick spirits. We have to accept the fact that something can go wrong with the smooth internal functioning of a man's body and soul, which has its origin within himself. We know that it is not caused by a wild goblin that has taken possession of us, but strange inner enemies can arise within our own minds or bodies, and we must consider them, and seek for their origin.

Too Many Hands on the Steering Wheel?

A complex human body can only function smoothly if the activities of all the individual cells and organs of that body are adequately supervised and controlled. Brakes must be applied here, greater effort must be made there, from moment to moment; everything must be completely co-ordinated. There is, for instance, a nerve center in the brain of every human being which works like a delicate relay thermometer or thermostat, and which is responsible for the regulation of body temperature. If the body tends to get too hot this center causes the blood-vessels just under the surface of the skin to open widely, so that blood is deflected to the surface of the body to be cooled by the air passing over the skin. At the same time sweating is turned on. The sweat evaporates from the skin surface, cooling the skin and the blood passing through the skin blood-vessels. The cooled blood goes on to wash around and cool more deeply-seated organs of the body. Conversely, if the body tends to get too cold, the temperature-regulating center closes down the skin blood-vessels, and cuts off perspiration. The layer of fat just under the skin now insulates the blood from the cold surface, and inside this insulating layer the muscles warm themselves and the blood passing through them by that involuntary activity which we call "shivering." The temperature-regulating center at the same time increases the amount of fuel or foodstuffs burnt up in the body to provide heat and energy. All these changes can be brought about by our temperature-regulating center, or thermostat.

The foregoing is only one small example of the co-ordinating mechanisms constantly at work in a complex human body. Skin blood-vessels are not only controlled by the thermostat. If a person receives a sudden shock, violent nerve stimulation results in that part of the nervous system which looks after skin blood-vessels and the internal organs of digestion and metabolism. As a result of nerve stimulation the adrenal glands pour adrenaline into the bloodstream. The adrenaline travels in the blood, and closes down the skin blood-vessels; this makes the person turn pale. The adrenaline also deflects the blood from the digestive organs to the muscles and brain, and the person is made ready for immediate thought and action, either of fight or escape.

But everyone knows, too, that skin blood-vessels are affected by emotions other than fright. Many of us will recall blushing from shame or embarrassment in younger days. When we blush, the skin vessels of our faces, necks, and throats suddenly expand.

These examples show what an infinite variety of commands can reach even such a simple body structure as a skin blood-vessel. All other organs throughout the body are constantly responding to elaborate systems of control. No organ is quiescent, all are constantly guided, so that the perfect balance of complete co-ordination is kept adjusted to the minute by minute changes brought about by the multitudinous outside influences of everyday life. In short, the whole body is alive, controlled in perfect balance, adjusting immediately and perfectly to our changing activities, in health.

Where Is the Fault?

When one considers what inner dangers might threaten us, one might be inclined to think first of all that in this entire complicated mechanism a little wheel was broken, something was no longer functioning, and this caused the whole machine to break down. But it is not a machine. There are no cogwheels, which can lose their cogs. Things do not wear out so easily in this mechanism of the body. What is used up is replenished. If, for instance, one thinks of the blood-cells, which are responsible for the important task of inner respiration, the transport of oxygen, if one looks at these blood corpuscles, one sees that they are constantly growing. The whole time new reserves are being thrown into the bloodstream and used-up elements are dissolved again. The individual cells are used for only about 130 days.

Now you will say, "All right, there really are no cogwheels. It is living material, which counteracts wear and tear by constantly renewing itself. But all this is held together by the nerves. These are cable wires, in which electric currents, electric signals dart here and there and keep everything going. Perhaps there are fires in the cable. Perhaps these nerves break. Perhaps this will cause a breakdown." Yes, that does happen: for example, when the virus of infantile paralysis attacks a body and completes its work of destruction in the nervous system. But that is an external illness—an assault by outside enemies of the body. The nerves, these white strands, which pass through the body, are the toughest, most resistant and enduring things we possess. A nerve is still capable of passing its stimulus signal when the muscle belonging to it no longer reacts to it because of overtiredness. Therefore it cannot be the cable wires in our body either.

Adapting Ourselves

What remains? How can we really visualize this "inner enemy"? It is not really the organs and it is not the nerve strands, and yet there must be something there. There only remains the highest activity of the nerves—that which takes part in the brain. This almost incalculable interplay from the automatic heat center to the feeling of blushing, from the quick heart-beat during a marathon race to palpitations at the sight of one's fiancée, from hunger to "unsatisfied" longing, from the normal intestinal movement to the panic experienced before an examination; in short, the "independence" of our mental world, which has borrowed from the emotions of our organs their means of expression.

For a wild animal the sight of the enemy results only in the emotion of terror, fright or rage. Under the influence of this emotion the whole body switches over to complete efficiency and alertness and readiness for battle; it makes the immediate decision between victory, successful flight, or being eaten. But, in human beings, fear can make itself independent.

In the vast complexity of the human mind the causes of such emotions can, so to speak, get lost and remain concealed. However, the character of the emotion is preserved. The guiding of the entire organism becomes warped. It no longer functions properly and there all of a sudden you have an illness—the most incalculable chain of human suffering; illness which may confront medical science with considerable difficulty, because the higher animals are no longer a "model" for us.

One cannot find an experimental animal which can develop high blood-pressure or a stomach ulcer on its own from purely psychological reasons. No animal is tormented by rheumatism. Of course domestic animals can get fat; of course the higher domestic animals can also be plagued by an "inner enemy" of that sort, although this happens to a lesser extent than with human beings. It is, for example, a fact that wild rabbits perish if kept in captivity. Cats kept in cages scarcely ever live many months.

This process of adapting can be overdone among higher animals. If they are moved to a too strange environment, nothing seems to "fit" any more and the work of their organs lacks the stimulus necessary for daily life. The normal welter of perceptions, of the sighted enemy and immediate action are absent in captivity. A caged wild rabbit lives defenseless in a state of constant fear. It cannot creep away and hide. The instincts, and the knowledge acquired previously during its existence in the wild state, no longer fit in. Its body is therefore wrongly guided, so much so indeed that it may be destroyed.

Our world is one of man-built towns and cars, trains and radios, and it has been proved that we human beings are very much more adaptable than any other animal on this earth. Our mental development is on a far higher plane so that we are always free to try out and take on new modes of life. The individual from an underdeveloped nation can adapt easily to the bustling life of a modern city. We "learn" infinitely more quickly than all animal creatures.

Our Own Cage

Our enemy, then, appears to be further inside us than in these direct connections between the organs of our body and our surroundings. The enemy is not among all the experiences, emotions, tastes, smells and sights associated with our habitat. There must be inner fronts within us which have just the same effect as cage bars on a wild rabbit. We can, so to speak, imprison ourselves in cages. There is so much for a human being to learn and it is such a long way from infancy to adulthood that he may well get stuck in a cul-de-sac and thus be prevented from achieving his final development or ambition. The aim, at any rate as far as human beings are concerned, is a completely trained intelligence, great mental agility, and physical soundness. Now, in these twenty or twenty-five or even forty years of trial and learning, there are culs-de-sac, where a person can get stuck.

Imagine a thirty-year-old person who treats his superiors with the defiance and brusqueness of a three-year-old child; he has got stuck in one of these culs-de-sac. He is long past the time when he had to use this method to get his own way with others. He should by now have learned more civilized techniques and he should also know just when to be abrupt and when to check himself. The failure to develop fully has become his inner enemy, leading from inside to the outside world, and determining his relationships with other people. There can be no doubt that these culs-de-sac, which can so impede us in later life, are caused by errors in our upbringing. It would be highly unusual for children to be born with a natural tendency to failure. Such a thought is quite contrary to our religious feelings as well as our scientific conception of living creatures as illustrated here. We shall hear later that there are hereditary defects of the mind and body, but we shall also find that their number is negligible compared with those defects caused by experiences.

Thus we come to the amazing formula that only man constitutes a danger for man. Our animal competitors, who vied with us for domination of the world, have succumbed to the invention of gunpowder. The smallest enemies of our race, bacteria, are in the process of liquidation at the hands of our chemical weapons. We ourselves are almost our only enemies. Let us hope that we can give each other peace and freedom from fear, starvation, disease and distress.

2. The Function and Anatomy of the Healthy Body

The previous chapter dealt with some of the ways in which a living body functions. First and foremost our bodies are a mass of cells dominated by the central organ, the brain. Cells are as indispensable to the body as bricks and mortar are to a house. So we must look at these cells a little more closely. If we did not understand what a cell was, we would not even understand anything so common and harmless as a wart on our finger. A wart forms when skin cells develop independently and get out of control. Without the knowledge of what a cell is we could not even understand the important processes of reproduction and birth. We have already discovered that unicellular organisms can lead an independent life, and that they can, in a primitive fashion, see, hear, taste, smell and move and must eat and reproduce themselves. The cells in our body are no longer able to do this. It is true that we have cells which are sensitive to light, but these are only to be found in the retina of the eye. With these cells we can neither hear, taste nor smell; our cells are specialized so that they can now only perform one function, but that they do brilliantly. This brings us to the amazing fact that the evolution of the human being has resulted in impoverishing the functions of our cells. One might almost ask why we are created with so many cells when, in a single cell (like the amoeba), all the functions are performed. It seems to be a retrograde step.

However, it will help us if we take the eye as an example and investigate the specialization of those of its cells which are sensitive to light. The animal composed of one cell can easily distinguish between light and dark and can also determine the direction of a ray of light, but it cannot see individual objects. Only by endless specialization and the division of many cells was it possible for an eye to be created. The eye is built like a camera. Its lens projects a picture on the retina which is the wrong way around just as it is inside a camera. Just as a photographic film picks up the varying intensity of the light that falls on it, so the single light-sensitive cells in the eye respond to the intensity and wavelength of the light coming into the eye, and report on it to the brain by means of a stream of messages which travel in the optic nerve. It is rather like television done in reverse. We can really see. We can in addition put a microscope in front of our eye and magnify objects so that we can see a single cell in detail. This the one-celled animal cannot do. It cannot recognize its own world, it can only react to light. It can swim away from the light or it can approach light and its sensitivity is as much as ours would be if we wore heavily frosted glass spectacles. It is our multitude of cells which helps to bridge the gaps between the indefinite sensation of light to definite vision and from the indefinite feeling of pressure to actual hearing. The cells of our body have had to lose their versatility in order to give to the whole body a higher degree of perfection.

THE PROTOPLASM OF THE CELLS

First of all, cells are so small that they cannot be seen by the naked eye. It was not until the discovery of the micro-scope three hundred years ago that we knew anything about them. Before that no one knew of their existence. If you were to ask what a cell looked like, I would have to be honest and say that I have seen thousands but cannot describe them. It is just as though I were asked to describe a plant and not a specific one like a parsnip, potato or a pine-tree. Cells under a microscope look just as different as these various plants. Neither their size nor their shape is standardized, and in this respect they differ from the bricks we use to build our houses. Therefore in answer to your question as to what a cell is like I usually have to say that it is composed mainly of protoplasm. This is a mixture of chemical substances, and is basically protein in nature.

Whereas there is only one substance like glucose, there are innumerable different kinds of protoplasm. They all have a rather similar composition but are not identical. They always contain approximately the same proportions of different atoms, which are the smallest particles of matter. The molecule is always composed of approximately 16 per cent nitrogen, and the rest for the main part is carbon, hydrogen and oxygen. The last two are the components of water; therefore this means that it is really just carbon, nitrogen and water. Even though the protoplasm molecules have practically always the same composition they are never really quite the same. Each kind differs in size and in the way its molecule is built up. This difference is so marked that, for instance, in the case of two brothers the same kind of cells contain different sorts of protoplasm. If for instance you wanted to take a piece of skin from one brother to graft on to a wound in the other, it would be a failure. Only one's own skin, that is to say the skin from, for instance, the inner side of the arm, will grow on one's own forehead, nose or anywhere else on one's body. The cells of one's body are uncannily sensitive and can recognize a strange skin at once. This brings the defensive cells into action, and our bloodvessels refuse to feed the foreign skin. All this is because no two bodies contain identical protoplasm.

The molecules of protoplasm vary just as much from one cell type to another as they do from one human body to another. Those in the outer layer of the cell, which we call the cell membrane, are different from those in the body of the cell, and these again differ according to activities and functions which they perform. The protoplasm of the nucleus is something quite on its own.

Now look at Figures 1 and 2. A cell usually has a mem-

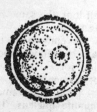

Fig. 1

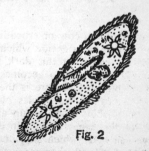

Fig. 2

brane, or outer covering, which surrounds its inner jelly-like protoplasm and prevents it from flowing away. The cell membrane has to act as both skin and bone. The protoplasm is often rather like the uncooked white of an egg.

CELLS

Almost every cell has a nucleus. This nucleus is in many ways the most important part of the cell, because the nucleus contains the chromosomes which determine the quality of the cell. Only nucleated cells can multiply and division of the nucleus initiates the cleavage of the cell.

But now let's really get down to the drawings. First of all an egg cell—the female seed. This represents the original of all cells. The female seed or human egg looks just like all other cells. But in Figure 1 it is impossible to distinguish between a human egg and that of a hedgehog, let alone those

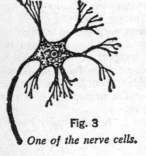

Fig. 3
One of the nerve cells.

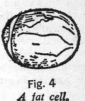

Fig. 4
A fat cell.

of an elephant, cow or crocodile. They all look the same but the chromosomes decide which it is going to be.

In the center of this dark nucleus is the embryo of the living being that is to become later a man, hedgehog, crocodile or pigeon. In there is the pulsing life force which will later determine the species of animal or human being, the colour of skin, blood group and physical build. The female part of the genes is contained in this minute nucleus. The large cell body which surrounds it contains practically nothing but food, which must last until the entire animal is able to eat independently or, as with us, the maternal body feeds the embryo.

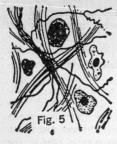

Fig. 5

Connective tissue cells. (The grass of the body which grows everywhere between the more delicate cell flowers.)

Bone cells lying within their walls.

Fig. 6

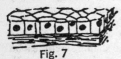

Fig. 7

A layer of epithelium that looks, on the surface, like a cobbled street. Many hollow parts of the human body look like that from inside.

Two kinds of white blood corpuscles. Like their ancestors, they can eat by tilting themselves over the edible object.

A red blood-cell—a blood corpuscle. It no longer has a nucleus and dies off in about 120 days.

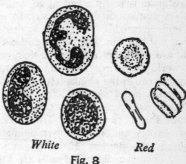

White   *Red*

Fig. 8

Fig. 9

And now a muscle cell which may be a collection of nuclei in a gigantically long, thin body of fiber.

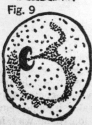

Fig. 11

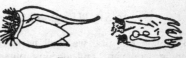

Fig. 10   A few more cells.

The *Plasmodium malariae*, for instance, which in India alone causes 3,000,000 deaths yearly. It is the cause of malaria.

Secondly, let us imagine the complete cell. It responds to light, pressure, heat and chemicals; it can eat, move, multiply by dividing, and can mate.

Thirdly there is an infinite number of incompletely specialized cells which later become more specialized and are classified accordingly.

All these are animal cells. You must admit that it is difficult to describe a cell. But perhaps these drawings may help you to conjure up easily a picture of a cell, just as we can all visualize a tree, regardless of the fact that there are many different kinds of trees. Each of us knows what a tree is, for we have all seen so many different ones in our lives. All the same we sometimes have difficulty in identifying a particular one as a shrub or a tree.

Just in the same way we shall know what a cell is after having looked at these pictures, and we shall sometimes be uncertain as to whether a certain formation, a muscle cell, for instance, is really a cell at all.

Every conception has its limits. In speaking of a tree or a cell, one invariably comes up against forms to which one cannot put a name. The words and definitions current in our world are much more inflexible than reality. We superimpose our world of words masking reality, which we can only glimpse through the chinks left open to us between our words.

For example, I have said that a cell always has a nucleus, but have drawn red blood-cells without nuclei, and have claimed that they are cells. This is because the red cells of birds, snakes and many other animals do have nuclei but those of man do not. However, in some forms of human illness, when the red blood-cells are formed too rapidly, they are thrown into the blood-stream when they are immature, and while they still have nuclei. Every red blood-cell has a nucleus during the period of its development in the bone marrow, and so it has a right to be classed as a cell.

Why One Has to Say "Usually"

To explain our title we shall have to dwell on something seemingly irrelevant and occupy ourselves with such mad things as semantics—this yawning abyss between words and what actually happens. But we want to try and come to an understanding, and for that reason I consider it important, not only to show drawings of cells, but also to explain why, in a book about human beings like this, one can only say "usually" and never "it is always like that." It is essential to exercise caution here and say "usually." Science demands that we think like that. Science will not allow us to behave like lawyers who frame the facts to their words instead of words to facts.

Language is merely an incomplete means by which the natural sciences may understand the "uncharted" world. We have all learned and practised the art of using words at school. We have been taught to believe in the omnipotence of the word, which cannot be shaken or twisted. And now I have to come and tell you that what I have to say may be shaken or twisted. I can only say it "usually" happens. In addition to that I must add that only when you have accustomed yourselves to thinking in terms of "usually" will you come to a complete understanding of the matter. For those who are inclined to doubt my words, I would say that I have proof to support the accuracy of my contention.

Nothing would appear to be more exact than the science of physics. The physicist calculates exactly how much weight the girders of a bridge may safely carry. And it is absolutely correct. One of the most stupendous achievements of this science is the atom bomb. For all the horror and threat it holds for us, nothing can alter the fact that it is a most impressive scientific discovery. But alas it, too, functions in an exceedingly exact way. It is sufficient to press a button to set the mechanism in motion. But this discovery would never have been made if the physicists had not learned to substitute the term "usually" for "always."

When an atomic bomb explodes, countless atoms are split at the same time or almost at the same time. What happens is like an enormously speeded up version of the disintegration of radium. In 1,580 years, exactly half of one gram of radium will have split, and after another 1,580 years, half of the remaining half-gram splits.

If one looks at a single atom in a gram of radium it is impossible to predict when it will split. It may happen in a second, tomorrow, in a year, or not for 10,000,000 years. A single atom is not subject to any laws of nature. The rigid law of radium-splitting is one of "usually." It only becomes absolute in the case of a virtually limitless quantity of atoms. Of these definitely half are no longer the chemical substance radium after a period of 1,580 years. Of fifty selected atoms it may just as well be twenty-five or forty, or even two.

Even the law of "usually" cannot be applied to such a small figure as fifty. Fifty single atoms exist without any law.

And so paradoxically enough we say "usually" when we know something for certain. It is erroneous to define something as positive and unchangeably valid. We shall also soon realize how quickly and easily we can become accustomed to thinking in terms of "usually" and how greatly it simplifies life for us. There are two important reasons why we should think in terms of "usually" rather than the more agreeable "always." First the nature of our human language causes us to mutilate the unbroken transitions in the world, and, secondly, the laws of nature are determined by numbers and not by the individual, with whom we are usually concerned.

CELLS OF THE BODY

We have looked at the cells of the human body. We know that they are not bricks or elastic bands, but living, functioning things. All of these three hundred million million cells have to eat and breathe constantly. Right in the interior of our bodies a constant stream of oxygen and food must be passed from the blood in order to maintain the working of this mechanism. Our cells, you see, are alive.

We know that these cells are scarcely able to live independently. Owing to specialization they have lost their ability to function alone and serve only one specific purpose. They are part of a plan; they perform functions which serve the whole body. Therefore it is only possible to understand their existence if one thinks of them in terms of the whole complete creature. Cells cannot be understood without their function, and woe betide us if they should ever revert to their former state of perfection. If they cease to perform their allotted functions, they can become our greatest enemy. They run riot and make it possible for cancer to complete the work of destruction, if the timely intervention of the surgeon's knife does not put a stop to their mischief.

HOW WE MOVE.
MUSCLES, BONES AND SKIN

Obviously, if a creature moves it cannot be dead. To be able to move is almost synonymous with living. All that moves and is capable of progressive movement can follow an objective and decide, to a certain extent, its own fate.

MUSCLES

Now, the solitary living cell or one-celled creature can move. It is able to do this by contracting and expanding the matter of which it is made. Or it can propel itself through

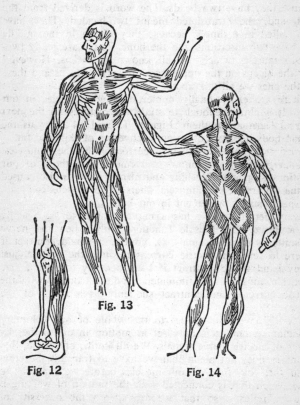

Fig. 13

Fig. 12   Fig. 14

water by setting little hairs on its surface in rhythmic motion. But the main quality of the protoplasm is always its ability to contract. And we, too, move like that. We have muscles and bones. In the muscles are to be found enormous quantities of muscle cells, of which we have seen individual ones in Figure 12. Their ends are attached to a bone by means of a sinew. If they contract, the bone moves in its joint. As is well known the muscle becomes thicker in the process. It becomes broader when contracted. What should happen to the cell mass otherwise? This is what happens when we play about with our biceps. They are called biceps incidentally because they have two heads. The word is derived from the Latin and when translated means two-headed. They have been called that simply because they divide in the middle and have two insertions into the bone. There are many two-headed muscles which are all known as biceps. However, only the biceps on the upper arms are visible to us and these are the ones we all talk about.

There are exceptionally numerous single muscles in our body. It is almost enough to study the pictures on the next page to learn about them. Figures 13 and 14 show us the human body deprived of its outer covering of skin and fat.

Every voluntary movement is performed by these muscles. But nearly every involuntary movement, like those of our intestines, stomachs, blushing and turning pale, is also caused by the contraction of muscle fibers. The muscle cells are the specialists of movement in our bodies.

Every decent muscle has a nerve, that is to say usually has a nerve. The muscle functions only when the nerve transmits its electric signals. Of course, it would contract if I were to send an electric current through the muscle, just as my hand would contract if I accidentally touched a live wire. The muscles are stimulated by direct contact with the electric current, and contract suddenly as a result of the shock.

What I have said applies to the whole of our voluntary muscular system. It is only set in motion in our bodies by means of electric nerve signals. We all know, of course, that voluntary does not mean that we have to transmit the command "lift your foot" to our muscles before we can start to walk. Much that is connected with the motion of walking is done by reflexes, so that we are spared the necessity of repeating the various commands. All the same the fact remains that all the muscles which come into play when we walk belong to the voluntary system. They only function when it is our express wish that they should do so. And that wish is transmitted from our brain to our muscles by means of nerve connections.

INVOLUNTARY MUSCLES

There are, however, muscles in our bodies which are subject to involuntary movements and which often cause us great embarrassment. We try our hardest to overcome this. We cannot simply say, "I want to turn pale now. The blood-vessels in my skin must contract." They will not do that. Only a quite different kind of nervous impulse will cause them to close the vessels and impede the flow of blood. When, for example, the sensory nerve endings in the skin transmit the sensation of cold to the brain, our reaction is one of annoyance. We say "there is a draft," and we feel uncomfortable. However, without our doing anything about it, the brain automatically transmits a command to the muscles in the blood-vessels of the skin which is the command to become pale by constricting the blood-vessels. So we have an involuntary muscular system as well as the voluntary one. These muscle cells are different from the monster on a previous page. They are long, spindle-shaped cells, each with a single nucleus. They are mostly connected to an involuntary nervous system which is in charge of all the organs. This system might be likened to a circuit of electricity. In this nervous system the involuntary muscles are not set in motion by definite individual signals, but they work together to fulfill some definite function. Some of these involuntary muscles, however, do work on their own to a greater extent—for example, when our stomachs rumble. The food we have eaten has caused a great deal of gas to form in the intestine. This has distended its walls, which are formed of muscles. These muscles signal to their neighbors via the nerves. The result is a worm-like, peristaltic movement of the intestine which drives the gas bubbles down through the undigested food, causing the rumbling noises.

The intestinal muscles are not voluntary, because we cannot make them work at will. Nevertheless they are subject to the commands of the involuntary nervous system. Little children wet their pants if they are frightened. Fear causes overactivity of those involuntary nerves which cause pallor of the face, fast beating of the heart, and the startled expression of the eyes. Other nerves of the involuntary system set the intestines in motion and increase the tempo of their movements just as flatulence does from inside them.

There is one important muscle which to a great extent looks after itself. It is the heart. Its muscle fibers are of a special variety. They have something in common with those of both the involuntary and voluntary systems. As is well known, the heart contracts rhythmically. Its "lub-dupp" is heard ceaselessly, but it beats more quickly if we are elated and more violently if we are going through emotional stress or tension. It must work harder if we take it into our heads to climb a mountain. It is only independent up to a point. It is harnessed to all kinds of good and bad emotions through the involuntary nervous system, and must obey the commands of all the working muscles. This last happens, for instance, when they cry out, "More blood, more oxygen. We are suffocating."

VOLUNTARY MUSCLES CONTRASTED WITH INVOLUNTARY MUSCLES

There are two different muscular systems in our bodies. One enables us to move and the other comes into play when our emotions are aroused.

Unfortunately, both systems sometimes work against one another. For example, during an attack of asthma the involuntary muscles of the more delicate bronchi stifle the air current and we feel suffocated. So then we have to use the voluntary muscles of the chest wall to make forced breathing movements in order to overcome the unfortunate activity of our involuntary muscles. We shall come up against the reasons for such conflicts in many cases of illness. More usually, during health, we find there is a wonderful co-operation between these two muscular systems. Suppose, for instance, that a person has received a shock. Perhaps a shattering noise has startled him. There is an unknown danger. Not only has his conscious attention been aroused by the din, but his nervous system has been shaken by the sensation of shock. Innumerable little involuntary muscles suddenly change their tension. The blood distribution alters throughout the whole body. The heart is stimulated to the maximum activity. Outer muscles, the brain and the heart are provided with a rich supply of blood at the expense of the other organs. The person thinks more quickly and his powers of coping with untoward circumstances are at their highest. He is ready for immediate action, regardless of what is required of him. This is an example of perfect co-operation between the two systems. A prolonged terror reaction is a sign of abnormality in the involuntary nervous system which controls the functioning of our body.

INVOLUNTARY MOVEMENTS

The involuntary muscles in our blood-vessels and internal organs have, of course, nothing to do with involuntary movements performed by the muscles of our limbs. Such "involuntary" or even "unconscious" movements are performed entirely by the voluntary muscular system. By this we mean trunk and limb movements which happen without our conscious awareness. The voluntary muscular system is also affected by nervous conditions which are not the equivalent of what is usually termed "conscious will." There are apparently short-circuit reflexes which circumvent our higher consciousness. For example, think of the way in which we instinctively raise our arm to shield our face and eyes when something suddenly comes flying toward us. We do not think that out. It just happens automatically.

These simple reflex movements which everyone knows about will help us to understand the reason for certain uncontrollable movements of the voluntary muscular system. Thus let us in future substitute the words reflex and unconscious movements for the words involuntary movement.

BONES

All visible outward movement is performed by the voluntary muscular system. But for all their perfectly constructed mechanism these muscles would be more or less useless if they were not inserted in a firm scaffolding.

Bones and joints are indispensable for movement. Architecturally the human skeleton is perfect, or would be, if it did not possess the drawback of having originally been constructed for a four-legged animal. Our tall spine is the weak spot in the human skeleton.

Fundamentally bones are nothing but ingeniously devised pieces of limestone. They are the work of the specialized bone cells which have transformed soluble calcium and phosphorus salts into insoluble calcium phosphate rods, enclosing themselves in the process. In a manner of speaking they have constructed a wall of bone, bit by bit, just as happens with a cement building. Under a microscope this bone is not really a piece, but still contains, even in its firmest parts, a narrow, soft network of cells, cell fibers and blood-vessels, for one cannot let the enclosed cells starve.

In the case of injury, i.e. broken bones, the whole building system becomes active, just as in the case of a growing child. In most cases the broken bones knit perfectly in an alternating process of reconstruction and demolition. Inside the mostly hollow bones (i.e. those containing soft marrow) is to be found a system of girders and supports which can compete with our Gothic cathedrals and most daring modern bridges. Engineers who have studied this system express their greatest admiration for the accuracy of the construction which was made without a draft or calculations and was designed to meet any demands that might be made of the body.

The bone system is completed by the gristly bits of the skeleton and firm, sinewy, fibrous ligaments. This elastic gristle covers all the joint surfaces, thereby acting as a kind of shock-absorber. The front parts of the ribs are also composed of cartilage which gives the whole chest its springy, elastic character. The springy tension of the rib cartilage helps breathing. This gristle is alive too and contains gristle cells.

The numerous firm ligaments—which include the joint sockets—are part of the muscular system. They keep our joints together, connect bones together, and give stability to the joints by preventing too free a movement.

But our skeleton would collapse without the support of muscular tension. When a person faints, his body sags because this muscular tension is not maintained. A skeleton of bones, gristle and ligaments cannot stand without the help of its living muscles.

FACIAL EXPRESSION

It is not only bones and sinews that are affected by muscles. Muscles do more than set gristle-covered joints in motion to enable us to hit, to run and to work. Whole groups of voluntary muscles betray our inner feelings and emotions. Whether our faces look tense and haggard, elated or sad, it is all the work of facial muscles which enable us to raise our brows, turn up our noses, laugh and smile, and which cause lines or wrinkles of worry and disappointment. All this is the "mimic" muscular system. These muscles or minute muscle fibers which run crossways over the tissue under our skin are alone responsible for our facial expression. They are muscles of the voluntary system, although we often experience difficulty in controlling them.

It would seem that involuntary impulses intervene on occasion and these betray our "true" feelings. Our features "go off the rails," as it were, which brings us once more to "usually." The voluntary facial muscles are subject in an astonishing degree to involuntary nervous impulses of an emotional nature, i.e. fear, terror, sorrow. These usually stimulate the involuntary muscle fibers in the skin vessels, intestinal wall, heart and other organs. The voluntary and involuntary systems encroach upon one another, as we all know, and that is why the facial expression of a person can be the key to understanding, an instinctive understanding, which renders words unnecessary.

THE SKIN

The skin overlies the muscles and is the organ of inner and outer contact between people, and also their protective armor against the outside world.

We find in it layer upon layer of cells, varying from that which is very much alive to that which is dead. The topmost outer layer of skin is composed of peeling, dead, horny cells, which are quite devoid of feeling. In places where there is a lot of wear and tear, as for instance, on the soles of our feet, this dead outer layer is especially thick, but constant friction causes it to wear away the whole time. As quickly as it peels off, it is replaced by new cells from beneath and these in turn are forced upwards until they become the dead outer layer.

FEELING

We all know from our childhood days that we can feel a great deal on our skin. There must be something amidst the cells of our skin enabling us to feel. We can feel by touch, we are sensitive to pain, heat and cold. These little bodies in our skin which enable us to touch and feel are really strangers. They are twisted nerve ends, offshoots of the brain which extend to the frontiers of our bodies' territory. The nerve cells are responsible for feeling in the skin itself.

The same applies to the receptive organs of the senses: the ends of the nerves of smell in the mucous membrane of the nose and the ends of the nerves of taste in the mucous membrane of the tongue, all communicate with the brain.

The well-known expression "mucous membrane" does not mean anything more than that the thin skin concerned should constantly be covered with mucus and kept moist. All hollow organs of the body have a mucous membrane. One can understand their need to be moist when one thinks of the unpleasant dry-mouth feeling which we have experienced. The mucus lubricates the membrane surfaces and prevents them from irritating each other when they rub together.

THE SENSITIVE NOSE

As is well known, we perspire through our outer skin. All over our skin there are little sweat glands, which give out salty liquid, and its evaporation helps to regulate the temperature of our body.

Similarly constructed sebaceous glands keep our skin and hair in good condition. They give out an odor which is peculiar to both hair and body. This smell, which in times of perfect health is not offensive to us, undergoes a marked change if one's health is in any way impaired.

If we human beings possessed the sensitive nose of a dog, we should probably be able to build up our whole medical science on our sense of smell. A gentle sniffing at the patient's door would suffice to enable the doctor to make his diagnosis without an X-ray or blood test. But as it is, we cannot achieve anything very useful with our sense of smell.

It would seem, however, that people who are quick on the scent make a point of disliking others and often succeed in this very well, which brings one to the conclusion that sensations of smell play a far greater part in human relationship than might be supposed. Like the subtle undertones of our speaking voices or the unconscious expressions on our faces, they, too, determine our instinctive feelings and actions.

All this arises from work done in the skin, and in their own primitive way our little glands help us to make contact with other people. Somewhere deep down inside ourselves we smell one another, just as our animal friends do, and we also possess the organs which provide the necessary smells by which others recognize us.

BREATHING OF THE SKIN

This is about the most important function of the skin, but I should like to explode one common fallacy. The skin does not breathe from outside. The outer layer of cells is dead and needs neither oxygen nor food. The inner cells, like all the other cells of the body, are provided with oxygen by the blood. Tight-fitting clothes or ill-ventilated ones are unsatisfactory for quite different reasons.

The quantities of perspiration which are being constantly and imperceptibly secreted moisten the skin and material, thereby increasing the material's powers of heat conduction. This makes it difficult and sometimes impossible to regulate the temperature of the body. Cold leads to chills, and heat results in an accumulation of warmth with all its unpleasant consequences, including heat-stroke. So one does not have to go about naked in order to be able to breathe through the skin. Our clothing should, however, be suitable. It should enable our bodies to regulate their temperature. Moreover, it is a fairy story to say that, in cases of extensive skin burns, death is caused by suffocation as a result of the skin's inability to breathe sufficiently. What is in fact fatal is the absorption from the burned tissues of certain substances destructive to the protoplasm.

It is a different matter with sunlight, and here I would like to add that there is sunlight even when the sky is overcast. When exposed to the sun, chemical changes take place in our bodies. For instance, the precursor of vitamin D, a deficiency of which causes rickets, turns itself into that valuable vitamin. Light and sun diminish our babies' need for cod-liver oil, a fact which I am sure they would not mind. But even our best source of vitamin D, cow's milk, is made more efficacious by ultraviolet rays. One could irradiate the milk before distribution. But one can also drink the milk as it is and lay the infant in the sun afterwards. Hence light treatment.

I Am Ashamed

The skin is not only a frontier and partition wall, but also a mediator between us and other people and the outside world. For that reason it is not surprising to learn that skin complaints are usually connected with these two things. Working with skin irritants, such as chemicals, can cause a rash which is repellent and disfiguring.

However, one often finds, in fact usually finds, that there is no adequate external cause for these symptoms. The reason for them is psychological. In the simplest case, for example, a certain substance contained in strawberries can upset the involuntary nervous system which can set up a hypersensitive reaction throughout the entire organism. The visible result is large red itchy spots scattered over the body—nettle-rash or strawberry hives. These processes are known and understood, but on the other hand the rash also depends upon the person's mental state.

From these simple symptoms, to which the term mental is applicable only in the "nervous" sense, we pass through various stages, finally reaching the purely mental skin afflictions. There is an unbearable "hysterical" itching which drives the patient nearly frantic so that he tears his skin to shreds with his nails. We all of us know and experience an occasional nervous itch. That can also have its origin solely in the mind.

There is scarcely a skin complaint where the mind is not involved, however remotely. Itching and scratching and being repellent are all signs that our mind is expressing itself in the shop-window of our body which is the skin.

When we torture and frustrate ourselves this may show externally, for example, if we blush for shame after some embarrassment, this can have far greater physical repercussions than we imagine and may cause skin ailments. The skin, therefore, in conjunction with the sensory organs, such as the eyes and the ears, and with the apparatus of movement, bones and muscles, helps us to make contact with the outside world. The skin and sensory organs transmit the impressions (from outside). But at the same time the skin acts as a shop-window to the body and gives other people the key to one's own inner life. Movement, too, can be expressive, as when we adopt poses, when we delight in dancing, fondle one another, adopt a threatening attitude; these are all the expressions of our feelings.

FUNCTION OF THE SKIN AND MUSCLES IN THEIR RELATION TO THE MIND

Being impenetrable and conquering the world go together. The strength of our muscles which we enjoyed testing in our youth and adolescence is the criterion of man's superiority. The seductive charm of the young girl with her pretty ways plays the same part in her growing up into a woman. The woman must acquire staying power and efficiency and the man must be sure of his mental and physical abilities.

Hysteria, as we shall learn, is neither a term of abuse nor one which is derogatory; on the contrary, hysteria is a widespread disease which is very difficult to cure. It is nearly always connected with the organs of our frontiers, with the apparatus of movement, the sensory organs and the skin. But that is not all. In the many cases of chronic illness involving these particular organs, as for instance rheumatism, one finds traits in the character and behavior of the patient which are all characteristic of hysteria. We have good reason to regard these nervous and hormonal deviations as the main cause of such complaints.

But now let us leave the patient and return to the subject of health, which is our prime objective. Apart from the question of sensible care and training, the health of our skin, bones and muscles depends on our mental health. It depends especially on such things as taking action when the need arises, but not always feeling obliged to do so; on letting off steam, if necessary, but not on tearing about in a blind rage; rather in wanting to live as a civilized human being; on being able to feel ashamed, but on ceasing to do so at the right moment; on not feeling ashamed, yet being able to exercise self-control, without being under a feeling of compulsion to do so. Only when we can do these things, will we be able to live happily and contentedly in our skin and restrain and protect it.

THE INNER WORKINGS OF THE HEART AND KIDNEYS

In the Old Testament we find the expression "to try out my reins and my heart," or to test a man by his heart and kidneys, and even today we still understand the symbolical meaning of the words which imply that before God we can have no secrets. It is exceedingly difficult to fathom why the ancient Hebrews singled out the heart and kidneys as being particularly valuable and impenetrable organs. Some people maintain that the expression derives from the time of animal sacrifices when the heart and kidneys were believed to have a special significance. That is as may be. Actually these old men hit the nail on the head when they used this double term, for these two organs are essential to the composition of blood and the regulation of its pressure. The heart is the motor for the circulation and the kidneys act as its overflow pipe.

WHY CIRCULATION?

As has already been mentioned many times in this book, all cells of the body have to breathe incessantly, i.e. they have to be provided night and day with oxygen. At the same time the carbon dioxide which forms when cells breathe must be disposed of. The same applies to the feeding of the cells. Soluble food is burned up when oxygen is introduced. The fundamental fuel of the cells is glucose. So you see our cells are not meat-eaters, but vegetarians. They feed for the most part on sugar which with the aid of oxygen they convert into carbon dioxide and water.

This burning-up process provides energy for the working of the cells of the whole body, but, of course, here again we must apply "usually." Brain cells, for example, will burn up amino-acids, especially glutamic acid, instead of glucose. However, generally speaking, glucose is the fuel which keeps the cells in working order.

Human beings and animals perish through inner starvation if their cells are deprived of the necessary quantities of foodstuffs. We shall learn exactly how quickly a person with too much insulin in his blood can lose consciousness for the reason that the cells no longer have sufficient fuel.

CIRCULATION

It is common knowledge that it is the blood which provides the materials for the inner working of our bodies. It takes oxygen on board in the lung and carries it into the left side of the heart. From there the oxygenated blood is pumped vigorously by the heart through an intricate network of pipes or blood-vessels. Its initial speed is about twenty inches a second.

What we feel as our pulse on the wrist is not the heart-beat itself, but a pressure wave. This moves at a speed ten times greater than that at which the blood actually flows. The pulse is something like a sound which moves like a wave through the air. We have all seen the plume of smoke from a distant engine and then heard the whistle seconds later. Pressure waves of sound move more slowly than the rays of light which transmit the visual picture of the smoke. Just in

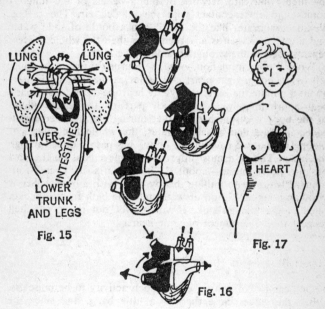

Fig. 15

Fig. 16

Fig. 17

the same way the blood flows more slowly than the pressure or pulse wave.

And that is why the heart-beat on the pulse wave can be felt on the wrist or ankle in split seconds, while the blood thrown out by the same heart-beat does not reach the tip of one's feet until after the third heart-beat. The return to the heart is even slower. The blood flows sluggishly back through the veins—those blue ones recognizable in our elbow—to the right side of the heart.

The right side of the heart, in common with the left side,

has two "pump chambers." The first one receives the blood which flows back from the body and with a little pumping movement helps to fill the right ventricle or pumping chamber. This then contracts—the whole heart is a muscle. The pressure which results causes the rear valve to close and the front one to open. The blood is compelled to flow out into the arteries of the lung. When the chamber is empty, its muscular walls relax, and the tension inside drops to zero. Now the higher pressure in the lung artery causes the valve door between them to shut. The blood passes on and is distributed among the highly intricate network of blood-vessels of the lung. It comes into close contact with the inhaled air. The carbon dioxide evaporates like the bubbles in a bottle of soda water and the vital oxygen is absorbed. And then the whole process repeats itself in the strong left side of the heart.

We call this circulation. A whole journey through the lung, left heart, body, right heart and as far as the lung again lasts about a minute, i.e. sixty to seventy heart-beats. At each heart-beat approximately a hundredth part of the entire blood of the body is dispatched, so that during one hundred heart-beats, i.e. one and a half minutes, the whole five quarts of blood (all that we have in our body) has passed once through the heart. This is a most impressive achievement on the part of our heart pump—about 10,000 quarts in twenty-four hours. Please try to imitate this by hand with a bucket. See if you can pour half a ton of water into the bath from a bucket filled at the kitchen sink. If you prefer not to do so, then respect the achievement of your heart!

HEART-BEATS AND HEART NOISES

One cannot, of course, expect such activity to be noiseless. When the valves close there is a little bang, and since the left and right sides of the heart work together in perfect rhythm, only two of the four closing valves can be heard—luh-dupp, the first sound from the two rear valves and the second from the two exit ones. These are the two noises which every healthy heart makes incessantly.

But when the valves are affected by illness, usually by rheumatism—when little knots or scars form on them—other heart noises can be detected. When, for instance, the edge of a valve is shrivelled and cannot close completely, a hissing sound can be heard during the pumping process. This is due to the fact that a fine jet of blood is leaking back under pressure. If a valve is stiff and cannot open completely, a similar noise can be detected, but this time when the blood flows in.

The doctor will listen carefully with his stethoscope for these noises which indicate valvular disorders. He can detect from the loudest point which of the valves is affected and from the time of hearing it whether a valve cannot close or open completely (Insufficiency or Stenosis).

ELECTROCARDIOGRAM. HEART STREAM CURVE

Always when a nerve or a muscle works, an electric current passes through the tissues. The tissues of our body are composed of sixty to eighty per cent of water and are excellent conductors, so it is possible to measure the changes in the electrical potential of the heart from any point on the body.

Electric currents flowing in the heart muscle can for that reason be led off from both arms, or from one arm and one leg, and be recorded in an electric measuring apparatus. These electric currents are equivalent to about a thousandth of the strength of those obtained from the battery of a flashlight. But they can be excellently recorded by means of sensitive modern medical apparatus. One must, however, dampen the layer of dry and greasy body skin to make conduction possible and all muscular movement must be suspended.

When currents flowing in the heart are recorded on a piece of paper which is drawn past quickly (a ray of light from the measuring instrument passes over photo paper) you have an electrocardiogram.

This method is unfortunately open to great abuse, for the electrocardiogram reveals much less about illness than one might imagine. One must not forget that one is measuring something which can vary greatly according to the patient's condition at the time. The heart is strongly affected by nervous influence, and this does not only apply to human beings, as we shall see from the following example.

If one injects a dog with morphine the poison brings about a change in the heart current curve. If this is kept up for eight consecutive days a strange reflex action takes place. The dog, now accustomed to the injection and its effects, has learned to "alter" his curve, and this amazing thing happens even when the doctor injects the dog with an empty syringe and a dry needle.

If a dog is capable of unconscious deception, how much more unreliable must such a test be in the case of the more complicated human animal.

BLOOD-PRESSURE

We have already learned something about the pressure wave of the pulse, and one might suppose that this has some connection with "blood-pressure," that nightmare of many a corpulent person. Now if you imagine a pump—our heart—which constantly pumps liquid into a tube: the pressure from within causes the tube walls to stretch until they are taut. As the walls of our blood-vessels are elastic, their width alters too as a result of increased pressure. The pressure wave of the heart-beat passes perceptibly into the artery which runs near the surface of the hand. If you put your finger on it, you can feel the vessel move. The blood flows on from the arteries to the smallest network of blood-vessels, those which wash round all the cells of the body, and then it returns to the heart.

The heart always pumps the blood more quickly into the big artery pipes than it can seep through the innumerable holes of the smallest network of vessels. For that reason there is always a considerable inner pressure in the arteries. If they are pierced in an injury, the blood fairly spurts out, because it is under pressure.

If there were no pressure head the blood could not flow through the minute channels of capillaries surrounding the cells. So without blood-pressure our cells cannot function. If our blood-pressure drops below a certain level, we faint because the nerve cells of our brain begin to suffocate. The blood flows too slowly to maintain their supply of oxygen. But if one lies down flat, one feels better as the blood traveling from the heart to the head does not have to climb and can start to flow again even when the blood-pressure is quite low.

Every heart-beat causes the blood-pressure to rise above its average, and then, before the next beat, it falls below its average. This rise of pressure occurs as a result of the pulse or pressure wave, and this rise may be as much as one-third of the average arterial pressure. When the pulse has passed, the pressure drops again, to the resting level, below the average. The peak value and the resting value are both measured, and are the two numbers about which so many people get anxious. Normal figures are 120/80 millimeters of mercury in young people. This means that the blood in the compressed artery would have spurted one and a half meters at the peak of the pulse wave, had the artery been severed. The pressure is measured in millimeters of mercury for convenience. Mercury is much heavier than water—about thirteen and a half times as heavy. If we used water in our measuring instruments they would be unnecessarily bulky.

To give an example—if we blow with all our might into a pressure measure, we can bring it up to 150 millimeters of mercury. A human heart can do, and does do, more than that. It can raise the pressure to 200 millimeters of mercury. It could even pump the blood more than three yards high.

Our blood-pressure averages are always changing, and these changes are not dependent on the pulse wave, although that goes on incessantly. Our blood-pressure is higher when we are standing than when we are sitting. It rises rapidly, but only for a short time, if we take a very deep breath; it rises much more than that if we are suddenly frightened. It rises too if we are in a rage, and stays high for a long time, and we feel that our throat is bursting. If we are sad and depressed, the blood-pressure is lower. When we measure blood-pressure we want both the body and the mind at rest. Any emotion changes the blood-pressure, and so the measurements we make sometimes simulate those found in illness when the illness is not really there at all.

REGULATING THE BLOOD-PRESSURE

If the blood-pressure fluctuates it must be regulated the whole time, that is to say, its actual level or height is adjusted by the brain. Of course we do not notice it, and we need not consciously think, now my blood-pressure must rise ten millimeters, or something to that effect. It happens automatically. When the blood-pressure rises, the blood flows more quickly through the body and the oxygen and food supplies for the cells are increased.

In the main artery which leads to the head are to be found nerve endings which are sensitive to acid. If the flow is too slow, too much acid accumulates. The nerves, sensitive to acid, signal this change to the brain, which promptly transmits nerve signals to speed up the heart and constrict the apertures of the smallest vessels through which the blood seeps. The heart, therefore, pumps more blood into the main arteries and the blood-flow gradually diminishes towards the ends of the arteries. The blood-pressure must then rise and the flow of blood is accelerated.

There are also to be found in the same segment of the artery to the head, nerve endings which are sensitive to pressure. They, in contrast to the other nerves, put a brake on the blood-pressure. The heart-beat slows down if the blood-pressure is too high. This provides us with a simple remedy for overcoming nervous palpitations.

If you press your neck firmly with both thumbs directly beneath the jaw bones, the pulse will slow down in a few seconds. By closing both the neck arteries, the blood accumulates, causing the pressure to rise. The nerve signal is given at once for the heart to apply the brakes.

If one does this when the heart-beat is slow, one can easily turn giddy. The heart and blood-pressure are so perfectly attuned that an artificial slowing down results in an insufficient blood supply to the tissues. However, when the heart-beat is quick and excited, this trick can be most effective in calming oneself down and restoring equilibrium. Of course, there are other nervous impulses connected with the regulation of the blood-pressure, but let these two most important reflexes suffice.

The more blood that is pumped into the main arteries, the higher the pressure. The vessels through which the blood seeps, the smallest arteries and capillaries in the tissues, are another important factor in altering the pressure. The wider these valves are opened the lower the blood-pressure.

KNOCK-OUT AND UNCONSCIOUSNESS

If a man is knocked out as a result of a kick in the pit of his stomach, he loses consciousness because all the small vessels are flung open. The blow involves a shock of the nervous system. The blood stagnates in the widely opened capillary vessels of the abdominal organs and not even the strongest heart can maintain a sufficient flow of blood. The nerve cells of the brain cannot get enough oxygen and the person loses consciousness. All this applies to other causes of fainting, which might be a visit to the dentist, having an injection, the smell of ether, or the sight of blood. The underlying nervous cause makes the smallest network of vessels open so that the mechanism regulating the blood-pressure collapses. Thus it is not the heart which fails; it is the blood trickling away too fast at the end of the pipe system. The heart works like mad to make good the loss. There is no doubt that we may faint for psychological reasons, and we shall hear later how and when this can happen.

HIGH BLOOD-PRESSURE

The opposite of a breakdown of the circulatory system is a rise of the blood-pressure, which eventually becomes what we know as "high blood-pressure." If the flow of blood has to be accelerated, this is done by raising the blood-pressure. There is constriction of the small vessels through which the blood trickles into the abdominal organs. The heart pumps harder, the blood-pressure rises, and the blood flows more quickly through the muscles. This spontaneous overactivity of the minute muscles in the walls of the smallest arterial blood-vessels constitutes the ailment known as "blood-pressure." It is a disease of the sympathetic nervous system, an illness which is often the result of psychological stresses.

Blood-pressure can, however, arise from other causes. If you narrow the blood-vessels which supply the kidneys in an animal used for experimental purposes, the blood-pressure rises. This is not a nervous reflex as in the case when pressure is applied by the thumbs to the arteries in the neck—the process which we have already described. The kidney, which now has an impaired blood supply, secretes a substance which constricts all the smallest arteries in the entire body. This is really a protective mechanism, for if all the blood did not flow at least once through the kidney every five minutes, the entire body would be in danger as the blood would no longer be purified. This is the basis of the high blood-pressure associated with most kidney ailments. The affected kidney is trying to provide itself with more blood, and the substance which it secretes for this purpose causes the blood-pressure to rise.

High blood-pressure generally is associated with a hardening of the walls of the arteries. Although the exact cause-and-effect relationship still is a mystery, there is growing evidence that high blood pressure may accelerate hardening of the arteries. And as the arteries become rigid, the high blood-pressure becomes constant.

All tissues deteriorate to some extent with advancing years and this effect shows itself in blood vessels as a hardening of the arteries. As a result of this increased rigidity of the blood vessel walls, the blood pressure of a 50-year-old person is higher than that of a 20-year-old person, assuming the individuals are otherwise healthy. Also, the blood pressure of a mature male generally is higher than that of an adult female, until the woman reaches the age of menopause after which her blood pressure may rise to a level that is higher than a man of the same age.

Normal blood pressure at different ages

Age	4	13	25	40	Over 50
Pressure	99/65	118/60	125/78	129/81	135/83

The figures on this chart represent the average blood-pressure of a person at rest and they should not be much higher. There is no strictly normal value for blood-pressure and even doctors vary in the values that they consider to be normal. If a patient's blood-pressure measures 190/100 once, it does not necessarily mean that he is ill. One can only call it high blood-pressure when the values obtained are consistently high. Even then, however, it may not be illness; it may be that the patient is one of those people who get very excited when they have a medical examination. Even otherwise normal persons may experience very high blood pressure readings during sexual intercourse or other exciting events.

LOW BLOOD-PRESSURE

This is scarcely ever a sign of an organic illness. It is nearly always psychological and low blood-pressure is seldom a symptom of heart trouble. People whose blood-pressure is lower than the figures indicated on the chart have a greater expectation of life than others.

RED BLOOD

We know something about the blood itself, which, as we have seen, is under constant pressure. It is a watery liquid tissue. It consists of 79 per cent of water. (Muscles are 76 per cent water and the kidney tissue 83 per cent water.) The watery tissue, blood, has less water than many firmer organs. This, of course, includes the water inside as well as outside cells—the red and white corpuscles. The volume of the corpuscles is roughly 40 per cent of the blood. These corpuscles float about together but they are not attached to each other.

The red blood corpuscles have almost only one purpose. They contain a red pigment, hemoglobin, which unites with the gas oxygen in the air of the lung and carries it into the tissues. In the tissues they give up the oxygen, and the blood then takes the carbon dioxide which has formed in the tissue back to the lungs. The red blood corpuscles can be called an organ of breathing. The most important constituent of hemoglobin is iron and approximately one three-hundredth part of hemoglobin is composed of iron. Almost all the iron in the body is to be found in this hemoglobin in the red blood-cells. Contrary to the usually extravagant behavior of nature, this iron is very carefully conserved. Only the smallest quantities escape from the body each day. The remainder is caught up again and used to replace old blood corpuscles which have been destroyed. Loss of blood means loss of iron to the body. The building of new blood-cells is one of the least difficult things to the body, but the necessary iron must be provided.

We have already said that 40 per cent of the blood is composed of red blood corpuscles. Then one liter contains roughly 400 grams of red blood-cells. One cubic centimeter contains 4½ to 5 million individual cells. That is the figure patients sometimes remember: 4½ million erythrocytes or red cells. That means that 4½ million erythrocytes are to be found in every cubic millimeter of blood. That is the normal content of the blood.

PERCENTAGE OF HEMOGLOBIN

Normally 16–17 grams of hemoglobin is contained in 100 cubic centimeters of blood. At a medical congress many years ago, exactly 16 grams in 100 cubic centimeters was fixed as the standard amount. Such a large amount of hemoglobin is called one hundred per cent. Anyone having only 10 grams of hemoglobin in his blood is described as having a hemoglobin content of 60–65 per cent of standard, which is written thus: Hb 60%.

WHITE BLOOD CORPUSCLES

It is not just the total quantity of white blood corpuscles which is important, because there are several kinds of white corpuscles, and each kind has individual functions to perform. The major function performed by white cells is to maintain order and cleanliness in the body.

When tissue cells wear out or are injured they break up, and the white cells, which can crawl out of the blood-vessels of their own accord, wander into the tissues and devour and digest the disintegrated pieces of broken-down tissue cells. White cells also remove foreign bodies. They come to the rescue, for instance, when a splinter gets under the skin. Millions of white cells collect round the splinter, and liquefy, forming pus which, when discharged, carries the splinter with it.

White cells are especially important when bacteria have invaded the body. They do the clearing up, and eat the bacteria. They carry within them substances fatal to germs and are, in a manner of speaking, like little penicillin factories, although they do not, of course, make penicillin itself. They are our main defense against infections. In a body where all the white corpuscles have been destroyed, death is almost inevitable. The person succumbs to infection and is killed by bacteria. Even the stupendous resources of modern medicine are only able to make good such a deficiency for a few weeks. At the end of that period either new white corpuscles have been made in the body, or the bacteria win, and it is all over.

The white blood corpuscles are most independent of all the cells in the human body. They can travel in the blood-stream, or creep out of the blood-channels into the tissues, and, like primitive one-celled independent creatures, swallow small objects and digest them. They follow their own laws of behavior more completely than is usual for the millions of cells that make up a complex animal, for the white cells receive no commands via the nerves. They instantly sense trouble, and trouble attracts them, so that they are to be found wherever anything is going wrong in the body. They deal with trouble automatically, in their own way.

The number of white cells in the blood-stream varies from hour to hour. They are always wandering off into the tissues, and coming back to the blood-stream again. A large number are always to be found in the blood-stream, keeping an eye, as it were, on conditions there, and guarding against untoward invasion of the blood-stream by bacteria from the intestines. They also remove fat globules from the small vessels of the intestine, and help in digestion.

THE KIDNEYS AND THE PURIFYING OF THE BLOOD

There are a great many substances in the blood, apart from cells. The blood-channels are the major roadways of the body. All food, oxygen, and waste matter flow along in the blood and are picked up by consumer or purifying tissues as they pass by. The chemical messengers or hormones of the body also travel by the blood-stream. Their function is to carry commands from one part of the body to another. Adrenaline is one such chemical messenger. It, for instance, is carried by the blood from the adrenal gland, and stimulates the liver to pour glucose into the blood-stream. This is of course only one of the actions of adrenaline.

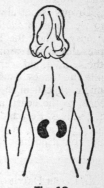

Fig. 18
The kidneys.

The kidneys are organs which purify the blood. Two wide branches of the main artery or aorta continuously deflect blood through the kidneys, which remove waste matter, and sieve it into the urine. These kidneys prepare urine, and in so doing dispose of waste matter, maintain a strict balance between the acid and alkalis in the blood, and keep a correct water content in the blood and body as a whole. We have two kidneys, and they lie one on each side of the spine, high up in the abdomen, just behind the stomach (Fig. 18).

These kidneys work night and day at their job, and do it very efficiently. They leave nothing that needs to be removed by blood-purifying tonics, a spa treatment. Such things may be very useful and stimulating at times, but not for the purification of the blood. Kidneys do that much better. A single kidney, working at half strength, is all that is really necessary to keep the blood clean, and it is fortunately very rare for kidneys to be so diseased that they fail in this function. If or when they fail, the poisoning that results cannot be cured by tonics, salts, or spa treatment.

True kidney failure is very rare. Much more commonly kidneys are made leaky by illness and are no longer able to keep valuable proteins of the blood from passing through the sieve by which they get rid of waste matter. The leakiness also disturbs their functions as regulators of the salt and water content of the body. Such diseased kidneys fail to get rid of excess salt and water, and so the patient swells up with a dropsy due to kidney disease. Accumulations of water occur first and to the greatest extent in the most delicate tissues—i.e. those which are most loosely constructed—such as the bags under one's eyes. As a result, the patient's face looks puffy and swollen.

Dropsy is not always due to kidney disease. It may be due to weakness of the heart, and is then called heart or cardiac dropsy. When the heart fails to pump properly, the blood-pressure is not properly maintained, and blood stagnates in the veins. Fluid seeps out from the capillaries and small veins into the tissues, causing dropsy. Cardiac dropsy begins, as one might expect, in the legs, since blood has to flow uphill from them to the heart, and so the blood will stagnate most easily in the legs. Feet and ankles swell in the course of the day, and go down again in the night while the patient is asleep in the horizontal position.

THE INNER DRIVING FORCE

The heart is by and large the "playing field" on which our nerves and emotions disport themselves. If we receive a sudden shock, the heart immediately goes faster, and beats more forcibly, and the blood-vessels constrict, causing the blood-pressure to rise. At the same time, every activity of the body unnecessary for prompt action slows down. The state of tension goes on, and we are keyed up in anxiety. Fear has snatched our steering-wheel, and is preparing to drive us to our greatest effort. Usually, during fear, urine formation is decreased. However, especially in small children, fear may cause a full bladder to empty. A state of anxiety makes us want to get things done as quickly as possible, and, once fear is in control, unexpected things may happen.

A very similar sequence of events takes place when we exert ourselves deliberately, but this time fear is not in control. The hundred-yard sprinter waits tense but collected at his mark. As soon as the shot is fired he is off at full speed down the track long before any surprise from the sound of a shot could have affected him. His own will-power has seized the steering-wheel and has thrown his body into action. Just as in an anxiety state, however, the heart beats faster and more forcibly, and blood-vessels constrict: the same hormones are poured out from the glands.

THE MIND AND ITS INFLUENCE ON THE HEART

We have already discussed the effect of fear and acute anxiety on the heart. Long-term anxiety states also frequently affect the heart. If you were to ask me what you should do in order to avoid this sort of heart trouble, I could only answer: do not be afraid. This does not mean that you should not fear real danger. It is perfectly normal for your teeth to chatter and for your heart to thump when bombs are dropping around you. However, when the time for action comes and steps have to be taken to rescue yourself or others in an emergency, the mentally normal person adjusts himself to the circumstances, and his will, rather than his fear, takes hold of the steering-wheel. It is not real dangers that cause anxiety states: these conditions are caused by the secret nagging fears that we all knew as children, and that we have not outgrown, although we think we have. We might even be annoyed were it suggested to us that we still had these fears, because it seems ridiculous to us. However, the anxiety associated with these fears may still be there, and continues to exist as far as the heart is concerned. This nagging, irrational anxiety is quite different from the sensible fear of air raids which vanished at the sound of the "All Clear," giving place to gay relief.

Hidden anxiety troubles us when we are well, but even more so in times of sickness. Then, if we are a prey to depression and secret fears, we feel more than just a little run-down. The heart mechanisms which were hitherto just about adequate for our needs break down. Water leaves the overfilled blood-vessels and penetrates the tissues. We become short of breath, and every step becomes an effort. We shall only regain security and confidence when we put ourselves into the hands of a capable doctor who will prescribe treatment to strengthen the heart muscle. We can help the treatment by putting aside our worries and our fears. If we have a fear we must acknowledge it, and not try to pretend that it isn't there. We should try to find the source of a hidden fear.

BREATHING AND DIGESTION

We cannot live without air to breathe, and to live we must both eat and drink. Oxygen, drawn into the body from the air taken into our lungs, is used to burn up food products. This provides energy for work, and for all our other pastimes. Solid unwanted food residues pass straight downward through the stomach and the intestines and out at the anus or lower opening of the bowel. Useful food products pass into the bloodstream from the intestine and then burned up or oxidized. Fats and starchy foods are converted to carbon dioxide gas and water by this process. Digested proteins are oxidized to carbon dioxide and water, and also form urea. All the carbon dioxide and some of the water leave the body in the air we breathe out, urea and nearly all the rest of the water leave the body in the urine. The lungs, the kidneys and the lower bowel are therefore all engaged in getting rid of waste matter, and are called organs of excretion.

THE LUNG AS AN ORGAN OF EXCRETION

An adult man breathes out 850 grams of carbon dioxide a day, and gets rid of about 60 grams of solids dissolved in two to three pints of water in his urine in the same time. Quantitatively then, the lungs are the most important organs of excretion. For every 100 grams (1 gram = $\frac{1}{30}$ oz.) of sugar or starch that we eat, 40 grams of carbon is converted to 146 grams of carbon dioxide which leaves the body by the lungs, while 60 grams of water is made. Only about 30 grams of this water passes through the kidneys into the urine; the rest is excreted partly through the lungs into the expired air, and part is lost through the skin, in the sweat.

The process of oxidation or burning up of useful foodstuffs is called metabolism. The end-products from the metabolism of starch or sugar are carbon dioxide and water.

Summary of the processes of the metabolism and excretion of sugar

Intake. 100 grams of sugar.

Metabolism   100 grams of sugar during metabolism use up 106 grams of oxygen, and give rise to 60 grams of water and 146 grams of carbon dioxide.

Excretion   146 grams of carbon dioxide is breathed out into the air. About 30 grams of water leaves the body in the urine, 15 grams leaves the body in the air breathed out, and 15 grams leaves the body through the skin.

Under normal circumstances, breathing is not regulated by the body's need for oxygen, but by the amount of carbon dioxide awaiting excretion. Nothing is more dangerous than an accumulation of carbon dioxide. All this means that we must abandon our views as to what are 'decent' and slightly 'indecent' organs, for the breath from our lungs, which most people consider to be pure, is the product of our major organs of evacuation. It is true that the air we breathe out does not smell offensive, yet the fact remains that it is extremely poisonous. If a living creature were put under a glass cover in a jar filled with exhaled air, it would die rapidly.

BURNING AND METABOLISM

Each day we use up about 1½ lb. of dry foodstuff, and at least 1½ lb. of oxygen. The oxygen is used to burn up the foodstuff or fuel. The burning of coal is a rapid process of oxidation, and generates a great deal of heat. The discoloration of the cut surface of an apple is a slow chemical process of oxidation, and energy is only slowly liberated, and is not apparent as heat. Our cells conduct the oxidizing or burning processes within themselves in a very controlled way, and have means by which some of the energy set free during the processes can be conserved, so that it is not all liberated as heat, and the body temperature can be kept at 98.6 degrees Fahrenheit (37 degrees Centigrade). About half the water formed during metabolism leaves the body in the urine, or exhaust, and the carbon dioxide (which is a gas) leaves through the lungs, or chimney, in the expired air. Breathing and digestion are inseparable.

It is easiest to measure how much we are burning from the chimney. We can find out how much oxygen is being used per minute, or how much carbon dioxide is being given off per minute, when the body is completely at rest. This gives us a measure of the basic energy requirement of the body when at rest, and this energy requirement is expressed in calories. One hundred calories represent the amount of energy equivalent to the heat needed to bring 1 liter of iced water up to boiling-point. There are standard basic energy requirements for human bodies of all ages, weights, and sizes, which are defined as 100 per cent. If then a patient is found to have a basal metabolic rate of 110 percent, it means that his basal oxygen and fuel consumption is + 10 per cent of standard. In actual fact, very few people are exactly standard in their basic energy needs, and the range of values found for perfectly normal people varies from − 20 to + 20 per cent, or even more.

The energy requirements of the human body can be supplied by any one of the three basic classes of foodstuffs, protein, carbohydrates (sugars and starches) or fat, but food is not only required for energy, but also for processes of growth, and of repair.

PROTEIN

If one leaves such things as meat, milk, eggs, fish, peas, et cetera, which contain protein, out of one's diet, disaster follows. Even if sufficient calories are provided in the form of carbohydrate and fat, absence of protein in the diet still leads to disaster. Food value cannot be measured in calories alone.

The human body cannot build up all the separate bricks which together make its complex proteins, and yet these proteins are vital constituents of all our cells. That is why we need 5 grams of nitrogen in the form of good-class protein each day. The 1,000 grams of nitrogen breathed in and out of our lungs a day is useless for this purpose, because we cannot absorb or use the nitrogen of the air.

Only a few kinds of bacteria exist among the countless number of animal and plant creatures which can use this air nitrogen to make protein. All life on earth is dependent on their activity, and it was not until early in this century that we learned to make ourselves independent of their activity. Now our factories produce artificial manures from the nitrogen of the air from which plants can make protein. Animals and people live on these plants.

Human lack of independence in nutrition goes even further. We are unable to make for ourselves some of the essential bricks of our own human proteins, and we have to obtain these bricks from the flesh of other animals, from fish, from milk or from eggs. We can get them from plant proteins, but animal proteins are the richer source. When we have eaten these animal or plant proteins we break them down by digestion into their component parts. These we rebuild in a different design to form proteins characteristic of our own species.

At first sight we might suspect that a finished, grown body should be able to dispense with the luxury of protein in the diet. But this would be an error. The human body is alive, and old cells are constantly wearing out and being replaced by new ones. Therefore we must have a continuous supply of protein with which to carry out these repairs.

In the space of 120 days or so, all of the body's 25 million million red blood corpuscles wear out, are broken down, and are renewed. Most of the iron they contain will be conserved and used again, but we have no mechanism by which we can exercise so strict an economy over the protein they contain. Every day we lose at least five grams of precious protein nitrogen through the kidney into the urine, mostly in the form of urea. This five grams of protein nitrogen has to be replaced, and the protein used in the diet to replace it must contain the essential bricks for the manufacture of our own protein. Those are bricks that we cannot make for ourselves. A proportion therefore of our protein food should be a good animal protein, rich in these necessary bricks.

DIGESTION

The process of digestion is more complicated than that of absorbing oxygen from the air, into the blood. A piece of bread which we have just eaten does not just dissolve and pass into the blood. All food substances have to be altered, and transformed into simpler substances, in liquid form, before they can be absorbed into the blood-stream.

The cooking, baking, and roasting of food is of primary importance. In this way we save our digestive juices work. Food which has been prepared in the kitchen can have greater nutritive value than raw food. During cooking, the hard indigestible cell coverings become ruptured, making the cell contents accessible to our digestive juices. When we bottle fruit valuable vitamin C can be preserved, but when fruit is stored its vitamin C content steadily decreases. Bottled cherries will still contain vitamin C at Christmas, but the keeping apple will by then have lost its vitamin C.

Thus cooking constitutes the first stage in human digestion. Moreover, cooked food is often more appetizing than raw food, and when the welcome smell of roasting penetrates to our nervous system via the nose, our mouths start to water. Less obvious, but equally important, is the fact that our stomachs do likewise, and so indirectly does the liver and the pancreas. These digestive juices, the saliva, stomach and pancreatic juices, bile from the liver, and juices from the intestine, contain enzymes or ferments which transform our food into a pap containing substances simpler than the original food, which we can absorb and use as fuel.

The saliva lubricates the food, making it easy to swallow, and starts the digestion of starch. When the food reaches the stomach it is subjected to the action of stomach or gastric juice which contains hydrochloric acid. The quantity of hydrochloric acid there is so great that were there no special protection it would damage the cells of the stomach wall. However, in the live body these cells are protected by a layer of mucus. None the less, there are good reasons for the repeated contention that one's own hydrochloric acid is in some measure responsible for stomach ulcers.

The real work of gastric digestion is not performed by the hydrochloric acid. The acid helps the pepsin enzymes, or ferments, in the gastric juice do their work. The enzymes are special protein molecules, which, without damage to themselves, smash up other complex molecules by first building water molecules into them, and then by tearing the water molecules apart, so that two smaller molecules are formed. These water-tearers act swiftly, so that after four hours a cutlet has been reduced by their action to small molecules which have dissolved in water, and the once cutlet is felt gurgling in the intestines.

The ferments could not act nearly so effectively were the food not first chewed in the mouth, and then well kneaded by the muscular movements of the stomach and intestines. The stomach is active throughout digestion. Waves of contraction pass across its strong involuntary muscular system, mixing the food with the ferments, and squirting the liquefied parts jerkily into the duodenum, which is the adjacent part of the small intestine. The stomach juices are acid, and the intestinal juices are alkaline. If the duodenal contents become too acid, the stomach door shuts. When the acidity has been sufficiently reduced, it opens again.

BILE OR GALL

Ferments from the pancreas are poured into the duodenum in the alkaline pancreatic juice to complete the chemical process of digestion. These pancreatic ferments are assisted by those secreted by small auxiliary glands found throughout the small intestine, and by bile.

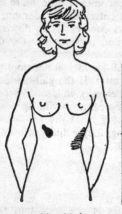

Fig. 19

Gall-bladder.

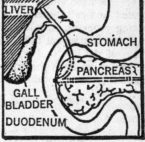

Fig. 20

Three-way bile.

Bile is the liver's contribution toward the process of digestion, and it is poured into the duodenum intermittently if the gall-bladder is functioning, continuously if the gall-bladder has been removed. Fat cannot be properly digested without bile, although the fat-splitting ferments come from the pancreas. But as we all know from observations of soup, little rings or balls of liquid fat form when melted fat is mixed with water. That is just what happens in the intestines. It would take a fat-splitting ferment a long time to tear its way through a fat droplet that measured several millimeters across, because the ferment has to stay in the water and so can only attack the outside of the droplet. However, special bile salts, found only in bile, greatly assist the action of the fat-splitting ferments by decreasing the size of the fat droplets, and by preventing torn droplets from joining together again.

THE GALL-BLADDER AND GALL-STONES

Bile made in the liver can pass straight down a bile duct or channel into the duodenum. However, if the bile is not needed at that moment in the intestines, it can also pass along a side opening leading from the main duct, into the gall-bladder. Once in the gall-bladder the bile becomes a little more concentrated during storage. When fat enters the duodenum, the gall-bladder contracts and expels its contents back down the side passage, into the main duct, and onward into the duodenum.

If the bile stays too long in the gall-bladder, it becomes very concentrated, and gall-stones may result. If the gall-bladder is not working properly, it quickly becomes inflamed, because bacteria thrive in stagnant bile. They cannot swim up against the current of the bile squirts coming from the gall-bladder, but once this organ stops performing, they achieve it only too easily, and make a habit of doing so.

ABSORPTION

We have seen how digestible foods are split into small molecules by the combined action of the teeth, saliva, stomach juice, the pancreatic and intestinal juices, and the movements of the stomach and intestines. These small molecules are dissolved in the fluid which lies inside the small intestine. The inner layer of the wall of the intestine is especially adapted to allow only the useful substances derived from food to pass through it into the blood-stream. Some of the unwanted substances are kept back within the hollow of the intestine, and never enter the blood-stream at all. The absorption of iron is peculiar; only a very small fraction of that available in the intestine is absorbed, and so injury of the intestinal wall can lead to anemia.

EXCREMENT

There is always a residue of indigestible material left from the food, and this passes out at the other end. However, this residue only accounts for a quarter of the total amount of the feces. One half of their whole bulk consists of bacteria and the rest of rejected, scraped-off surface cells of the intestinal walls.

The contents of the small intestine are liquid, and it is here that digestion takes place. When the contents of the small intestine pass on into the large intestine or colon, water and products of digestion are continuously absorbed, and so the final excreta are solid or nearly so.

The contents of the human intestines teem with bacteria: they grow there. These organisms are not only cadgers, picking up the crumbs which fall from the rich man's table; they also help the digestive processes of the human being by secreting ferments which destroy the cellulose of plant fibers. Our own ferments cannot do that for us. The bacteria also make chemical substances which we can use, but cannot make for ourselves in our own bodies. Vitamin K is made by the bacteria in our intestines, and is absorbed by us from the intestines for use in our bodies. Without vitamin K we might bleed to death when we cut ourselves, because vitamin K is necessary for blood coagulation.

If all the bacteria in our intestines are killed by modern germ-killing medicines, the bowels become loose, and the intestinal wall becomes irritable. The result is diarrhea. Bleeding can be prevented by giving vitamin K prepared commercially.

In a healthy body the bacteria are not allowed to spread from the hollow of the intestine where they do useful work for us. But when the body is run-down, and its defenses are weak, these intestinal bacteria not infrequently give trouble by spreading to the gall-bladder, to the urinary bladder, or to the kidneys, where they set up protracted inflammation. The most important of these intestinal bacteria is called *Bacterium coli*. One of their unpleasant characteristics is a habit of producing skatol, a chemical responsible for the smell of feces; in addition, they are gas-formers. It is the bacteria and not we ourselves who make the intestinal gases. It is a pity that otherwise useful organisms have developed these unpleasant habits.

THE CAECUM AND THE APPENDIX

The small intestine opens into the large intestine in the lower part of the right side of the abdominal area. The caecum hangs downward from just below this junction, as a short wide sac ending in a narrow finger-like appendix. This appendix has a blind end, and is believed to be a relic of the past. Our animal ancestors must have had a large appendix or blind-ended intestinal bag in this position. Cows and rabbits have them still, and use them for a place where bacteria can really get to work undisturbed to digest the cellulose of grass, converting it into sugar. The cow then absorbs the sugar, and the bacteria start again on the next batch of grass. Human beings have, however, given up eating grass, and the appendix remains as the only and a rather pathetic portion of the grass-eater's equipment; it has no recognizable function nowadays.

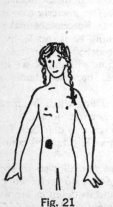

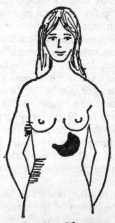

Fig. 21
The appendix.

Fig. 22
The stomach.

Sometimes the intestinal contents accumulate inside the appendix and ferment, and cause a pain in the lower right-hand side of the abdomen. This we call appendicitis. Operations for the removal of the appendix used to be very fashionable, but experience has shown us that, in adults, a great many cases of appendicitis will clear up without operation. However, if an appendix is obstructed, and its contents suppurate, there is danger, and an operation is necessary. A neglected suppurating appendix may rupture, and then the inflammation may spread throughout the whole abdomen, producing what is known as general peritonitis. It is the doctor's job to decide whether or not an operation is necessary when the appendix is in trouble.

Peritonitis used to be a greatly feared complication of appendicitis, and doctors nearly always advised operation lest peritonitis should ensue. Nowadays, peritonitis is less dangerous than it was because we have an effective range of germ-killing drugs with which to save the patient. The result is that operations for removal of the appendix are less fashionable than they used to be. Twenty years ago nearly everybody had had an appendix removed at some time or another, and tales about these operations were regularly exchanged across tea-tables. But in these days, the appendix is regarded as a curious and useless human organ which reminds anatomists of prehistoric days.

HUNGER AND LOVE: THE MIND AND ITS INFLUENCE ON THE STOMACH

The better a thing tastes, the more easily we digest it. But the influence of our senses and our emotions on our digestive apparatus does not end there. When an animal is hungry it just wants something to eat. That can happen to a man too. But man's emotions are more complicated and varied than are those of animals. We can hunger after love, adventure, or a thousand other things—at least, that is what our language tells us and it is somehow true. The trouble is that our emotions are too varied and complicated for the simple, primitive, animal-like design of our human body. Right back from childhood all our emotions have taken place on and through the same nervous apparatus. As babies our only concern when we were hungry was to get our milk in sufficient quantity as soon as possible, whether from the breast or from the bottle. We came to associate not seeing, hearing, or feeling our mother with being hungry, and here we have our first example of overlapping emotions. Hunger has overlapped with a need for mother. Longing was synonymous with hunger. The foundation is the same in both cases, even when one is adult.

Thus, later in life, our more tender feelings and emotions play on our digestive apparatus. If life becomes tough, and we have to "swallow the pill," it has repercussions on our digestive apparatus. These repercussions are invariably accompanied by secret, perhaps even unrecognized, longings for help and protection which are not exactly compatible with our proud conception of independent manhood. In patients with gastric ulcers the stomach is in a continual state of excitement. The juice flows all the time, night and day, and not only when one is eating. The stomach is behaving as if we were hungry the whole time. We may be longing for something, not necessarily for food.

If you asked me how to keep one's stomach healthy, I would reply, "Eat sensibly, and preferably only when you feel like it. Always enjoy your food, and don't be too strict with yourself or others. If, like most other people, you have to drive yourself on in the daily round of work and worry, try to find time to be 'soft' and to let others do a bit of worrying about you. Remember that our bodies demand that we distinguish between night and day, and between self-abnegation and self-indulgence."

NERVES AND HORMONES

UNBREAKABLE NERVES

Nerves are the only things which never really break down in our bodies. They are the most efficient, enduring, and undemanding things we possess. If you take a nerve and the muscle belonging to it from an animal's body, and put them into a suitable solution containing food that they can use, and subject the nerve to electrical stimulation, that nerve will go on transmitting work signals to the muscle for hours. The nerve will still be signalling long after the muscle has ceased to respond.

Nerves are virtually inexhaustible. Muscles tire, but nerves never break down or collapse. They are always alert and ready for work. Many are active all the time. Even at night the reflexes of breathing and heat regulation and numerous other automatic functions do not rest. There is a continual stream of activity along these nerve routes.

Even our dreams show us that our brain works at night while we are asleep and all the "windows" are closed. Undigested experiences, wishes, disturbing emotions, and censored impulses are kept away from its most sensitive layer during our conscious or waking hours, but often form dreams while we sleep.

When we dealt with the muscles we learned about the two nervous systems—the voluntary and the involuntary one. We learned that involuntary movements are always transmitted by voluntary nerves to voluntary muscles. Everything which moves visibly is ordered to do so by the voluntary nervous system. Correspondingly there is also a "voluntary sensory-nervous system." That is, of course, an idiotic term, but it only means that feelings or sensations are also transmitted along the paths of the central nervous system, which looks after the muscles and skin. These are the feelings which penetrate our consciousness—and what we know as nerves. A good touch on the piano, or sensitive finger-tips, are just as much a part of this nervous system as the pain from a wound or any sensation of heat or cold. The nerves which run from all the special sensory organs, from the eye, nose and mouth to, for example, the brain, also belong to this "conscious" system. Everything that we experience, feel, see, hear and perceive in the outside world and are consciously aware of in our body and its organs, works through it too.

NERVE ROUTES

The voluntary nervous system is made up of the biggest nerves in our bodies. We not only transmit our commands to our muscles through these nerves, but also, through them, we receive messages from the outside world as it impinges on any part of our body, all the way from the top of our heads, down to our big toes. Some of the fibers in these voluntary nerves are the biggest fibers found anywhere in nerves, and these transmit their signals at a greater speed than do narrower fibers. All the fibers in these voluntary nerves are remarkably well protected by their own individual insulating sheaths. The sciatic nerve is the major voluntary nerve to the leg, and it is almost as thick as one's little finger. When we feel or move anything below the knee, signals run to and fro through this nerve, either to or from the brain and spinal cord.

There are no cells in these voluntary nerves, only fibers,

and these fibers are offshoots of cells which are situated in the spinal cord. These nerve cells in the cord can be as much as a tenth of a millimeter in diameter, but most of them are smaller than that, yet the nerve fiber attached to them may be a whole yard long. By comparison we can imagine, in the extreme case of the sciatic nerve, a football extending into a 2,500-yard length of rope, or 200 miles of cross-country electric towers leading from a power station 35 yards high.

Those nerve cells in the spinal cord act rather like the points in a railway shunting yard, and these points intersect the network of fibers leading to and from other nerve cells in the brain. In a way the spinal cord can be regarded as a nerve itself just because it is the great main road of communication between the brain and the outer nerves of the voluntary nervous system. The cord is a bridge over which all messages, except those travelling by some special nerves of the head, must pass.

The nerve cells in the spinal cord are collected together toward the center of the cord, and are surrounded by the fibers. When the cord is cut across, the fiber part looks white, and the cell part grayish. The pattern made by the gray part is rather like a central butterfly; the cells in the front or ventral horns of this butterfly are occupied in switching commands from the brain to the muscles. So you see, those front cells are not only points, but signalmen too. If these front horn cells become sick and do not function, the muscle they direct becomes paralyzed, as in poliomyelitis.

SPINAL FLUID AND LUMBAR PUNCTURE

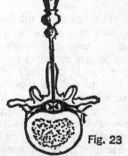

Fig. 23

Doctors never puncture the spinal cord, at least, not intentionally. When a spinal or lumbar puncture is performed, a cannula is pushed just through the coverings of the cord, into the fluid which fills a fairly wide gap between the cord itself and its coverings. This fluid space extends from cavities in and around the brain right down to and beyond the bottom of the spinal cord.

The fluid in this space is really filtered blood which contains food for nerve cells. It also protects the brain and cord, which are very sensitive, from jolts and knocks, for they float in it like a ship with many anchors. This fluid is made inside the brain, where there are special blood filters which not only make the spinal fluid, but also hold back harmful substances and bacteria as well as the blood-cells. However, these filters get damaged when a person has meningitis; bacteria can enter the fluid, and the composition of the fluid also changes.

The spinal fluid alters in composition differently according to the type of illness that has occurred in the nerve tissues, and the changes in the spinal fluid often take place early in the course of the disease, before much damage has been done to the sensitive nerve cells. That is why doctors are always so anxious to do a lumbar puncture, to draw off some of the spinal fluid, and to examine it both chemically and microscopically. They can, as a result, often get information which enables them to prevent further development of the disease by early treatment. They can also inject suitable curative agents into the spinal fluid, knowing that they will spread throughout the fluid space, and reach the brain, if they make their solutions of the correct density for this purpose.

Lumbar puncture is, as we have seen, a very useful operation. It is also a very harmless one. At times it may cause headache for a few hours, especially if the patient has got up too soon, or has not lain quite flat for long enough after it. Any liquid the doctors draw off is replaced very quickly. Lumbar punctures, then, are not dangerous, and should not be feared. Perhaps the most unpleasant thing about them from the patient's point of view is that you cannot see what the chap in the white gown behind you is doing to your back.

DEGENERATION OF THE SPINAL CORD AND BAD MODE OF LIVING

A rather widespread belief that masturbation can cause damage to the spinal cord is completely erroneous. Those old wives' tales are just nonsense. Parents should never threaten their children with disease of the spinal cord as a punishment for masturbation, because, in doing so, they are telling them a lie which can cause untold harm in later life. The harm caused is not physical but mental, as we may learn from the section on "Education and Health." Morals certainly should be taught, but they should not be based on lies.

Apart from the fact that lies should be avoided just because they are untrue, lies have a nasty habit of catching up with us.

Degeneration of the spinal cord is most commonly caused by one of three diseases. First, it may result from untreated pernicious anemia; secondly, the person may have got a disease called disseminated sclerosis, which can cause temporary paralysis, sudden loss of bladder control, and a variety of other symptoms. Both these diseases require the help of doctors. Thirdly, it may be the belated consequence of the infectious disease, syphilis. Syphilitic degeneration of the spinal cord is often called tabes dorsalis, and usually turns up ten to twenty years after infection, when the germ has not been destroyed by timely treatment.

Syphilis is contracted as a result of infection, and can be passed on to the next generation. Infection can happen just as readily to a person who indulges in sexual intercourse at a single time as it can to one who is dissolute and promiscuous. Only the chances of infection are greater when there is promiscuity, and not the susceptibility to the germ. It not infrequently happens that a faithful wife is infected by a normally faithful husband who had had perhaps only one lapse, and has been infected by another woman. Just because of their clean mode of life, no thought of venereal disease enters their heads when trouble begins, and so they do not come for treatment. By the time they have realized that treatment is necessary, the disease has become widespread. Such people are therefore more likely to develop tabes than is a loose-living person who is expecting trouble, and who submits to treatment at once. Tabes does not develop if the disease is properly treated early in its course.

THE VEGETATIVE NERVOUS SYSTEM

The voluntary nervous system, which is concerned with conscious movement and sensation, has already been described. We have, however, nerves other than those of the voluntary nervous system. These other nerves are those which supply our blood-vessels, our hearts, and all our internal organs, and which cannot be directly influenced by the will.

This involuntary nervous system is also called the vegetative nervous system, because it looks after all our internal organs responsible for digestion, growth, and development. Its job is not to regulate growth, but to supervise the activity of all these organs, which it guides and checks, so that their activities synchronize. For instance, if the heart suddenly has to work harder, the vegetative nervous system sees to it that the blood-vessels which go to the heart muscle widen; as a result, more oxygen in carried to the heart muscle, and it needs that oxygen.

This vegetative nervous system is more primitive than is our voluntary nervous system. The vegetative systems of both man and animals act in the same way, and express our moods and emotions in our organs. In so doing, the vegetative nervous system adapts the activities of our internal organs to our life outside. We have already had examples of this (see page 57).

We cannot normally force ourselves to weep. When we do weep in sadness it is the work of the vegetative nervous system. Some born actors can learn to weep at will, and so can some children; it is done by imagining oneself to be really sad, and so creating a mood of sadness so successfully that the vegetative nervous system responds, and tears flow. With practice, a skilled actress can produce this mood at will and very quickly, and with further practice no more will-power is needed to make the tear glands run than to lift one's arm deliberately. Even so, she must still do it by adopting the mood of sorrow, even if she is so practised that this initial step is almost effortless.

Just as one can imagine and artificially induce an emotion, so one can gain control over the activity of one's stomach, blood-vessels, heart and most internal organs. This is the basis of an Indian fakir's training. Similarly, Eastern psychiatry includes special sorts of relaxation exercises in the treatment of patients. But such treatment is by no means infallible and is always liable to go wrong if not properly directed.

An example of such untoward results is that of a woman suffering from cardiac trouble. She made her son, who was at the start of his medical training, give her a stethoscope (of course one with a tube), and she began to listen to her own heart-beat. She grew more and more frightened and her heart responded by beating wildly. This she heard, and so she was more frightened still. In the end she lay in bed for months with the stethoscope over her heart and became incapable of performing the smallest task. Eventually she was removed to a hospital, where she was strictly forbidden to listen to her heart-beat; the harmful effect of such a practice on her condition was explained to her, and she was given no other treatment. After a short time her heart-beat became more regular and she was able to get up and resume her domestic duties. She recovered completely.

One can cause frightful harm through one's vegetative nervous system, especially if one sets about it with one's conscious will and insufficient knowledge.

SYMPATHETIC AND PARASYMPATHETIC NERVES

The vegetative nervous system is divided into two parts. These are called the sympathetic and parasympathetic nerves —these, incidentally, are idiotic and antiquated terms, which date from the days when nothing was known about the functions of the vegetative nervous system. The main parasympathetic nerves are called the 'vagi' (the wandering ones). This term has also been handed down to us from a time when nothing was known about the matter. The sympathetic nerve system has nothing to do with the human emotion of sympathy. On the contrary—it is most violently excited when a person flies into a rage.

A sympathetic and a parasympathetic nerve lead to nearly every organ, and guide the organ, almost as if they were two reins to a horse's head. One applies the brakes and the other drives the organ on to further work; between them they maintain the balance. The sympathetic nerves prepare the organs for fight or flight. When excited they stimulate the heart muscle, and relax the arteries which carry blood to the heart muscle; they make the small vessels of the skin constrict, while those to the voluntary muscles slacken. Their opposite numbers—the parasympathetic nerves—are by no means sleeping partners. Parasympathetic work differs in each organ. It excites here and applies the brakes there.

All this seems at first confusing, but it is readily understood from the point of view of effects and emotions. The sympathetic nerves are always in the ascendancy when external effort, i.e. work and activity, is demanded. A typical example is rage.

The parasympathetic nerves are always in charge when one is quiet, or asleep, and during the process of digestion. Whenever there is something to be done inside—when the digestive juices and intestinal movements are in full swing, then the parasympathetic nerves are issuing their electrical commands. They also predominate during tissue repairs, and during convalescence after illness. One feels lazy and tired and peaceful after having eaten. The things that aggravate and annoy one become agreeably blunted. One feels in the mood for love. All that is represented by parasympathetic activity. Emotion and mood are unquestionably connected with the activity of the vegetative nervous system, which normally is independent of "cold" reason. Apart from its activity in moods and emotions, we don't notice anything about the vegetative nervous system. It works quite unconsciously. When we feel palpitations, this sensation does not emanate from the heart. It is conveyed by nerve endings of the central nervous system, which are sensitive to pressure. Only these reach our consciousness. For this reason pains from internal organs can be felt in the most improbable places. For instance, cramp of the heart, or anginal pain, is often felt on the inside of the left upper arm; an inflamed gall-bladder on the right shoulder; a stomach ulcer on a spot on the skin on one's back. These are transferred pains. Impulses coming from the organs or viscera are only consciously appreciated after they have been transferred in the spinal cord to the voluntary nervous system. These impulses are then relayed to the brain through the voluntary nervous pathway. The conscious brain, however, interprets them as having arisen in the voluntary nervous system at the level at which they entered these pathways. So the brain imagines the pain in the place from which voluntary sensation entered the cord at that same level. As a result, gall-bladder pain is not felt over the liver, but in one's right shoulder instead.

The impulses of the vegetative nervous system, however, are controlled by the brain in a primitive manner, but they do not penetrate our consciousness. They are dealt with by automatic parts of the brain, at a level lower than that of consciousness.

Much is, however, performed by the vegetative system half independently. In the chest and stomach areas there are to be found point systems in the form of nerve plexuses. Some of you will have encountered the names "solar plexus" or "kidney plexus." These are not small, independent, separate brains. They are all joined to the large strands of the sympathetic and parasympathetic nerves. They look after the organs' activities in sections. For instance, the "solar plexus" is in a state of greater excitement during the process of digestion than during a fast. A lot of nonsense has been perpetrated with the name "solar plexus." It has nothing to do with the sun and it certainly has no connection with the supernatural. It is just a point system of the vegetative nervous system which helps in the control of the interplay of stomach juices, intestinal movements and blood distribution in the stomach. When these all work together in perfect harmony, we have a pleasant feeling of well-being.

MODERN LIFE

The vegetative nervous system does, as we have seen, reflect our moods and emotions on to our internal organs. These emotions are in large part our response to the world as we find it.

Life in former times went at a more leisurely speed than it does today, and the public was not, in those days, expected to exert much self-control. In olden times one simply drew one's sword if one was annoyed badly, or threw a stone at somebody if annoyed less badly. There was room in the world to keep out of the way of unwelcome visitors. Nowadays we have to behave in a more civilized fashion, whether we like it or not. That would be quite healthily restful for our vegetative nervous systems and organs, if only we really were civilized and liked behaving nicely. Not many of us do. So when we are behaving beautifully, we may be suffering great internal frustration. If we cannot find outlet for this frustration, and divert it to some useful channel, it can on occasion and quite without our knowledge create an unrecognized mood in the back of our minds which is forever expressing itself on our organs through our vegetative nervous systems.

Such unrelieved frustration can result in diseases caused by disbalance in the vegetative nervous system, such as a tendency to high blood-pressure, gastric ulcer, and many others. We can regain balance in our vegetative nervous systems when we find new outlets for our feelings and cease to be obliged to restrain ourselves so much.

HORMONES

The nervous system is not the only signaling system in the body. There are in addition chemical messengers, or hormones, which are manufactured by glands called "glands of internal secretion." These glands store the hormones and release them into the blood-stream as they are needed. The hormones, in turn, activate a second chemical messenger known as cyclic AMP, which speeds up or slows down special body functions. An example of a hormone is insulin, which is made by special cells of the pancreas. Insulin is released into the blood-stream which carries it all over the body. As insulin contacts cells of the liver and muscles, it activates cyclic AMP in those cells to increase storage of glucose. The cells do this by converting the glucose into a complex substance, resembling potato flour, and called glycogen. The glycogen is deposited as little granules inside the storage cells. While this is going on, the insulin has caused other body cells to take glucose from the blood-stream and to burn it up for the provision of energy. Insulin therefore causes both an increase in the rate of storage and in the rate of utilization of blood glucose for energy, and so the blood-sugar level falls. If the blood-sugar gets too low, specialized cells in the adrenal gland liberate their hormone, adrenaline. Adrenaline has an effect on blood-sugar opposite to that of insulin. It makes the liver cells convert their glycogen back to glucose, and pour that glucose into the blood-stream.

A substance very like adrenaline is released from the tiny end fibrils of sympathetic nerves, inside the organs they supply, whenever an impulse or message travels down those nerves. This local chemical messenger produces the effects of sympathetic nerve stimulation in the organ. However, this locally released adrenaline-like substance is very quickly destroyed locally in the organ, and does not enter the blood-stream as does adrenaline manufactured by and liberated from the adrenal glands. Similarly, parasympathetic nerves liberate another local hormone acetylcholine, at their endings, whenever they are sending messages to an organ. The acetylcholine causes the organ to obey the command of the parasympathetic nerves. As soon as the command has been obeyed, the acetylcholine is destroyed inside the organ, and so it never enters the blood-stream. Atropine, the poisonous substance in Deadly Nightshade, prevents the actions of acetylcholine liberated at the parasympathetic nerve endings, and so paralyzes the parasympathetic nervous system. There are times in medical practice when we want to block the effects of parasympathetic nerve action: it is then that atropine becomes a very useful drug.

If we inject adrenaline into the blood-stream, we get effects that resemble powerful but short-lived stimulation of the whole sympathetic nervous system. Similarly, if we inject acetylcholine into the blood-stream, the effect is exactly like that of widespread stimulation of the parasympathetic nervous system. In health, the activities of the sympathetic and parasympathetic nervous systems are nicely balanced, and balance between them automatically adjusts to the needs of our lives from day to day, from hour to hour, and from minute to minute. Quite frequently, however, in medical practice, one meets patients whose real trouble is a disbalance between these two parts of the vegetative nervous system. In treating this disbalance drugs acting like adrenaline or like acetylcholine are very useful, because, by using them, we can weight the scales in favor of the weaker part of the vegetative nervous system. Alternatively, with drugs such as atropine (which damps down the effects of an overactive parasympathetic nervous system) we can simply tone down the over-efficiency of one or another member of this vegetative couple. We get the best results of all of course if we can remove the cause of disbalance, because then we leave our patients' full powers of minute-to-minute adaptation to life's needs intact.

One example of hour-by-hour adaptation of the vegetative system of life can be taken, using adrenaline. Just as a short-term supply of adrenaline is thrown out from the suprarenal glands into the bloodstream to prepare us for quick action when we are in a rage, or frightened, so the feeling of keenness or deep interest calls for a supply of adrenaline, but this time at a slower and more sustained rate. We are all acquainted with the fact that we get tired very easily when engaged on a boring routine job; not so a scientist who is completely engrossed in some fascinating problem, and who is oblivious of all else. The blood-sugar, and the amount of blood flowing through one's brain, are insufficient when one is bored, but the excitement of the chase will keep the scientist going, because it will cause the steady liberation of adrenaline, and he will work on by the hour, and thoroughly enjoy it, once he is interested.

The Pituitary

The pituitary gland is a queen among glands, and lies inside the skull just below the brain, with which it is connected, and by which it is controlled.

This gland produces a phenomenal number of hormones, and nearly all of these are hormones whose sole function is to guide the activity of one of the other internally secreting glands of the body. For instance, the thyroid gland is controlled by the thyrotropic hormone secreted by the pituitary. The work done by the thyroid gland varies strictly in accordance with the stimulus (thyrotropic hormone) which it receives from the pituitary. The more thyrotropic hormone secreted by the pituitary, the harder does the thyroid work. You will therefore not be surprised to learn that the cause of thyroid disease is very rarely to be found in the thyroid gland itself, because the thyroid just obeys the pituitary.

The following glands all depend on the guidance of the pituitary gland: thyroid, parathyroid, adrenal, sex glands, milk glands, and the insulin-secreting part of the pancreas.

Each of these glands responds to one or more individual

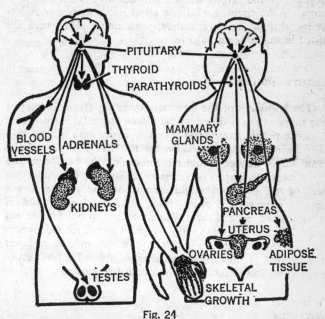

Fig. 24

Influence of pituitary.

hormones secreted by the pituitary, and the sole function of each of these pituitary hormones is the guidance of that one particular gland.

Apart from its work as a controller of other glands, the pituitary secretes three hormones into the blood-stream which affect the body as a whole:

The growth or metabolic hormone.

The antidiuretic hormone, which reduces the amount of water escaping from the body through the kidneys into the urine.

The uterine hormone, which causes thrusting movements of the uterus or womb, especially during childbirth.

The activities of the pituitary gland are summarized in the figures on the opposite page.

Hormones are always present in the blood, and health depends on the perfect balance between all the different hormones in the circulation. If one gland is overactive, or underactive, this balance is disturbed, producing results which are listed in the table on page 89.

BEAUTY AND FORM

The hormones of the internally secreting glands determine the shape of our bodies, and the places where fat is stored.

Some people tend to get fat more easily than others: in a way hormones are responsible for this too. Fat people who want to get thinner should remember that the body can, and does, convert sugar to fat for storage. Starving is a dangerous way of trying to lose weight, because the body must have a regular supply of protein (meat, fish, milk, eggs) and of vitamins and mineral salts. We cannot live on our fat deposits only. The sensible way to lose weight is to reduce the amount of sugar and starch in the diet to a minimum, and to lower the amount of fat, to eat lean meat or fish with fresh green vegetables, and to substitute fresh fruit for puddings.

VITAMINS

The human body is always undergoing change. Tissues wear out, and are silently demolished and reconstructed, during perfect health. These processes go on continuously, and the mate-

THE EFFECT OF HORMONES

GLAND	TOO LITTLE	TOO MUCH
Thyroid	Lazy, stupid, dull-eyed, eyebrows disappearing. Skin dry and doughlike. Body temperature low. "Myxedema."	Over-excitable, vacillating, popping eyes, and tremor of hands. Skin moist and body temperature slightly raised. "Thyrotoxicosis."
Parathyroid	Too little calcium in the blood. Cramps of hands and feet. "Tetany."	Too much calcium in the blood. Bone ailments.
Adrenal cortex	Muscular weakness, bronzed skin, susceptibility to illness, nausea and vomiting. Low blood-pressure. "Addison's Disease."	Obesity, fat neck, moon face, loss of sexual appetite.
Adrenal medulla	Does not occur.	Rare form of intermittent high blood-pressure. "Phaeochromocytoma."
Sex glands	Loss of sexual appetite, cessation of monthly period, changes in shape of body; above all, flattening of the upper thighs. Lack of courage and fear of the future.	Increased sexuality is only very rarely caused by hormones. It is much more often an expression of a mental state, in the presence of perfectly normal sex glands.
Milk glands	Feeding difficulties.	Enormous breasts composed of fat rather than of glandular tissue.
Pancreas	High blood-sugar. Sugar in urine. "Diabetes mellitus."	Tiredness and confusion, leading to loss of consciousness.
Pituitary	Underaction of all dependent glands—stunted growth and underdevelopment. Obesity common. "Diabetes insipidus."	Overfunctioning of dependent glands, gigantism.

rials used for reconstruction, although in part derived from the products of demolition, are in large part provided by the food we eat. That is why a diet for a human being must contain protein, some fat, some starch or sugar, minerals, and vitamins.

Vitamins are chemical substances that we cannot make in our own bodies, and yet cannot do without, although we need only very small amounts of them. Some of the vitamins are found in abundance in animal fats, or fish oils, e.g. vitamins A, D, and E. Others are soluble in water and occur in fresh fruit and vegetables, e.g. vitamin C.

Lack of vitamin A makes a person susceptible to infections. Lack of vitamin D may result in rickets. Lack of vitamin C causes scurvy. Vitamin B_{12} is needed for the building of red blood cells in the bone marrow. Absence of vitamin B_{12} results in pernicious anemia. Pernicious anemia generally develops in people who have inactive stomach linings, and who are, in fact, eating just as sensible a diet as their neighbors who do not get pernicious anemia. The people who get pernicious anemia are those whose stomach linings are deficient in a hormone-like substance which turns the precursor of vitamin B_{12} into the finished substance. We can treat them by giving them the finished article B_{12}, or by giving liver or liver extract, because all animals store B_{12} in the liver.

LIVER AND SPLEEN

The liver is the chemical factory of the body. The foodstuffs we digest and absorb are carried at once to the liver, for inspection as it were, before being dispersed throughout the body. Some of the products of digestion are stored in the liver for future use; others undergo chemical transformations which make them suitable for use by other cells before they are passed on; potentially dangerous substances such as alcohol and nicotine are made non-poisonous in the liver, provided that the amount absorbed does not exceed that with which the liver can cope; other substances already suitable for other cells are allowed to pass straight through the liver without change. In other words, the liver acts as a chemical filter which prevents the blood from being contaminated by poisons, and also provides the blood with the right mixture of foodstuffs for the body cells.

The spleen is the largest lymphatic gland of the body, and works both as a huge lymphatic gland, and as a blood sieve and reservoir. Lymphatic glands act as bacterial filters. When painful swellings occur in the armpits or in the groin as the result of a festering finger or toe, we know that the swollen glands have sieved out the invading bacteria, and that the in-

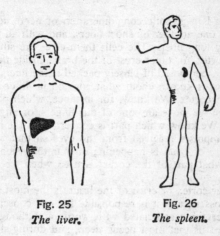

Fig. 25
The liver.

Fig. 26
The spleen.

flammation is a sign of the battle being fought out in those glands between the white blood corpuscles and the invaders. Similarly, the spleen swells and performs the same functions when widespread infection of the blood-stream has taken place. The spleen also filters old worn-out red blood-cells out of the blood-stream, and breaks them down, while the bone marrow replaces them with new, younger ones.

THE BRAIN AND ITS PECULIARITIES

Over and over again throughout our journey through the body we must have noticed how all routes lead to and run into the brain. The brain is the highest seat of authority in the body, which holds everything together, dominates, and guides. The most human aspect of man is his thought, and this is entirely a brain process.

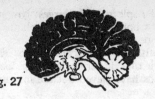

THE CONSTRUCTION   Fig. 27
OF THE BRAIN

The brain is a gigantic conglomeration of nerve cells connected with one another by short fibers, and with all parts of the body by long fibers. The cells themselves are situated in the gray "cortex" or outer crust of the brain. Inside this is the white matter, composed of closely packed nerve fibers.

Quite a lot is known about what goes on in different parts of the brain cortex. We know, for instance, which part of it is used when we move any one of our fingers, or any part of our bodies. We know which part is concerned in the interpretations of impulses received from the eyes so that we get a visual picture of what is happening on our television screen. We know what part of the cortex is used when we learn to read.

The upper cortex or crust of the brain is the most sensitive tissue we possess, and it is responsible for our consciousness, and for everything associated with words and thought. This is the part of us that most needs sleep, and during sleep it is inactive and cut off, so that we have no recollection of our sleeping hours. Feeling and emotion, even if they result from thought, take place at a lower level in the brain. There are large collections of cells embedded in the white matter which are associated with feeling. Other similar but smaller groups of cells form the highest controlling centers for the vegetative nervous system. Lower still in the brain are cell groups concerned with the maintenance of breathing, the regulation of body temperature, and the control of blood-pressure.

The activity of the pituitary gland is also controlled by cell groups in the brain. A female rabbit only sets free an egg cell from the ovary for fertilization when it is necessary. If it is mated, nervous impulses from the sex organs travel upward through the spinal cord and reach the vegetative nerve cell collections in the depths of the brain, and cause them to secrete a hormone-like substance which travels through a local blood pathway to the pituitary gland. The effect of this hormone is to make the pituitary gland liberate a hormone which acts on the ovary, causing it to eject ripe eggs so that fertilization becomes possible.

In humans, eggs are thrown out of the ovaries in a regular monthly rhythm, but this rhythm can be interrupted as a result of nervous activity. For this reason one can never completely rely on the occurrence of non-fertile days (see page 309) shortly before and after a monthly period.

The activity of the vegetative cell heaps in the depths of the brain never ceases for they never sleep; neither does the pituitary.

If the whole of the higher cortex of the brain were removed the patient would not die, but he would become like a sleeping person; he could not learn or know anything, and he would be doomed to vegetate throughout his existence. When an operation called a leucotomy is performed a small part of this higher cortex is detached from the underlying brain. The patient usually becomes duller, but he soon finds his feet again, and can usually earn his own living. Leucotomy also makes him a less positive person, and more easily led. The operation of leucotomy is sometimes undertaken in mental patients to make them able to continue their life at home with their families, and to earn their own livelihood.

THE HUMAN AND ALL TOO HUMAN ASPECT

And that is all that we need to know about the structure of the human brain. We do not need to describe these nerve processes as physical happenings. They are our consciousness. We perceive them directly. They are our thoughts and emotions, which involve the whole body through the nervous system. We do not need to learn that we think, feel, desire. That is a fact—the basis of our existence, as it were. That is all us, and we call it I, or ego.

We know, however, as well, that there are forces right down inside ourselves which sometimes overpower us. They run away with us. We talk about "It," but if we look into the matter more closely, we see that this "It" is sometimes anger, sometimes love, sometimes pain. We are disposed to regard these impulses as something alien, something for which we do not wish to assume responsibility. "My hand slipped. I did not mean to hit so hard," we say, as though our hand were something independent.

And if we take a closer look, we find that this "It," or id, which annoys us from time to time is somehow connected with the driving force in our life. These are apparently impulses which we cannot at the moment make use of—they do not fit into our scheme of things; otherwise we should use them to feed our thoughts and wishes. They are demands which come from our organs. Think of the imperious way in which hunger can disturb our peace to assert its rights.

This feeling is closely akin to "I." We say, "I am hungry," and no one denies us this right. We can admit to being hungry; but in the case of love it is much more difficult—and with anger, too. We are sometimes reluctant to admit these, even to ourselves, for these are deep feelings, which we are apparently unable to control. And up to a point that is correct. The love for another—for a wife and child—may conflict with the love of our own ego and our desire for self-preservation, but this instinct which draws us to another person is unquestionably there and it may turn up in a thousand different disguises. It cannot be denied or removed, inconvenient though it may be from the point of view of our social etiquette.

And so the instincts come up against two difficulties. First the ego, which says, "No listen, perhaps not now and not here. That is not expedient. I should have difficulties and trouble. I am afraid of that." Pure expediency. Pure self-preservation. The ego has no objection to fun and pleasure in itself.

This is the primitive part of the ego; it is no more complex in man than in animals, and is related to the ability of our pets to learn to retrieve sticks and to scratch gently at the door.

But we also have inner cage-bars in the form of the moral law inside us, and this exerts a forceful restraining influence on our instincts. It is this which makes co-existence possible. Its actual form differs with each individual because it is dependent on the person's cultural background.

It is not innate, but is rather something which has grown into us. The form prevalent in an Oriental culture may be quite different from one occurring in a particular community in Europe or America, for instance. An individual raised in an American family may adopt a Christian code of behavior, regardless of his personal religious beliefs, while a person who grows up in the Orient may be influenced by Buddhism.

Only when the moral law—the inner cage-bars—becomes so powerful that we are driven to falsehood and hypocrisy, does the harm begin. Then we become alienated from our instincts, and so from ourselves. The forces deep down inside ourselves no longer support us, but turn against us, and we cease to understand them. We suppress them on the principle that one cannot be what one is not allowed to be.

Let us think back to the time of our grandfathers before the first world war. Public morality was unjustly harsh on women. They were not even permitted to show any signs of sexual feeling in their own marital bed. "A decent woman has no feelings at a time like this. She must perforce tolerate the beast in man." And what was the outcome of this over-strict moral code? Amusing and spicy stories which are still a source of delight to us today. That was the answer of healthy people who were able to escape in secret from the cloying power of extreme morality.

One may well be indignant about it and say "disgusting," but what of it. What was worse was the other extreme; the hysterical woman whose repressed sexuality found an outlet in the most impossible disguises. People who could not snap their fingers at this over-rigid moral code, who sought to live according to the principle of "one cannot be what one is not allowed to be," became ill.

One can restrain all one's instincts and urges without detriment to oneself. But one cannot ask what is illogical and impossible—for example, permitting marriage and then refusing to allow the woman to enjoy carnal love. One can live as a monk and sublimate one's desires in something higher and nobler. This can be done, even if it prove difficult. It is not impossible, but in order to be able to do this, one must be mentally very stable, and not many people are. Nevertheless, there are individuals who can meet such extreme demands without harm to their health. All who have succeeded in this have had to face up to their instincts. The Christian ascetics did not repress their temptations, but deliberately set about overcoming them. One has only to look at the descriptions which St. Hieronymous left behind to understand what is meant.

3. Man and His Food

The digestion of food begins in the stomach, and continues in the intestines. As the food is broken down (digested), soluble substances that the body can use for energy production, for growth, or for tissue repair, pass into the bloodstream. Insoluble substances (roughage) and soluble substances that remain unabsorbed pass into the feces.

SUPERSTITION

From time immemorial man has attached special significance to the choice of foodstuffs for his physical and mental well-being. In far-off days this was carried to the extreme; people were cannibals because they believed that by eating their opponents they could invest themselves with their powers. Some primitive people chose to eat the heart, some the brain, and others the testicles of their enemy as spiritual food. We know now that one cannot acquire mental or spiritual force in this magical way.

However, in turning our backs on superstitions about food, some have gone to the other extreme, and think of meals as necessary evils that are just a means of taking in fuel for the stove. This idea is quite wrong and does a great deal of harm. Others make up modern superstitions about their diet and become vegetarians or eat only raw foods or protest against the use of artificial fertilizers, etc. Whole food sects have come into being—superstitious communities who have built up their own sacred health doctrines on a grain of half-truth.

NATURAL GOODNESS

Usually doctrines on nutrition are based on the basically correct assumption that our food which has been prepared and refined in factories has lost its "natural goodness." Modern food certainly differs from that eaten by our simple-living forbears. Nowadays flour is ground too fine, rice is polished, and sugar lacks the mineral substances and juices of the sugar-cane or sugar-beet. Civilization and technical skill have sought the land "flowing with milk and honey," and have produced refined sugar. Honey is in point of fact just what originates from quite ordinary refined sugar in our small intestine—i.e. a mixture of glucose and fructose. In the blood the fructose too becomes glucose, which is the fuel of our cells.

Man has always had a sweet tooth and has apparently always instinctively set great store by sweet things. We talk of an especially delicious kiss as being sweet—a girl is sweet. So sweetness appears to be a very desirable thing.

HAVING A SWEET TOOTH

There is a possible and very prosaic explanation for this. Sugar is the easiest and laziest way of augmenting our fuel, because it affords the body the minimum amount of work, for it is virtually already digested. Therefore, since we living creatures are disposed to take the line of least resistance, we have an inclination for sweet things. Just as we all secretly long to be millionaires—and that, frankly speaking, amounts to nothing more than wanting to do nothing—so our taste craves for sweet things—for idleness. The Italians have a saying, "Dolce far niente," which means sweet idleness, and there we have it in a nutshell.

One cannot even defend our sense of taste by claiming that this craving for sweet things is, in fact, an instinctive search for the vital vitamin C, since under primitive living conditions fruit (the source of vitamin C) was the only sweet food. Nowadays that is not so, for the humble turnip contains ten times as much vitamin C as a fresh apple. Plums and pears contain even less than apples. Even the potato contains as much vitamin C as most kinds of fruit. In fact, fruit cannot be compared with any green vegetable as a source of vitamin C.

BASIC FOODSTUFFS

(1) Sugars

The body needs fuel, i.e. glucose and fat; these provide the bulk of our calories. The amount of energy necessary daily for medium-heavy work is provided by 15 oz. glucose.

This quantity can be found in

    15 oz. sugar,
 or 2½ lb. bread,
 or 6¼ lb. potatoes,
 or 10 oz. fat.

But we need not waste time worrying about the fuel supply. We always get enough glucose if we have sufficient to eat, for all food either contains glucose or can be transformed into glucose by the body.

(2) Protein

The body needs protein to keep itself in repair. All cells contain proteins which cannot be replaced by anything else. One ounce of our body protein is broken down every day and has to be rebuilt. Therefore, whether we work, play, or rest, we need 2 oz. first-class animal protein, or more of second-class plant protein, every day. First-class protein is best obtained from meat, fish, eggs or milk. There are 4 oz. first-class protein in every pound of meat, fish, cheese, heart, lung, kidney, or liver and also in 8 pints of milk, whether skimmed or full cream.

There are 3 oz. second-class protein per pound of peas, lentils, beans, or soya beans, but this plant protein is inferior. One must have at least 3 oz. daily, unless one also eats small quantities of first-class animal protein. The very small amounts of protein found in flour, rice, and potatoes are important since we consume large quantities of these foods.

Amino-acids

Every protein, no matter what its origin, is composed of amino-acids—these are chemical compounds containing nitrogen. Our liver can manufacture many of these itself, out of sugar and nitrogen, and does so too. But eight or ten of these amino-acids it cannot make, and these therefore must be present in the protein foods we eat, if health is to be maintained.

These essential amino-acids are more often present in animal flesh than in plant proteins, and that is why we have to eat double the amount of plant proteins to replace animal proteins if we want to remain healthy. But we can mix both kinds of protein, and this is important because the plant protein is cheaper. We can take some amino-acids from them provided that we also get the essential amino-acids from meat.

To put it simply, we can eat anything and everything. We are just as well off as vegetarians, grazing in the meadows, as we are as beasts of prey, living on roast joints and fat. But it is always bad to be one-sided. A mixture of an animal and a plant diet is, in the long run, the best guarantee for a well-functioning body.

(3) Minerals and Salts

Sugar and amino-acids are not the only substances required by our body. It also needs minerals. Ordinary salt is included among these. In inland countries where this is in short supply it is the most popular condiment and one can literally crave for salt. In some parts of Africa, people and animals long for it, and it is probably man's oldest article of trade. For thousands of years it has been used as barter between people living on the coast and those inland. A completely saltless diet is incompatible with life. It is, of course, a good thing to cut out any addition of salt to food in cases of heart and kidney ailments, but complete salt deficiency is catastrophic. Incidentally, a diet is not salt-free even if the housewife uses no salt in the kitchen. There is salt in almost every unprepared animal and plant food, even if they do not taste of it. Harm begins only when one chooses food to live on which is extremely deficient in salt.

It must be remembered that two pints of cow's milk contain one gram of salt. The five grams of salt which we require daily are present in ordinary food, without our having to worry about it.

(4) Calcium and Iodine

Another thing that matters is a sufficient supply of calcium and, in inland districts, iodine. It is only in districts far from the sea that the field and garden fruits and water may be deficient in iodine.

We need one to two grams of calcium a day in our food. More is not harmful. Calcium preserves our elasticity and powers of resistance. When calcium is deficient in the blood, cramp results. The calcium content of our food has no connection with hardening of the arteries. Calcium deposits in damaged blood-vessels are the result of disease and are not due to the calcium present in the blood.

In the adult an especially rich supply of minerals is only required for the building of bones when these are broken, and in pregnancy. Children always need a diet that is rich in minerals.

Minerals and metallic salts are used as component parts of

important substances—for example, iron in the coloring matter of the blood, and iodine in the hormone of the thyroid gland. Also, salts help the kidney to distribute the water correctly in the body. With the exception of iron, there is, however, practically no shortage of supply.

(5) Vitamins

However, the vitamins are much more important than minerals. We have already heard about them in the chapter on substances in the blood. Their number is fairly large, and they are designated by letters of the alphabet; A, B, C, D, etc. There are also vitamins with numbers after their name; B_1, B_2, etc. The name vitamin is a misnomer. It originated because the first vitamin to be discovered belonged to the chemical substance group of "amines." It was a vital amine. Most vitamins are, however, not amines, but this was not known at the time.

If glucose is our coal and protein the furnace—then vitamins are the draft. They kindle the flame of our life-processes. Each vitamin has its own significance in the body. Where certain ones are lacking, definite deficiency diseases result. Each vitamin has its own special significance for the health of individual organs or organ systems. They protect them from faulty working, as is shown in the table opposite.

These are the most important vitamins, and we must be particularly careful to get enough of them.

The one that we need in the largest quantity is C. We need fifty milligrams of this daily.

Of other vitamins we need less than a milligram a day. But for all that they are none the less important. Only with fat-soluble vitamins, particularly A and D, is an excess harmful. But an excess is not likely to occur just by eating food rich in vitamins. Yet a surfeit can occur if one takes vitamin tablets as well; for this reason take only the prescribed dose.

Vegetables are the main source of vitamins B and C in our food, as they are cheap and plentiful. They are richer in vitamin content than fruit. Liver cannot be surpassed, as far as vitamins are concerned. Milk and egg yolk are also rich in vitamins.

Vitamins are not as easily destroyed by boiling and frying as one might imagine. Most of them are chemically very stable. The substances which are destructive to vitamins are usually rendered ineffective by heat, so that cooked vegeta-

EFFECT OF VITAMINS

VITAMIN	DEFICIENCY	PLENTIFUL SUPPLY
A	Poor night vision, and hardening of the skin, including the transparent skin of the eye. Coarse, shaggy hair. Unhealthy mucous membranes (mouth, nose, windpipe, urinary tract).	Healthy skin and hair. Protects against infection.
B Group	Nerve pains and muscular weakness, nervousness, beri-beri, pellagra.	Proper functioning of nerves.
C	Tiredness, bleeding gums, susceptibility to infection, scurvy.	Increased resistance to infection, cold, and other harmful things.
D	Rickets in children.	Correct metabolism of bones and calcium.
E	Sterility (in animals).	Fertility (in animals).

bles retain their vitamin content longer than fresh ones, when stored. So do not be afraid of cooking them. Freezing is, of course, the best way of preserving foodstuffs, since the vitamins are not destroyed by the cold and all chemical changes are checked—in short, everything remains as though they had just been gathered.

Vitamins are not contained only in the husks or peelings of fruit and vegetables, as many people believe. This belief derives from the time when the first vitamin was discovered. Among East Asian peoples, whose staple diet is rice, illnesses caused by a deficiency of vitamin B_1 arose as a result of the introduction of machines for "polishing" rice. Hitherto the people had found the necessary amount of vitamin B_1 in the incompletely husked grains of rice, for, as in all other kinds of grain, vitamin B_1 is to be found predominantly in the husk. For that reason whole wheat bread is to be recommended; it also contains bran. It is not more nutritious than white bread, but richer in vitamin B_1. If anyone prefers white bread he can get his supply of vitamin B_1 elsewhere. One should look at the section on vitamins (pages 106–7) in order to see how one can accommodate one's requirements to one's own personal taste. But please do not be hard on your palate for the sake of vitamins. One need not eat apple peel if one does not like it, since the cabbage we eat at lunch contains an adequate quantity of vitamin C.

In the same way one should not overburden one's intestines with indigestible pea and bean pods. It is not the vitamins which are important in peas, but the abundance of protein they contain. The cellulose husks provide cattle fodder. Cows

SUBSTANCE	WHAT HAPPENS TO IT	WHEN THERE IS A SURPLUS	WHERE TO GET IT FROM
Sugar and fat	Used in muscles, nerves and glands. Work and warmth.	Stored as fat and glycogen.	Potatoes, bread, flour, butter, margarine, oil.
Protein	Replaces wear and tear.	Stored as muscle.	Meat, skim milk, fish, peas, flour.
Minerals	Building into substances, regulation of water in the body.	Excreted. They cannot be stored.	Milk, water, potatoes, cheese, meat (iron), etc.
Vitamins	Substances which keep the life processes at their highest strength.	Excreted when they cannot be stored.	Fruit, vegetables, fish, milk, meat, coarse flour, in all natural products which have not been too much altered.

have a special stomach, different from ours, in which bacteria turn this cellulose into valuable glucose. If we give our intestinal bacteria this stuff, we just get flatulence.

For all this we must not despise our intestinal bacteria. Although they produce troublesome gases, they also produce a number of vitamins, which make us somewhat independent of our diet. They are responsible above all for the vitamins of the B group. Eating yogurt is considered to stimulate these valuable qualities. Yogurt is a special kind of sour milk, which anyone can easily make at home. It keeps one's bowels regular and helps the intestinal bacteria to preserve their youthful freshness. The aging bacteria are passed out and constitute the major part of our excreta. And so by keeping our bowels regular, we keep our own vitamin factory in good condition and working order.

Yeast is a very good source of B vitamins.

So, all in all, four groups of substances play a part in our nutrition:

(1) Fuel, which is glucose (fats also come into this category).

(2) Life substance, which is protein.

(3) The "scaffolding," which is the minerals, salts and metals.

(4) The spark to burn the fuel, which is the vitamins.

MODERN NUTRITION

WHAT CAN A HEALTHY STOMACH STAND?

A healthy stomach can stand anything, or practically anything. Our digestive apparatus is an exceedingly versatile instrument, through which our body supplies itself regularly with fuel and food. It is quite immaterial what the stomach is offered, provided there are sufficient proteins and vitamins. Eskimos exist mainly on seal blubber and the flesh of fish, but they take an occasional tidbit in the form of a spoonful of the contents of a fish's stomach. Their vegetables thus are half-digested seaweed, which gives them the minerals and vitamins they would otherwise lack. They keep fit and their skins are beautifully clear and healthy since blubber and fish flesh contain large quantities of vitamin A. We Americans could not live like this without long years of practice and preparation. We shudder at the thought of the taste of this natural diet! Give me a decent chop any day!

Some races live almost entirely on rice. One must not forget, however, that they constantly long for a decent bird, or even a roast rat. These people do not live voluntarily on rice. The protein in rice is really more valuable than that in wheat or rye. But no one lives on it alone. A morsel of meat, a drop of milk or an egg go down with it. Nobody lives entirely on rice—not even in China. That is a myth, even if it is one which is very widespread.

Other races regard as delicacies food, the mere thought of

which makes us shudder. This shuddering can be carried too far sometimes. In 1934, during a famine in Russia, people in the Ukraine declared emphatically that potatoes were poisonous, and could be used only for making gin. And so they starved, surrounded by plenty of potatoes. We think this odd, just as a South Sea Islander would think it odd to see us turn away in horror from his dish of roast rat.

BUTTER OR MARGARINE?

There is the idea that expensive butter in any form is superior to a good, modern margarine which has been enriched with vitamins. Margarine is the legal name for any mixture of eating-fats. They are mixed in such a way that a melting-point suitable to the time of the year is found and the mixture can always be easily spread. There are no "pure" fats. Even butter made fresh from cow's milk is a mixture of many chemically different fats. One can make margarine so that its taste is indistinguishable from that of butter. However, the flavoring agent is often added in too large a quantity and this gives the typical "margarine taste" which so many people do not like.

As everyone knows, butter that is kept for a long time goes rancid. It doesn't improve margarine to keep it, although it keeps much longer than butter, for it contains substances which prevent it from going bad. Nevertheless, one should always try to buy the freshest margarine possible. For those concerned about cholesterol levels in their diets, butter as well as margarines with large amounts of animal fats contain higher levels of cholesterol than all-vegetable fat margarines. And cottonseed oil margarine contains a greater proportion of saturated fats than corn oil margarine.

SKIMMED MILK, TOO

The view that cream builds one up is equally erroneous. It is nonsense. It is only fuel in concentrated form and it is easily digestible. The valuable part of full cream milk is the skimmed milk, not the cream fat. A wise and discerning person will only use fresh full cream milk for drinking and skimmed milk for cooking.

In the same way cheese which has been made from skimmed

milk is, as a source of protein, superior to that which has been made from full cream milk. It is one of the cheapest and most concentrated forms of valuable animal protein. Cheese also is a good source of calcium and protein for many people whose bodies lack the enzyme necessary for digesting milk.

TABLE OF FOOD VALUES

A study of this table will enable a housewife to spend wisely. The best principle to adopt is that of buying cheap sources of fuel instead of expensive ones, so saving the money for valuable proteins:

FOOD	PERCENTAGE OF PROTEIN	PERCENTAGE OF FUEL, SUGAR, FAT, STARCH	WATER PRESENT IN EACH POUND	VITAMIN CONTENT
All kinds of lean meat .	90	10	12 oz.	Predominantly B
Fat meat	25	75	8 oz.	" "
Pickled pigs' feet, salt pork, etc. . .	1	99	1½ oz. approx.	
Heart, liver, lung and other variety meats	65	35	14 oz.	Predominantly A
Ham (smoked) . . .	25	75	5 oz. }	
Bacon (fat)	5	95	2 oz. }	" "
Sausage, salami . . .	20	80	3 oz.	
Milk (full cream) . . .	20	80	14 oz.	All vitamins
Skimmed milk	45	55	15 oz.	" "
Cheese (full cream milk)	approx. 25	approx. 75	8 oz.	B
Curd	75	25	12 oz.	" "
Butter	0.3	99.7	3 oz.	A, D
Margarine	0.3	99.7	3 oz.	A, D, E added
Eggs	30	70	12 oz.	Many vitamins A, D, B
Fish (cod, sole, flounder, etc.) . . .	90-97	3-10	13 oz.	A, B, D
Herrings, carp, etc. . .	50	50	12 oz.	Much D
Eel	15	85	10 oz.	A, B
Crab meat	85	15	12 oz.	
White bread, mixed wheat and rye bread, whole wheat, noodles, macaroni, semolina . . .	13	87	3-6 oz.	B
White rice	10	90	2 oz.	Scarcely any vitamins
Oatmeal	17	83	2 oz.	B
Peas, lentils, beans . .	30	70	2 oz.	A, B
Spinach	50	50	15 oz.	Very much A, C
Salad (lettuce, endives, etc.), cucumber . .	35-40	65	15 oz.	Much A. Little C
Asparagus	45	55	15 oz.	C
Mushrooms	40-50	50-60	15 oz.	D
Leeks	30	70	15 oz.	C
Cabbage (including cauliflower and brussels sprouts), green beans .	25-35	65-75	13 oz.	A, C
Carrots, celery, beetroot, turnips	10-15	85-90	13 oz.	Carrots have A. Otherwise C
Onions	12	88	15 oz.	C
Potatoes	9	91	13 oz.	B, C

First Work It Out and Then Buy

Well, work it out and go on working it out. It is quite easy. Always keep the average of the protein value around twenty per cent, and always mix in animal protein. Small quantities of bacon improve the pea and bean protein, and skimmed milk improves potatoes. Proteins can be fried, salted, peppered or smoked without any harm to themselves. On the contrary, the more they are cooked or fried and the better they taste, the greater their value. One thing, of course, should never be done with meat, and that is to throw away its own natural juice, but I do not suppose that anybody does that.

A housewife who goes into this chart closely and follows its instructions conscientiously, will soon get a good idea as to what are cheap sources of protein. She will bear this in mind when she goes shopping at the market and in this way she can do a great deal for the health of her family.

Only in the supply of vitamins has fat its own modest value. Vitamins A, D and E are more easily absorbed from food when fat has been used in cooking.

The simplest thing for us would be to take a vitamin cocktail every day, in order to insure that nothing is lacking. Another very good thing is to take a tablespoon of wheat germ each day. This is rich in vitamins of the B group and contains also the vitamins E and A. Apart from this it tastes good and can be used in many different combinations.

Just as with proteins, so one can look out for vitamins, when shopping, until this becomes second nature. If one knows the list, one can "see" the vitamins without having to think about them.

Vitamins

(1) The vitamin which is important for skin and beauty: Vitamin A.
Present in large quantities in
        Cod-liver oil. Eel. Egg yolk. Fish. Carrots. Spinach. Salads. Parsley. Green cabbage. Tomatoes. Apricots. Butter. Fortified margarine.
Plentiful in
        Green peas. Dates (preserved ones too).

(2) The vitamins for protecting the nerves: Vitamins of the B Group.

Present in large quantities in

Brewer's and baker's yeast. (Beer contains less than nothing, since alcohol consumes the body's B supplies.) Wheat germ. Liver. Kidney. Heart. Peas. Beans.

Also found in

Meat and fish. Bread. Cheese. Egg. Spinach. Cabbage.

Traces in

Whole milk and skim milk.

(3) The vitamin of resistance: Vitamin C.

Found in

Lemons. Oranges. Strawberries. Red currants. Green peas and beans. Potatoes. Asparagus. Radish. Kohlrabi. Cauliflower. Tomatoes.

Traces in

Rhubarb. Turnips. Onions. Fruit (with the exception of grapes, pears, cherries and plums). Mushrooms. Leaf vegetables.

(4) The calcium vitamin: Vitamin D (Healthy bones).

Present in large quantities in

Cod-liver oil. Herrings. Fat fish.

Also found in

Egg yolk. There is a little in butter, liver and fortified margarine.

(5) Vitamin E

Present in large quantities in

Wheat germ and vegetable oils.

Also found in

Milk, eggs, muscle meats, fish, cereals, vegetables.

(Vitamin E is considered an essential nutrient in humans but its exact function has not been determined.)

WHAT A HEALTHY PERSON SHOULD EAT

(1) Plenty of protein. A person who does hard physical work does not need to increase his consumption of protein. The wearing out of his body is no greater than with someone in a sedentary occupation. The person who does hard physical work needs more fuel and vitamins. There does not appear to

be any danger of getting fat. All fuel is constantly used up. On days of extreme muscular strain (for example, ten hours' mountain climbing), almost four times the amount of fuel is consumed in energy burned against the energy which could normally be drawn from food intake during a day. Even by excessive eating the energy lost cannot be replaced immediately.

Where heavy muscular work is involved, more fat should be eaten, as it is a more concentrated source of energy than starch or sugar.

(2) A more than plentiful supply of vitamins. Regardless of the nature of one's work or occupation, one can never get too many of them. Every person needs a lot of vitamins. We can make vitamin D ourselves only in sunlight. Those who work out of doors need less in their food. Manual labourers or those doing hard physical work, use up more vitamins, especially of the B Group and vitamin C.

What we eat too much of: Potatoes, bread and flour products. Pure sugar.

What we eat too little of: Vegetables containing a lot of proteins and vitamins.

What we overrate: Butter. Full cream milk. Fat meat. Fruit, white flour and bread.

What we underrate: Skimmed milk. Margarine. Vegetable oil. Cabbage. Fish. Vegetables. Whole wheat flour and whole wheat bread.

What we might use in addition: Wheat germ. Yogurt. Calcium tablets. Vitamin preparations.

SPECIAL DIETS

FOOD FOR PEOPLE WITH DISEASES
OF THE GALL-BLADDER

People who suffer from disease of the gall-bladder have difficulty in eating fat. Now, one can live entirely without fat, but where the bile does not flow, the vitamins A, D, and E cannot easily be absorbed. One should take, in addition, vitamin D, preferably as a medicine, vitamin E in wheat germ, and vitamin A with carefully selected vegetables. Go on trying. It is not only the gall-bladder which is sick. The mind, too, is involved. One's taste and ability to digest food are in one's frame of mind. People suffering from gall-bladder trouble can dispense with fats, including expensive butter, provided their vitamin supply is ensured. This makes life far simpler for them.

PEOPLE WITH WEAK STOMACHS

People who suffer from chronic gastritis feel sick after some foods and sometimes have to vomit. They often have stomach-ache, especially after "rich" food. It is scarcely possible to give a general list of dishes which these people cannot digest. It varies with each individual, and what agrees with one, does not agree with another. Each one has times when his stomach behaves well, then, when the spring or autumn comes, the fun begins again. In the summer and winter these people are usually better. All the same they would be well advised to exercise caution and confine themselves to "light" food. This is invariably poor in vitamin content.

The diet which these people select for themselves must be improved upon. Harm is always caused if there are too few vitamins. Experience has shown us that these people are most likely to suffer from a deficiency of vitamin C. So study the vitamin chart and go on trying to find a way out of the "impasse." Chop or mince the vegetables, boil them thoroughly, or drink the liquid which has been drained out of them. Vitamin C must be found, otherwise one will never get really fit again, nor one's stomach either. Lack of this vitamin worsens the ailment. It is a good thing to take vitamin C in tablet form as well. One should get one's doctor or druggist to recommend a preparation which is easily dissolved, so that one can take it in a drink or in food. In tablet form it tastes pleasant, but it does not always agree with people in this concentrated form.

If, as is usually the case, the gastritis also affects the upper part of the intestine, there is the added danger of poor absorption of iron. The iron in the food does not enter the blood in proper quantity. Anemia from lack of iron results. Oatmeal, bananas, salad, spinach, cheese, herrings, kiln-dried flour, hazel-nuts, chocolate and whole wheat bread provide the iron. Bananas and the vegetables already mentioned kill two birds —vitamin C and iron—with one stone. If need be, iron can be taken additionally in tablet form.

In all stomach and intestinal disorders an adequate supply of vitamins is of paramount importance in the diet. This supply is always endangered and vitamin deficiency is the first danger. One must choose one's diet oneself and, by consulting the protein and vitamin charts, do so while at the same time bearing in mind one's own and one's stomach's personal dislikes. This varies with every sufferer, and each person can watch out for this and judge this best for himself. Pain and discomfort, diarrhea and constipation guide him with the charts to good health. The only thing is to try things out and experiment with new combinations and methods of preparing food. This, too, has to be learned. Let us take an example:

(1) Finely chopped spinach is served with fried potatoes and fried egg. This does not agree with the person.
(2) The next day or the day after, the same quantity of spinach, prepared in exactly the same way, is served with boiled potatoes. No ill effects.
(3) After a time spinach and fried potatoes. No ill effects.
(4) Spinach, hard-boiled egg and fried potatoes. No ill effects.

So it was the combination of fried egg, spinach and fried potatoes, but in other combinations the fried egg can be digested. All these things have to be found out and the results of one's experiments should be written down in a little notebook, otherwise one gets muddled with all the different dishes. But it is only by experimenting like this that one can overcome the vitamin-deficiency problem, even if it takes months before one hits on the right diet. And after a year at the most one should have another shot at the so-called "indigestible" dishes. They may suddenly agree with you as things may have changed in the meantime. If you do not do that and do not keep a little notebook, you get more and more worried about your food, until you are living only on vitaminless starch and superfine flour which is very low in vitamin content—in fact, one is only half alive.

As soon as you are better, you must try to build yourself up. You should try and see whether vegetables which do not agree with you are any easier to digest if prepared with milk, above all skim milk. But don't throw away the vegetable water. Milk usually makes things easier to digest and should not be underrated as a provider of vitamins either. However, it does not contain sufficient quantities of vitamin C to help anyone with stomach trouble to get right again.

The worst possible thing is to let matters slide and to lose heart. You should not resign yourself to the idea that you cannot eat this or that, for stomach-ache and complaints occur for reasons that are quite unconnected with eating. The root of the trouble may be in the mind and nervous system and it just happens that the pains come after a meal. You tell yourself that it must have been the celery for lunch as the attack came on just afterwards. One cannot rely on such an isolated piece of self-observation. Only after endless trials and experiments, which should be recorded in a notebook, can you really find out something about your own diet. It is highly interesting and everyone will discover to his amazement how many "indigestible" things he is really able to digest.

ENVIRONMENT

One thing a person suffering from stomach trouble should never do, under any circumstances, is to gobble his food in a tense atmosphere. He must take time to eat his meal in peace. He must remember that his ailment depends on his mood at table and that he is of more use to his family and business if he takes time to enjoy his food and keeps fit. For stomach sufferers eating is sacred. Nothing is so important that it should be allowed to interfere with it. He must be free from worry, and serious conversations about money and other troubles are forbidden at table. Anyone who starts these topics is doing him harm.

DIET IN SICKNESS

This is not inflicted upon one as a punishment, and living on a diet should never have the sad associations of childhood when one was told "you were naughty, so you won't get any stewed fruit." If a doctor prescribes a diet, it must be prepared with greater care and love than meals when one is fit. It must be as tasty as possible within its own obvious limitations. However, anything that has been forbidden must under no circumstances be eaten. Otherwise the diet is useless. It is no good saying "A little won't do any harm." That won't do. "A little" is an uncontrollable amount. A diet for a sick person should never be chosen from diet cookery books. It is something to be prescribed by the doctor and is adapted to the circumstances of the individual case. A sick liver might need a diet which is rich in proteins just as much as a healthy one. Only the doctor in charge of the case can decide which kind of diet is the right one for the particular case.

LIVER DISEASE

In all liver complaints, fat is bad for you. Alcohol and nicotine are even more harmful in these cases. When diseased our chemical factory, the liver, is working only at half strength. It is no longer able to deal with poisons as it used to and it suffers if it is driven on to do unnecessary work. As far as diet is concerned, we must cut out fat in liver complaints. We know that fat is not vital, in fact it is harmful for a sick liver or gall-bladder. The rest has to be left to the doctor in charge of the case. Never fool about with a proteinless diet: it is dangerous. Remember the vitamins. The more, the better, and that goes for when you are ill even more than when you are well.

KIDNEY AND HEART DISEASE

In hypertension, and kidney and heart complaints which may result in dropsy. Doctors often prescribe a diet which contains very little salt. Salt is cut down, not because it is "poisonous" and therefore harmful for even a fit person, but in order to assist the damaged kidney or kidney that is not receiving sufficient blood, to cope with the distribution of water in the body.

We have already discovered that it is very difficult to construct a diet free from salt, since all natural products contain it. So one must select those natural products which contain least salt and give up all idea of a "pinch of salt" for seasoning.

Things that must not be eaten in a diet when salt is forbidden

Salt meat and smoked meat. Sea fish. Fried and smoked fish. All kinds of sausages. Meat extract. Canned meat and fish.

Cheese. Milk. Salted butter and margarine. Bread and cake. Celery. Spinach. Sauerkraut. Endives.

To achieve anything one must get down to below 2 grams a day. And here are the grams of salt contained in every 3 oz. of the following substances:

Meat extract	10–18	Margarine	1.5
Salt meat	7–10	Milk	0.16
Smoked meat	6–9	Sauerkraut	0.75
Ham	5–9	Bread	0.5
Canned meat and		Sea fish	0.3
fish	3–10	Celery	0.25
Sausage	2–10	Spinach	0.2
Cheese	2–4	Mustard	2.6
Butter	1.0		

Things that may be eaten

All kinds of fruit, all vegetables with the exception of those mentioned above. Unsalted butter, margarine and bread. Also flour, starch. Noodles. Potatoes. Egg yolk. Lard. Jam. Honey. Fresh meat and freshwater fish. Cream diluted with water.

Even in these natural products there are noticeable amounts of salt. For example, 1 lb. of baking plums contains 0.1 gram; 1 lb. of animal or freshwater fish flesh, 0.5 gram; and vegetables containing little salt, 0.3 gram. However, if one keeps to the food indicated, one can say that one is living on a diet with very little salt. A single helping of salt on one's plate can ruin everything. That is the equivalent of 2 grams—one's maximum for the day. So if one takes a "pinch" of salt (½ gram) four times, all one's efforts are unavailing as that too amounts to one's daily quota of 2 grams.

So living on a diet containing very little salt does not only mean that one must refrain from using salt to season one's food, but that one must only use natural products of very low salt content. The same rule applies to products containing sodium, a component of salt. Most canned or prepared foods contain salt (sodium chloride) or another sodium compound such as sodium saccharin or monosodium glutamate.

Special diet is just as much a medical measure as prescribing medicines or drugs and neither should be used indiscriminately or at the mere suspicion of illness.

THE UPSET STOMACH

We all know what this means. From a medical point of view, not only the stomach is affected, but also the intestines. One's stomach hurts, one feels miserable, and often there is diarrhoea. Either something has disagreed with one, or one has caught a chill or something like that.

In the matter of diet, nature is very accommodating. At first everything is utterly nauseating, and so only drinks are acceptable. For one whole day only tea—ordinary tea, lemon tea. If you want to make quite certain, you can stay for two days on this "tea diet." After the "tea diet" one cannot, of course, go straight over to boiled beef and carrots! One's stomach needs a strict diet to help it to get back gradually to normal.

(1)   Strict diet

DRINKS: Tea. Cocoa. Vegetable water.
SOUPS: Barley. Rice. Flour soups. Broth containing little fat with rice and noodles.
MEAT: Minced. Only finely chopped meat of chicken, veal or fish without skin.
OTHER SOURCES OF PROTEIN: Up to one pint of skimmed milk. Finely chopped hard-boiled egg.
BREAD, CAKES AND PUDDINGS: Toast. Stale white bread. Sweets and puddings which contain little fat.
VEGETABLES: Potatoes mashed with skimmed milk.
FATS: If absolutely necessary, 2 oz. butter.
FRUIT: Only fruit juice sweetened with sugar.

From this one can gradually pass to a medium and then a mildly strict diet. The following can be taken as well as the items given in the strict diet.

(2)   Medium diet   (3)   Mildly strict diet

DRINKS

Whole milk. Sweetened fruit   The same as 2.
juices. Mineral water. Wine.

SOUPS

Cauliflower and carrot.

Milk foundation and all vegetables indicated below.

MEAT

Calf's brain. Chopped and fried beef. Boiled ham. More fish.

Lean pork. Game. Liver. Kidney. Anything simmered in its own juice or roasted in good fat. A lot of fish.

OTHER SOURCES OF PROTEIN

Soft eggs. Light omelettes. More milk. White cheese.

Scrambled egg with butter. Use eggs for cooking and milk and skimmed milk powder. Cheese.

CAKES AND PUDDINGS

Crackers. Cakes with little fat content. Semolina pudding with milk. Rice pudding.

Milk and plain rolls. Light bread that is not too new. Wheat bread. Puddings with milk, butter and eggs. Soufflés with rice and semolina.

VEGETABLES

Spinach. Cauliflower. Tender carrots.

Beetroot. Asparagus. Salad. Green peas. Cabbage. Tomatoes. Potatoes.

FATS

Good butter and good margarine in large quantities.

Vegetable oil.

FRUIT

Plenty of fruit juice. Apple purée. Purée of pears, plums. Raw scraped apples. Raw strawberries. Raspberries.

Bananas. Oranges. Grapefruit. Tangerines. All kinds of stewed fruit.

Everything should be chopped finely and be as well cooked as possible.

Eat calmly and without haste. No serious topics at table. Frequent small meals neither too cold nor too sour. Lie down after the main meals with a hot-water bottle on one's stomach. With all these diets the following are forbidden: beer, gin, sour wine, all sharply spiced, smoked and sour food, sausages, fat pork and mutton, meat and raw salads, mayonnaise, lard, all leguminous plants, food which has been cooked in a lot of fat (fried potatoes and doughnuts), raw and unripe fruit, cabbage, celery, radish, cucumber, paprika, mustard, garlic, new bread, ice-cream as well as all iced drinks.

All this for a sick stomach! Of course, if one's stomach is not severely upset, one need not carry out the whole program from the "tea diet" to the other three diets over a period of fourteen days. One must adapt it to one's own personal needs. But there are cases when a stomach should "go slow" for a long time and it is a good thing for the housewife to have a somewhat varied menu but all the time paying attention to the vitamin chart for it is easy to go short of them. A chronic stomach sufferer should never make a habit of sticking rigidly to a diet for years on end.

BUILDING YOURSELF UP

Being fat is not synonymous with fitness and vigor. Fat is the body's fuel reserve for lean days. Anyone who chooses a diet that makes him fat is endangering his supply of proteins, for the stomach's capacity is limited. It can take either the fat-making fuels, sugar and fat, or else those with ideal quantities of protein.

Those who are too thin, must eat more. If the appetite is poor, it is a good thing to take vegetable oil, especially olive oil, with salads and all food. Fat is a concentrated fuel. In 1 gram of fat there is as much fuel as in 2 grams of sugar or in 4 grams of bread or in 10 grams of potatoes. Anyone who eats little must increase the fat content of his diet, but he must never limit his amount of proteins, nor endanger his vitamin supply. By taking large quantities of vitamin B_1 in tablet form and vitamin A he can stimulate his appetite.

But one thing is most important. Anyone who stays thin, in spite of eating more food more often, should be medically examined. Something is wrong with his inner glandular system or digestive apparatus. Or there is a mental reason for his lack of appetite, which is the commonest cause of being thin. In this case psychotherapeutic treatment should be carried out, as little can be achieved just by giving more food.

GROWING CHILDREN

When children are growing quickly and when they are adolescent, nothing is worse than cream, butter and filling puddings. They do not build them up, but, at the best, tend to make them fat, which is unhealthy. There is only one substance for body-building and this is protein, which should be as lean and tasty as possible. It should also contain as much vitamin D as possible (though without a doctor's prescription this should not exceed 5,000 units a day), as well as all the other vitamins. The fuel for one's daily requirements is taken in with the food. Don't worry about fat. Worry about health and beauty.

AFTER SEVERE ILLNESS

Exactly the same applies to the process of building oneself up after severe illness and operations, or after a fracture. First and foremost, protein losses, which can be very great, must be replaced. The body's need for glucose is always met. All foods contain fat, sugar and starch. One need not worry about them. A rapid increase in weight is not a sign of a speedy recovery, but usually of wrong and unhealthy food. The lost quantities of protein are built up slowly. True recovery is a slow business and is retarded further by a fattening diet, which prevents the body from building up its lost substance. Fat is the last thing which should be replaced again. So regard any rapid increase in weight with suspicion. Ask yourself where the fault in your diet lies and study the protein and vitamin charts.

WHAT SHOULD FAT PEOPLE EAT?

Nobody puts on weight unless he eats too much, but there are vast differences between the quantities of food which various people can eat without becoming fat. We all eat more than we need. But most of us don't actually deposit the surplus food. We dispose of the surplus, without storing more than a small quantity of reserve fat. A person whose glandular system and whole inner mechanism function all right keeps his weight steady even if he consumes a moderate surplus of food. It is only dangerous if the protein part of the surplus is under 20 per cent; if carbohydrates and fats are predominant. One should realize how small is the quantity of food necessary to meet the minimum calorie demands of a person doing no work:

5 dry rolls.

Or ¼ lb. crackers.
    1 piece of cake with whipped cream.
    2 rolls.
    1 oz. butter.
    5 boiled potatoes with a little sauce.

This meets the fuel requirements of a non-working person, but there is a terrible lack of proteins. One can't reduce on "I'm not eating anything, only dry rolls and dry potatoes." Nothing is less effective or more harmful to one's health. A slimming diet consists of eggs, skim milk, meat and vegetables containing a lot of proteins and vitamins. A feeling of hunger is a sign that one is eating the wrong food. It shows that in spite of the surplus amount consumed the really necessary substances are lacking. A daily ration for a person reducing is as follows:

In the morning: A boiled egg, a half-slice of toasted whole-wheat bread, ⅙ oz. butter. A glass of milk, into which a heaped dessertspoonful of dried skimmed milk powder has been stirred, and a glass of fruit juice (grape-fruit, tomato, orange juice without sugar). Instead of milk, yogurt from skimmed milk can be taken. Also, if desired, a small cup of black coffee without sugar or milk.
    In between, if hungry, nibble a carrot or drink a glass of vegetable water or eat a tomato.

Midday:. A large piece of lean meat, roasted, boiled or grilled (½ lb.). It can also be fried liver, or chopped lean meat with pepper and salt. But it must be ½ lb., and no bread or potatoes with it. Only vegetables which can be chosen from the chart. A cup of black coffee may be taken with it as above.

In the afternoon: A glass of fruit juice or vegetable water with 2 tablets of vitamin C and a spoonful of wheat germ, which have been mixed with a little skimmed milk. Take 2 drops of vitamin D and 10 drops of vitamin A (in cod-liver oil).

In the evening: 3 oz. lean meat, a hard-boiled egg with raw salad (but please no oil). Tea with lemon.

Before going to bed: A glass of skimmed milk, which

has been thickened with skimmed milk powder. A teaspoon-ful of sugar may be taken with it as a reward.

This plan must be adhered to for fourteen days. At the same time the protein and vitamin charts should be consulted and the menu varied. Cheese can be used as an alternative to meat. Salt is not harmful. Sugar and fat intake must be watched. Vegetable water appeases feelings of hunger. Vitamins may be taken additionally in wheat germ, as described above and in the form of vitamin C tablets.

So one can live really well on a reducing diet. One does not only slim, but one keeps fit as well.

Not everybody will be a sylph immediately after the fourteen-day cure. He must take breath and pause. But no cakes or sweets should be eaten during this time. The protein and vitamin charts must always be kept in mind. You can have a rest, but there must never be less than 30 per cent of proteins on an average in your diet. Otherwise you go downhill again. The rich protein diet tastes better than the other one and one is not so anxious to give it up again.

And now a warning about alcohol in any form. Alcohol is as much a fuel as is sugar. One always imagines that what one drinks does not count as food. This is wrong. It is alcohol that increases (without our realizing it) the number of surplus fuel calories. A half-pint of 100-proof liquor is a quarter of a day's ration of fuel for a person doing light work.

Therefore: No alcohol.
           No nibbling between meals.
           Go easy with sugar, bread, potatoes and fat.
           Eat one's fill of proteins and vitamins.

4.   Poisons

Poisons are substances foreign to a healthy stomach and its only protection against them is to vomit, which is what happens if a person has drunk too much alcohol. It is an automatic means of self-protection, but, as civilized man has had to learn to control this reflex, he has robbed his stomach of this natural defense. Perhaps if this were not so, cases of intoxication would be rarer. Anyone who drinks five double whiskies within an hour, one after the other, is likely to find that alcohol has become an acute poison.

ALCOHOL

This takes an intermediate place between a poison and a food. Alcohol is used by the tissues to produce energy, and in fact does produce nearly twice as many calories per gram as sugar does. On the other hand, it can be a deadly poison and deaths from drinking pure alcohol are not unheard of. It is possible for a man to drink himself senseless, lie down and never wake up. This really has nothing to do with how much he can take or what he is used to, as was seen during the war with healthy young men. What is significant is the concentration of alcohol, the weight of the person's body, and what is already in the stomach when the alcohol is drunk.

The first signs of alcoholism are known to everyone: tipsiness, vomiting, giddiness, and lack of co-ordination with double vision. In more serious cases there is low blood-pressure, through poor circulation, and from this even death may follow.

Some people are excited after only a small quantity of alcohol. The amount drunk may be so small that it would not affect the average person, and this pathological intoxication has nothing to do with real alcoholism. In the first case a few drops of alcohol seem to bring on this state of excitement and it happens particularly to people who are usually quiet and controlled, perhaps too quiet and reticent. With this pathological intoxication they suddenly become just the reverse. They get into an unusual state of excitement which they cannot check and which they do not afterwards remember

All this goes to show that alcohol works specifically as a poison to the nerves. First of all the higher centers of the brain are affected. The moral part of us and our ego lose their control, which is not always very gratifying, but most of us do not lose control completely. People who are patho-logically intoxicated go completely out of control at the least provocation of alcohol. It is as if they had a psychological earthquake. Their reason and ego are apparently blotted out and their memory disappears. Only with exceptional psychotherapeutic methods can these people be made to remember what happened to them at the time. It is not alcohol alone which brings about this irresponsibility. It depends upon the personality, and the degree of intoxication is dependent upon past experiences, especially when feelings of anger have been suppressed. It also depends upon other psychological factors and upon the patient's need to free himself from his inhibitions. The wish to free oneself from the fetters of the ungratifying realities of life and the restraint imposed by one's inhibitions is the reason for the passion for alcohol with its devastating results among the Western peoples.

One of the more serious effects of excessive consumption of alcohol is the disturbance of diet which results. Alcohol can be used as a fuel by the tissues, and so, when large amounts are habitually taken, requirements of ordinary food become less. Appetite is further reduced by the irritant effect of excess alcohol on the stomach, producing a distaste for food. (Furthermore, the confirmed alcoholic with a limited income tends to spend his money on drink rather than on food.) All these factors result in an inadequate intake of protein, which can cause serious damage to the liver, especially when continued for several years. The breakdown of alcohol by the tissues (as a source of energy) uses up large quantities of vitamin B_1. As the dietary intake of B_1 is also low in these people, their bodies become very short of the vitamin. This deficiency causes damage to nerves and even to the brain itself.

It is not easy to cure a chronic alcoholic, since the craving for drink is often based on serious psychological difficulties. Drunkenness is a form of temporary escape from our worries and troubles and the habitual drunkard is the type of person who is unable to face up to life's problems. Hence psychotherapy is an essential part of the treatment, and in most cases the intake of alcohol has to be gradually reduced rather than abruptly stopped.

It has even been suggested that one should prepare for any protracted festivities by taking extra vitamin B_1 (in the form of yeast) beforehand: but there is probably no real need, since it is only the habitual heavy drinker who becomes deficient in this vitamin. The best method of dealing with the hangover that may follow these occasions is to rest quietly, taking aspirin if there be headache, with abundant fluids in the form of tea, coffee or milk. If a very large quantity of alcohol be taken in a short while, the person may become seriously ill, and even unconscious. In such cases a doctor must be called: in the meantime, the patient should be kept warm. If he is vomiting, the head should be turned to one side, so that the vomit does not block the air passages.

NICOTINE

While the amount of nicotine absorbed from moderate smoking is harmless, it should be realized that this substance is poisonous when taken to excess. Really heavy smoking, especially in someone not used to tobacco, produces nausea, vomiting, sweating, trembling, and dryness of the mouth. In severe cases there may be mental confusion and muscular weakness. Habitual heavy smokers tend to lose their appetite, owing to irritation of the stomach. However, all effects of excess smoking completely disappear after a few days' abstention from tobacco.

Nicotine speeds up the heart-rate and so palpitations may be noticed as an effect of smoking. These are harmless to people with healthy hearts, but sufferers from heart disease, and especially those with angina pectoris, are well advised to curtail smoking. Patients with arterial disease of the legs (see page 252) should be absolutely forbidden to smoke, as the condition is greatly worsened by nicotine.

CAFFEINE

This substance is present in tea and coffee, but only in small amounts. The stimulating effect of these drinks is due partly to their warmth and flavor, but also to their caffeine content which may be considerable if the brew is strong as in espresso coffee, or, especially, if the drinker is unaccustomed to the beverage. In larger doses caffeine is used by doctors as a useful stimulant, as it quickens the heart, raises the blood-pressure and increases the flow of blood through the brain. There are many popular but erroneous beliefs concerning harmful effects of excessive tea- and coffee-drinking. Any untoward symptoms are more likely to be due to lack of sleep (since caffeine induces wakefulness) rather than a direct effect of the drug.

DRUG ADDICTION

The consumption of alcoholic drinks in moderation is regarded without disfavor by most people, and an expert acquaintance with them is even considered a social accomplishment. Only excessive drinking, or antisocial behavior under the influence of alcohol, is frowned upon by society. Yet it must be realized that even among the moderate drinkers there are some people with psychological difficulties who turn to the stimulant and narcotic properties of alcohol as a means of escape from their depression and their problems. These people are, however, tolerated by society. It is only those who use other drugs to attain the same ends who are regarded as lawbreakers.

The commonest drugs of addiction are the opiates: opium, morphine, and heroin. Although marihuana and hashish, which are derived from the cannabis sativa plant, and cocaine are classed with narcotics as illegal drugs, cocaine is rarely addictive. Marihuana and hashish are not considered addictive.

The serious effects of drug addiction are two-fold. First, people who come under their influence and acquire a craving for them, find they need larger amounts as time goes on, to produce the same euphoric effect. Eventually they are taking such quantities as to make them seriously ill. Secondly, crime is encouraged, since addicts find it difficult to earn enough money to pay the high prices demanded by illegal vendors and resort to theft or robbery to obtain the money. Curing an addict is a lengthy business, since sudden withdrawal of the drug causes illness. Treatment may consist of doses of a substitute drug, methadone, which is gradually reduced over a period of time. Drugs called narcotic antagonists, which can counter effects of opiates, may be used on certain occasions. But treatment also requires intense psychological care.

CARBON MONOXIDE

A poisonous compound in some heating or illuminating gas is carbon monoxide. Carbon monoxide also may be produced by a defective gas appliance such as a hot water heater. Pure carbon monoxide is odorless, but frequently a sharp smell due to other gases accompanying the carbon monoxide can serve as a warning. However, plaster in the walls of a room may absorb the other gases and let the odorless carbon monoxide seep through. Cases of poisoning have occurred this way.

Carbon monoxide is also produced whenever combustion takes place in a limited supply of oxygen. An example of this is a fire in a grate when the chimney is partly blocked and all doors and windows closed. Another well-known danger is that of running the engine of a car in a closed garage.

Whatever the source of carbon monoxide poisoning, the symptoms are always the same. At first there are headache, giddiness and mental confusion and there may be a feeling of weakness and nausea. Later the sufferer may become quarrelsome and even attack his rescuers. A curious apathy develops, so that a person may realize he is being poisoned, but does not bother to do anything about it (such as opening a window). Eventually there is a loss of consciousness, paralysis, and cessation of breathing. The carbon monoxide absorbed into the blood turns this bright red, so that the patient develops a cherry-pink color.

First Aid. It is very important to get the patient into some fresh air. If breathing has stopped, artificial respiration should be applied. Medical aid should be summoned and an oxygen mask applied to the victim's face as quickly as possible. The victim also should be taken to a hospital where special drugs to stimulate breathing and cleanse the blood of carbon monoxide can be administered.

When fresh air or oxygen has been given in time, recovery is rapid, though the patient may have a headache for some days afterwards. Fatalities do occur, but in patients who recover, no harmful after-effects are seen.

OTHER POISONOUS GASES

These are usually encountered only as the result of accidents in certain industries.

HYDROGEN SULFIDE is one of these gases and is familiar as the cause of the characteristic smell of a bad egg. Industries in which this gas is either produced or used include certain metallurgical processes, the manufacture of matches and of artificial silk, tanneries, glue factories, sugar refining and breweries. In small quantities, this gas causes irritation of eyes and nose, with secretion of mucus. If a large quantity be suddenly inhaled, unconsciousness and death from asphyxia may result.

First Aid. As for cases of carbon monoxide poisoning. Long-term effects of repeated exposure are conjunctivitis (reddened smarting eyes), nasal catarrh, cough, headache and indigestion.

PRUSSIC ACID (hydrocyanic acid) is a highly poisonous liquid which quickly vaporizes. It may be accidentally produced in the laboratory when hydrochloric acid comes into contact with potassium cyanide. It has a characteristic smell of bitter almonds. Inhalation of the vapor or swallowing the liquid (or potassium cyanide) usually causes immediate death. If the dose be not lethal, there is collapse with much weakness, cramp and shortness of breath.

First Aid. When potassium cyanide has been swallowed, give diluted hydrogen peroxide to drink and encourage the patient to vomit. If recovery occurs, there are no permanent after-effects whatsoever.

PHOSGENE and NITRIC OXIDE are produced in certain chemical processes, such as dye manufacture and nitrogen production, and from some types of fire-extinguishers. These gases have an intense irritating and destructive effect on the lungs.

The effects do not occur until some hours after inhalation and comprise an irritating cough, with frothy sputum and shortness of breath. The patient becomes blue in color.

First Aid. Keep absolutely at rest until removal to hospital. On no account should artificial respiration be attempted: this will only cause further damage to the lungs. Some relief may be obtained from a steam kettle.

CHLORINE, HYDROCHLORIC ACID VAPOR, FLUORIC ACID VAPOR, SULPHUR DIOXIDE and TRIOXIDE, AMMONIA, ARSENIC TRICHLORIDE, PHOSPHORUS TRICHLORIDE, PHOSPHORUS OXYCHLORIDE and FORMALDEHYDE (all of which are used in chemical industries) are gases with sharp, choking smells, irritating the nose and lungs. Fatalities rarely occur since they give ample warning of their presence by their smell, but enough may be inhaled to produce an irritant cough and painful breathing.

First Aid. As for phosgene poisoning. Long-term effects of inhalation are nasal catarrh and cough.

It is most important that every person employed in any of these industries should be acquainted with these possible risks, so that he can inform his doctor of the possibility of poisoning should he be taken ill. His family should also be aware of the risks, so that they can tell the doctor if the patient is too ill to talk. The correct treatment may depend largely on the doctor's having all the facts in his possession.

INDUSTRIAL SOLVENTS

These substances are liquids which easily vaporize (e.g. petrol), and the poisonous effects which occur are due to inhalation of the vapor. There are many such substances used in industry, including carbon tetrachloride, trichlorethylene and tetrachlorethylene (all used in "dry-cleaning"), benzene, ether, acetone or ethyl alcohol, ordinary alcohol, and many others. A detailed list would be pointless since most of them are known by trade names. They are used, among others, in quick-drying paints and varnishes, in rubber manufacture, in leather and shoe factories, and in the preparation of explosives. Trichlorethylene is the basis of a popular stain-remover used in the home. Methyl alcohol (wood alcohol) is found in methylated spirits and also occurs in illicitly distilled alcoholic beverages.

Symptoms common to many of these substances include a state closely resembling drunkenness, and recovery may in fact be attended by a severe "hangover"! The drinking of wood alcohol can cause blindness.

Long-term results of continued exposure include loss of appetite, indigestion, lack of energy, and headaches. Later the nerve fibers which convey sensations are damaged, resulting in impairment of sight and hearing and loss of feeling in the hands and feet, with an unsteady or staggering gait. In some cases there may be impotence, mental derangement, jaundice and anemia, with minute hemorrhages into the skin.

Precautions. The various regulations devised as safeguards in industry must be strictly observed. Care should be taken that safety devices in factories are working properly. Warning signs (such as a suspicious odor) should never be disregarded. Do not do varnishing unless a window is open in the room. Don't keep stain-removers where it is warm (i.e. near the stove).

First Aid. Strong coffee if the patient is still able to swallow; artificial respiration if consciousness has been lost. In any case,

and try to keep him awake by talking, and movement. In all cases, send for a doctor.

ANILINE, NITROBENZENE, NAPHTHALENE

These liquids can be absorbed through the skin during handling as well as by the lung when present as vapor. They are used in the manufacture of dyes and explosives.

Symptoms of acute poisoning are a bluish color of the skin, mental confusion, and the passage of blood-stained urine.

Long-continued exposure to these substances causes a skin rash at the site of contact, anemia, and damage to the liver with resulting jaundice. Asthma and urticaria ("nettle-rash") may occur. When exposure is prolonged over some years, growths may develop in the urinary bladder.

First Aid. In acute poisoning, send for a doctor immediately. If the patient is unconscious, apply artificial respiration. If the victim is conscious, strong coffee may be offered as a stimulant.

Precautions. The safety regulations laid down for the industry must be observed. Strict attention to personal cleanliness and to cleansing of working clothes will guard against repeated contact. (See also the section on industrial solvents.)

SNAKE POISON

This is rare, but can follow being bitten by a rattlesnake, copperhead or moccasin. The area becomes swollen and discolored and there is a feeling of weakness, breathlessness and fever.

First Aid. A tourniquet should be applied above the bite on a limb (to prevent poison entering the general circulation). This must be temporarily loosened every half-hour. A doctor should be seen as soon as possible, so that he can inject anti-venom which counteracts the venom. Do not give the victim alcohol or any stimulant.

FIRST AID IN POISONING

In most cases of poisoning in which the substance has been swallowed, vomiting should be induced. This can be done by tickling the back of the throat with the fingers or a feather, if available. (It is inadvisable to provoke vomiting when a strong acid or alkali, or a petroleum product like kerosene, has been swallowed: in such cases, drinking water or other bland fluid helps by diluting the poison.) If there is faintness or collapse, hot strong coffee may be offered as a stimulant to a person who is conscious. If breathing has stopped or is feeble, apply artificial respiration.

With all cases of apparent poisoning the doctor must be summoned with all possible speed. Any remaining tablets, powders, liquid or their containers must be kept for the doctor to inspect.

5. Parasites

Parasites of the smallest species are man's last enemies among the living creatures on earth. They alone of man's living enemies have survived under civilized conditions. Shot and shell have given us dominance over large animals, but for eighty years our doctors, chemists and chemical factories have waged war on these minute parasites. This battle is now going more and more in our favor. We are trying to rid ourselves once and for all of these tiresome creatures and so establish our supremacy over all living creatures. We shall see in the next chapters how far advanced our chemical weapons are and what each of us can do in order to defend himself against these menaces.

INTESTINAL WORMS

In the course of their development some species of worm have made a specific point of living in the intestinal canal of humans and animals and feeding on the pre-digested food there. All these particular worms lay their eggs outside and the first part of their development takes place in the open air or in the flesh of another living creature. With such worms the greatest danger of spread from one person to another is in countries where human excreta are used for manure. There has been a decline in worm infestations ever since artificial fertilizer has been used on an increasing scale.

TAPEWORMS

SOURCE OF INFECTION. Meat or fish eaten raw. Cattle and pigs are infected by eating grass contaminated with human excreta. The tapeworm embryo settles in the cattle or pig flesh. If this meat is afterwards eaten raw, the embryo develops into a tapeworm in the human small intestine.

SYMPTOMS. General weakness. Loss of appetite. Nausea. Vomiting. Headaches. Loss of weight. Sometimes pale complexion. In one's stool one may notice detached segments of the worm—they look like pieces of white ribbon.

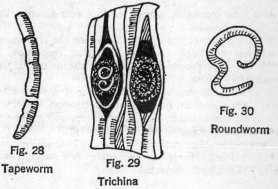

Fig. 28
Tapeworm

Fig. 29
Trichina

Fig. 30
Roundworm

The freshwater fish tapeworm causes severe anemia and bowel obstruction: freshwater fish should be cooked thoroughly.

TREATMENT. Purging and chemicals which poison the worms, under medical supervision. The doctor's diagnosis is made after the stool has been microscopically examined.

PREVENTION. The one certain method is never to eat raw meat. The embryos may be seen when the meat is inspected, and meat which contains them is declared unfit for consumption.

THE DOG TAPEWORM

In this case the worm lives in the intestine of dogs, and human beings are the carriers of the embryonic stage of the parasite.

SOURCE OF INFECTION. Dogs' excreta. The eggs of the worm, after being evacuated by the dog, may adhere to the fur. Handling the dog then results in transference to the human. The eggs develop into large cysts in the liver, lungs and elsewhere: they may attain the size of a grapefruit.

SYMPTOMS. These depend on the organs invaded.

PREVENTION. Scrupulous washing of the hands after contact with animals, especially before meals.

TRICHINA

A minute species of worm, which forms capsules in pork and human muscles.

SOURCE OF INFECTION. Pork containing the trichina worms which has not been declared safe after inspection. Meat, which has been properly cooked or smoked, no longer contains living trichina.

SYMPTOMS. Severe, at times fatal illness. A week after eating the infected meat, diarrhea or constipation, extreme tiredness and nausea. Later high fever, severe pains and swelling of the muscles. Rash similar to nettle-rash.

TREATMENT. The patient will require hospital treatment.

PREVENTION. Do not eat raw pork or raw sausages, or meat which has not been inspected.

THE ROUNDWORM (*Ascaris*)

A large worm similar to an ordinary earthworm, measuring up to sixteen inches long. The eggs develop in damp soil contaminated by human excreta. From the small intestine they pass into the blood. They continue their development in the lungs and then migrate back into the intestine via the throat. There they develop into the adult worms.

SOURCE OF INFECTION. Vegetables, salads and fruits which

have been grown in infected soil and eaten raw. This condition is common only in countries like India where human excreta are used as manure. Children can become infected through playing with earth.

SYMPTOMS. As with tapeworm. Sometimes nettle-rash, anemia, attacks of cramp, sight disorders. In the beginning bronchial catarrh occurs. Worms in the stool. Illness occurs only with heavy infestations.

COUNTER-MEASURES. Can usually be got rid of easily by drugs. Medical supervision is essential, since too strong doses of the worm medicine are dangerous.

PREVENTION. Cleanliness. Ascaris worms have become rarer since the standards of general hygiene were raised.

HOOKWORM AND THREADWORM

These worms, found in warm, moist areas of the United States, can enter the body through the skin of the feet. Hookworm causes anemia, heart diseases: threadworm causes gastric distress. The preventive measure is to wear shoes.

PINWORMS OR SEATWORMS (*Oxyuris*)

The most common intestinal worm in our climate. Quarter- to half-inch long. Occurs in children. Passed directly from one human being to another.

SOURCE OF INFECTION. Food which has been handled by persons with worms and who have not washed their hands.

SYMPTOMS. A harmless ailment apart from the itching of the buttocks, especially at night. (The worms come out at night and lay their eggs.) Small, white wriggling worms in the stool.

COUNTER-MEASURES. Owing to the highly infectious nature of the eggs, cures are not successful unless scrupulous hygienic measures are also adopted.

Here one can help oneself better than any doctor. The affected child must wear tight pants in order not to get any eggs on his fingers when scratching, and should keep the finger-nails cut short. He must wash his hands with soap and a nail-brush most frequently (ten to twenty times a day), especially after going to the toilet. He must also wash his hands after washing his buttocks and genitals. The doctor will provide drugs and a mercury ointment for application to the buttocks.

PREVENTION. Personal hygiene. Cleanliness.

Anybody who becomes infested with these worm parasites nowadays must have disregarded the laws of personal hygiene or the regulations pertaining to "Meat Inspection." One can protect oneself almost completely against parasites like this if one does not eat uncooked meat, or unwashed vegetables and fruit; if one never sits down to meals with dirty hands; if one uses absolutely clean dishes and utensils, if one does not make a habit of touching one's lips and nose with one's fingers; if one uses one's own napkin; in short, if one is a really clean person. With our average standard of hygiene the danger of worms is not very great.

We can eat raw vegetables and salads without running undue risk, since the practice of using human excreta in growing vegetables is practically unknown in this country. An occasional roundworm cannot harm a healthy person. The worm usually dies a natural death unnoticed and is passed out with the excreta. In the country the danger is greater than in the town; not because country people are less clean than those in towns, but because the hygiene services (bathrooms, running water) are of necessity less adequate.

6. Infectious Diseases

THE REALM OF MICROBES

The whole of the earth's surface is densely populated by an endless variety of one-celled living creatures. An invisible world of tiny creatures (microbes) fills the air which we breathe, grows on our skin, lives in the milk which we drink, and in the rivers, lakes and seas of our earth as well as in the chinks in the brickwork of our houses and in the ground on which we stand and in which we grow our food. This realm of microbes reaches to all frontiers; it penetrates every cranny and utilizes all scraps and waste. It is the living mass between the large, visible living creatures. Wherever they see a possibility to live, these small creatures congregate, multiplying with enormous rapidity, and when the foodstuffs are exhausted, they retreat again just as quickly and go into a decline and die.

Most species of these microbes feed on the remains of other creatures, humans, animals and plants. They ferment and decompose organic substances. But among them were species who caught the nitrogen in the air and introduced it into life on earth. All animal and plant life was founded on this achievement of some kinds of earth bacteria until man learned to build his nitrogen factories.

As has already been mentioned, most microbes live on the remains and excreta of large and small animals and plants. They break up everything which they can use. Harmless bacteria penetrate all accessible cavities in the body all the time. The intestines and mucous membrane of the respiratory passages, as well as the cavity of the mouth, are constantly covered with bacteria. So the microbe world does not only advance as far as the outer frontiers of our body, but it reaches the inner frontiers as well and does quite useful work. Our intestinal and skin bacteria live usefully together with us. The intestinal bacteria synthesize some vitamins for us and the skin bacteria cleanse our surface of many waste products.

Our body has an extraordinarily effective method of preventing microbes from penetrating its real interior. All microbes which try to get inside are killed off. Our bloodstream is "poisonous" for all bacteria. Our lymphatic glands are slaughter-houses and are inserted at all danger-points. (The tonsils are a similar bastion of defense.) Our white blood corpuscles consume masses of bacteria each day.

There is, however, a diminishing number of microbes which, provided conditions are favorable for them, are able to exist in the interior of our living body. Sometimes the body's living and chemical wall of defense breaks down and they penetrate its interior and an infective process is set up in the living tissue.

These are the germs of infectious diseases. They comprise the most minute virus bodies and the one-celled creatures, bacteria and protozoa. The body's normal powers of defense against these pathogenic micro-organisms are not always adequate and so illness results. The main thing is the body's attempt to destroy the microbes which have invaded it. At the beginning the damage to the tissues is usually slight. The illness represents a struggle between the defense of the body and those of the microbes. New kinds of "counter-poisons" or anti-toxins are produced by the cells of the body in order to counter-act those of the bacteria and to destroy the bacteria. The whole body switches over to defense against infection.

FEVER

Fever is part of this process of adjustment and it occurs in nearly all infectious illnesses. It is not the result of bacterial poison, but an automatic reaction of the heat-regulating center in the brain. This part of the brain center, which belongs to the vegetative nervous system, causes the temperature to go up in all cases when cell and protein disintegration are taking place and above all when foreign protein is destroyed. If one injects milk, which is free from bacteria, under the skin, this brings on a temperature as well, because the milk protein is destroyed by the body. It is the same with the destruction of bacteria. In many cases a temperature is good for the body as it accelerates the work of the nerve tissues and hormones, while almost all bacteria have their greatest vitality at temperatures of up to 99 degrees Fahrenheit. So by this rise in temperature the body becomes stronger and the bacteria lose strength. (Chickens and other birds can be inoculated with the germs of some human diseases only if the creatures are put in cold water. A bird's body temperature is between 102 and 104 degrees Fahrenheit—a temperature at which the germs can live only with difficulty. So one has to cool the bird's body temperature, in order to give the germs a chance to grow.)

A temperature is not so much a sign of illness as of health. It represents the increased work of the body when removing harmful products which get into the tissues. In cases of infection it shifts the power ratio between the germs and the human body in favor of the body. An adequate temperature reaction only occurs in a body with healthy defense powers.

Properly functioning adrenal and pituitary glands are essential for this. A temperature also does not occur if the body is suffering from a serious lack of vitamin C. Vitamin C is used for all defense activities of the body, not only when there is a temperature. So it is of paramount importance to supply the body with sufficient quantities of vitamin C in all infectious illnesses.

A temperature is an active achievement of the body. The

heat center sets the "thermostat" at a higher level. The normal temperature of 98.6 degrees Fahrenheit is felt as a "subnormal" one; one feels chilled. It is just the same as when one stands naked for too long in the cold. One's muscles start to tremble uncontrollably; this muscle activity accelerates the formation of heat in the body. The cold person makes up for loss of heat in this way and the feverish one raises his body temperature by shivering to a higher one, as dictated by his heat center. A drop in temperature is also an active process. By breaking out into a perspiration the body cools itself and the temperature goes down. We all experience this in health when our heat production is increased as a result of great physical exertion. Feeling chilly and shivering are the body's method of achieving a higher temperature. A feeling of heat in the face and breaking out into perspiration indicate that the sick body is causing the temperature to drop.

FOOD FOR PEOPLE WITH A TEMPERATURE

Special attention should be paid to this. We know that a feverish body has a greater demand for vitamin C, which must be met. For this, orange, lemon and grapefruit juice are particularly suitable. For preference one should take the vitamin in tablet form as well. The tablets can be stirred into the juice and they can also be easily dissolved in yogurt.

Moreover, a light diet should be selected, in order not to overburden the body by giving the intestines too much work. Sufficient liquids must be taken and there must be an ample supply of all the vitamins since the body cells need more of these when there is a temperature. In this case the digestive organs are not able to absorb so well, while the demand for fuel is greater. Hence the fuel supply must be maintained with carbohydrate foods which are easily digested by a sick person.

FEVER AND THE HEART

It is said that fever affects the heart. That is not quite correct. The heart-beat is accelerated because the body temperature is higher. The tempo of the heart-beat, according to a natural law, is accelerated if the temperature rises. If the normal rate is 60–70 beats a minute at a temperature of 98.6 degrees Fahrenheit, then 100–120 beats a minute at a temperature of 102 degrees is also a normal process and does not indicate any abnormality of the heart.

There are, however, some infectious diseases (for example, diphtheria, scarlet fever and typhoid) in which bacterial poisons actually damage the heart-muscle. It is these poisons which affect the heart, not the fever.

The temperature is the body's declaration of war on bacteria or other harmful things which have invaded it. It is therefore pointless to try to lower the temperature except by treating the infection. Only the doctor can decide whether a very high fever is harmful in any particular case. In cases where a very high temperature persists (over 103 degrees), the doctor may order sponging with tepid water. In any case, a damp cloth applied to the forehead may make the patient feel more comfortable.

GERMS

An infectious illness does not consist only of passive suffering, but also calls into play the active defenses of the body. The outer lines of defense have been taken unawares and representatives from the invisible realm of microbes have invaded the body. The illness reflects the body's struggle to remove these disturbers of the peace in its interior.

The individual kinds of germs differ in their ability to cause harm. There are some which can only penetrate the interior of the body when a person is in a weak condition. A typical example is the common disease of pneumonia. The causal germs are to be found on the mucous membrane of most people's throats, without causing harm. But if bodily resistance is lowered (e.g. by severe chilling) pneumonia may result. There must thus be a preliminary condition favorable to this illness, which otherwise only occurs with bedridden patients whose reserves of strength are low. The body must be "ready" for the illness. So inflammation of the lungs is not strictly speaking an "infectious" illness, but an internal complaint, in which bacteria are involved.

As opposed to this there are illnesses which only few people are able to resist. They are caused by germs described as very virulent (virus = poison). Even a small number of them can cause illness, once they enter the body. These virulent germs are able to multiply rapidly in the human body, despite its defenses. Plague is one of these illnesses, as well as measles, scarlet fever and diphtheria.

In all infectious illnesses the number of microbes that invade the body is of importance. The tubercle bacillus, for example, is inhaled in equal quantities by all dwellers in any particular locality. In one town, for example, only a small percentage of people actually contract T.B.—those with poor resistance to the tubercle bacteria. But in another town T.B. may be more common. This may be due to there being more sources of infection, i.e. more people with T.B. who are not in a hospital or sanatorium. Thus on the average more bacilli are inhaled and so a larger proportion of susceptible people become ill.

IMMUNITY AND INOCULATION

A person who has recovered from an infectious disease usually (but not invariably) becomes immune, i.e. cannot again contract that particular disease. The body has "learned" in the first illness to produce the appropriate antitoxin with which to combat the germs. This can also happen quietly, without an acute illness developing. Almost all healthy adults in a large town have had T.B. in this quiet way and in many cases are thus immune for the rest of their lives, provided this immunity is not weakened by ill-health, poor diet, or serious overwork.

Inoculation is an attempt to imitate this very mild illness by injecting into people weak or dead germs or bacterial toxins. Statistics testify to its success. The incidence of smallpox, for example, among vaccinated people is much lower than in unvaccinated. Here again the law of "usually" must be applied. In general the inoculated person is better protected against the illness, even if he should get it: he will have a much milder attack.

WHO BECOMES INFECTED?

Two things are essential for infectious illness. Firstly, a human body which is "ready" for illness (i.e. whose resistance is low), and secondly, a sufficient number of microbes. If we imagine that in an auditorium a shower of microbes rains evenly down on a hundred people for a whole hour, thirty people would be completely unaffected, fifty would become slightly ill, and twenty seriously ill. This has nothing to do with the virulence of the germs, but only with the powers of resistance or readiness for illness of the individual people. Increased virulence or numbers of germs would, of course, alter the percentages.

All of us are subjected to an experiment like this every day and hour, and most of us succeed, apart from a few small blunders, in passing this test for sixty-five or seventy years. We only become infected when we are unfortunate enough to get an overdose of germs, especially if our reserves of strength are temporarily low. So there are a lot of "whens" and "ifs" involved.

MICROBES WHICH MAKE US ILL

The microbes which cause disease are as different from each other as are all other living creatures of the earth. Some can live out of doors, in water or in dry dust (i.e. typhoid bacteria in water and tubercle bacteria in dust). Others, on the other hand, can only exist in the human body and can be transferred to another person only by direct contact. This is true above all of the venereal diseases, syphilis and gonorrhea. The measles virus, too, cannot exist in the open air. Infection only occurs if a child breathes the same air as an already infected person.

With some infectious conditions, the disease can be spread only by some animal acting as a carrier. Malaria is an example of this. Should a mosquito bite a person suffering from malaria, the germs get into the mosquito, which then carries them about without itself being affected. The next person to be bitten will, however, become ill with malaria. The mosquito is referred to as the "insect vector" of malaria. The insect vector of typhus is the louse. Plague is a disease involving rats, fleas and humans. Both rats and humans become ill and the flea is the vector.

On account of the vast differences in mode of life and habits of the various species of microbes, preventive measures are also varied, ranging from the extermination of rats and vermin to washing one's hands!

WHY CHILDREN'S ILLNESSES?

A number of very infectious illnesses are the fevers of childhood—measles, scarlet fever, chicken-pox and diphtheria.

They are so infectious that pretty well everyone picks up some quantity of their germs at some stage in his childhood. Adults are usually immune, either because they have actually had the illness, or because their bodies have in a quiet way produced the necessary substances for defense as a result of contact with a few germs, insufficient to cause illness. Hence these diseases are usually seen only in children. The general standards of hygiene in the past decades, however, have produced the rather unexpected result of prolonging the age at which one can catch these illnesses. We have made things so difficult for all germs that more and more people go through childhood without succumbing to these typical children's illnesses. So that as adults they are still susceptible to scarlet fever, German measles and diphtheria.

So it is seen that there are no hard and fast rules about infectious diseases and one must always use the word "usually" in describing their effects. For example: Infectious diseases "usually" leave one immune after recovery. Inoculation "usually" protects a person from infection. Measles, chickenpox, etc., "usually" occur only in childhood. Fever is "usually" a healthy reaction of the body, and is not of itself harmful.

VIRUS DISEASES

Let us start with those illnesses which offer the most stubborn resistance to our chemical weapons. These illnesses are caused by the most minute creatures, which are a cross between inert chemicals and living creatures, and which have become visible to us only in recent years. Yes, we have been able to photograph these uncanny creatures with the beam of an electron microscope only since the 1950s. A few years before that, we had concluded that they existed because we were able to transfer some infectious illnesses to animals by bacteria-free material. A culture could be filtered through china clay without the filtrate losing its infectious power. No microbe could squeeze its way through the fine pores of the china filter. But the liquid which filtered through was able to reproduce itself in the animal's body. So it was obvious that we were dealing with a "poison" that was living, which is how the name virus originated.

The first one to be identified, in 1935, was a rodlike virus causing a disease of tobacco plants. It was an astonishing discovery that something which could be crystallized out like any ordinary chemical substance was also a living organism, capable of reproducing itself. Viruses seem to be living protein molecules without any ordinary cellular structure. Lack of structure seems to be no drawback to life nor to reproductive ability: they can multiply with positively explosive rapidity, and the tobacco virus could lay waste vast fields of plants at incredible speed.

This is the reason why virus diseases are so infectious. The virus species have other irritating qualities. They can apparently change more easily than other organisms. We have observed over and over again that a virus disease of animals can spread to people. They adapt themselves easily. There are usually several species which cause similar illnesses. This is the case with "flu." An attack of "flu" does not make one immune to the disease, because there are several varieties of "flu" virus.

The fact that they are such simple creatures renders our attack on virus illnesses more difficult. Unlike bacteria, they live by using the oxygen and metabolic substances produced by the body cells they have invaded, instead of having an independent metabolism.

Therefore we can poison them only by poisoning our own cells, and that is impossible. It has been done in animal experiments. For example, if one deprives monkeys of vitamin B_1 and thus produces an illness due to lack of the vitamin, they do not become paralyzed when inoculated with the virus of poliomyelitis. Of course this cannot be applied to human beings. There would be no point in protecting ourselves from one disease by causing another. But perhaps our future weapons for overcoming virus diseases may be forged from the results of these experiments.

Further hopes for chemical weapons against the small virus species derive from advances in protein chemistry. The virus of tobacco mosaic disease has been split chemically and resynthesized again. There may, therefore, be methods of manufacturing "sham" virus molecules, harmless and inert, to compete with the live viruses in body cells.

In order to live and multiply, the virus needs a living fertile "soil," whether this be a human or animal body cell, or even a bacterial cell; it needs a living "virus carrier." At present, we are able to deal only with some of the larger species of virus by using drugs. But one natural defense against viruses is a substance, called interferon, which is manufactured by invaded cells. It seems to block the ability of the virus to multiply. The growth of most viruses also is prevented by antibodies formed by the affected person. This is best illustrated by the fact that most virus illnesses leave one immune to that disease for the rest of one's life.

Not all viruses are equally small; only a few are single molecules. Some are so big that they are almost the same size as bacteria, and are visible under the ordinary microscope. Typhus and psittacosis (parrot disease) are two examples of diseases caused by organisms intermediate in size and nature between viruses and bacteria.

The law of "usually" can again be applied in general to the following:

Virus diseases are usually highly infectious.

Virus diseases usually leave one immune.

Most drugs are ineffective against virus diseases.

Only the body can form substances which prevent the growth of the virus.

Viruses are usually very resistant to chemical disinfectants and to cold.

All viruses are destroyed by boiling.

THE COMMON COLD

This virus illness and its symptoms are well known to us all. The medium-sized virus is almost always present in large numbers. Actually, there are more than 100 kinds of common cold viruses and the symptoms also are produced by many other kinds of viruses, including the disease organisms associated with influenza.

INFECTION. If nasal washings from a case of common cold are instilled in the noses of volunteers, about 50 percent become affected. On the average, this happens from 18 to 48 hours later. Although some persons feel a cold "coming on" a few hours after being chilled, experiments show that chilling of the body surface will not by itself induce a cold. The general state of health and nutrition of the individual do not appear to be factors in susceptibility to colds.

IMMUNITY. Although immunity apparently cannot be acquired, it is likely that a person can become immune to one kind of cold virus, but that does not protect him from infection by one of the other many kinds of cold viruses.

TIMES OF DANGER. The damp cold seasons are the most likely periods of infection and age seems to be a factor, with children under 5 most susceptible, followed by young adults.

SYMPTOMS. Running nose, slight fever of short duration. Often headache. Sore throat and bronchial catarrh and tracheitis. Secondary invasion by bacteria may produce pus in nasal discharge or sputum. Measles, whooping-cough and epidemic flu begin with a cold.

TREATMENT. The usual domestic remedies, which have stood the test of time, are best. Rest in bed, hot drinks and aspirin. Nasal drops containing ephedrine can be used to relieve the running nose. These are not cures; they merely help to deal with the tiresome secretions.

PREVENTION. At times when colds are prevalent, take plenty of citrus drinks. Dress warmly and try to keep dry.

INFLUENZA (Epidemic flu)

This epidemic illness is caused by a medium-sized virus and a mild attack can hardly be distinguished from an ordinary chill. Chill, i.e. cooling of the body, does not play so important a part as with a cold; a considerable proportion of epidemics occur in the summer. The illness can develop into pneumonia.

INFECTION. Droplets coughed or sneezed into the air by other cases. In times of epidemic many healthy people carry the virus in their mucous membranes and constitute a danger to susceptible people.

TIME BETWEEN INFECTION AND ONSET OF SYMPTOMS. One to four days.

TIMES OF DANGER. Especially winter, but epidemics occur during other seasons also.

IMMUNITY. Protection following an attack is of short duration only.

SYMPTOMS. Usually begins suddenly with a temperature between 100 and 103 degrees. General feeling of illness with headache and pains in the limbs and the small of the back. Running eyes. Hoarse voice. Dry cough.

TREATMENT. Mild cases are treated as a cold. In serious cases a doctor is essential.

PREVENTION. Just as with colds, one must protect oneself from vast quantities of virus. Don't let people cough and sneeze at you. Infected people should remain at home to avoid spreading the disease. Influenza vaccine injections should be administered once a year, preferably in the autumn.

PARROT DISEASE (Psittacosis)

An illness similar to influenza. Several other respiratory diseases, including encephalitis and cryptococcosis, are transmitted to humans by birds.

MUMPS

A virus infection of the parotid gland in the cheek.

INFECTION. Conveyed from person to person by droplets when speaking, sneezing and coughing. Patients are especially infectious at the beginning (before any swelling), but remain infectious for some time after recovery.

TIME BETWEEN INFECTION AND ONSET OF SYMPTOMS (INCUBATION PERIOD). Two to four weeks.

TIMES OF DANGER. More frequently in the winter than in the summer.

IMMUNITY. Long-lasting after recovery.

PREVENTION. People who have not had mumps should not visit sufferers from the disease unless the former have received vaccination against mumps.

SYMPTOMS. General feeling of illness. Temperature up to 101 degrees. Headache and earache and pains in the neck. Soon characteristic swelling of the parotid gland. The ear lobes protrude. With adult males inflammation of the testicles may occur and can lead to infertility, but is rare.

TREATMENT. Bed rest, aspirin, hot poultices to the face if the swellings are painful.

MEASLES

Usually only in children. Very infectious. Small virus, which dies off very quickly in the air.

INFECTION. Almost only through direct contact with an infected person (droplets when coughing, sneezing and speaking). Cases are infectious two to three days before the appearance of the rash until shortly after the rash comes out. Healthy carriers play no part in transmission.

TIMES OF DANGER. It occurs at any time of the year.

TIME BETWEEN INFECTION AND ONSET OF SYMPTOMS (INCUBATION PERIOD). Ten to fifteen days.

IMMUNITY. Lasts one's whole life.

SYMPTOMS. For the first three to four days the illness is like a cold, with catarrh and a temperature. Conjunctivitis. Whitish specks may appear in the mouth. On the third to fourth day there is a rise in temperature and the appearance of a rash. This begins on the head behind the ears. The face is affected, including the region round the mouth (which remains free in scarlet fever). Spreads to body, upper arms and thighs until the entire body is covered. As the rash spreads the temperature goes down (unlike scarlet fever). Sometimes the accompanying "chill" symptoms are serious.

TREATMENT. Keep warm and at rest. It is not necessary to darken the room unless the eyes are very inflamed and irritated. Very young or feeble children should be injected as soon as possible with gamma globulin serum from convalescents. Measles is not so harmless as is usually imagined. It is always advisable to call the doctor.

COMPLICATIONS. Pneumonia. Inflammation of the middle ear. All this makes medical treatment imperative.

PREVENTION. Patients need not be isolated after the rash has gone. When there are several children in the family they are never isolated in time, since the illness is infectious before it is recognized. Several live virus measles vaccines are available.

GERMAN MEASLES

This is predominantly a disease of children and may be confused with measles (germane = related to). It is a mild illness with rapid recovery, and is alarming only when occurring in a woman in the early months of pregnancy, since there is a risk of harm to the unborn child, which may be born deaf. However, German measles in adults is very uncommon.

INFECTION. As with measles. The epidemics often occur just before or after a measles epidemic.

INCUBATION PERIOD. Two to three weeks.

IMMUNITY. Usually throughout life after recovery.

SYMPTOMS. The day before the rash appears, there is a general feeling of malaise with shivering and loss of appetite, and sometimes a slight rise of temperature. On the next day the rash appears and for two or three days spreads from the face over the whole body. The spots are small and pink and unlike the blotchy rash of measles. There is usually no coughing nor running nose and eyes.

TREATMENT. The patient should stay in bed for a short while. A woman who is pregnant and gets German measles must go to her doctor.

PREVENTION. Keep infected children away from other people. Vaccination in childhood is recommended; pregnant women and certain other older individuals should not be vaccinated.

SMALLPOX

A severe and often fatal virus disease. It used to be very prevalent in Europe as well as other parts of the world prior to the widespread practice of vaccination. In countries such as Holland, Switzerland and India where vaccination is not compulsory, small epidemics occur from time to time among those who have not been vaccinated.

PREVENTION. The whole population should be vaccinated at least twice in their lives in order to guarantee immunity from epidemics. People who were vaccinated a long time ago may still catch the disease, but it will take a milder course than if they had never been vaccinated and is unlikely to leave pock-marks behind. Vaccination is carried out with a weak strain of virus and the vaccine is taken from calves which have been innoculated with smallpox. The virus, after living in the calf, becomes altered so that it is not harmful to human beings. Vaccination against this disease is very effective.

CHICKEN-POX

Predominantly a disease of children which is usually mild.

INFECTION. As with measles and German measles, etc.

INCUBATION. Eleven to twenty-one days.

EPIDEMICS. In the cold months of the year.

IMMUNITY. For life after recovery. Herpes zoster (shingles) may occur with chicken-pox symptoms in persons who have recovered from chicken-pox.

SYMPTOMS. The disease usually begins suddenly with a high temperature and small red spots. These are found at first on the face and head and they become like small blisters and gradually dry up. The spots, which even occur in the mouth, may be seen in their various stages all over the body as they do not develop at the same time. Unpleasant itching occurs as they dry up. With adults the disease is rare but can be severe.

PREVENTION. As with measles.

TREATMENT. Rest in bed if necessary. The chief thing is to try and stop the child from scratching, as this may leave scars behind. Calamine lotion may be used to overcome the itching. The fingernails should be kept short.

HERPES (Cold Sores, Fever Blisters)

A virus disease of the skin and mucous membranes where groups of watery blisters are found, especially on the lips.

INFECTION. The virus is a normal inhabitant of some people's mouths, but does not cause disease except with some other illness, usually an ordinary cold, but also with pneumonia.

INCUBATION. Two to three days.

IMMUNITY. None.

SYMPTOMS. Only those of the precipitating cause, i.e. a cold or pneumonia. Soon after the onset of these, a group of small blisters appears on the upper lip.

TREATMENT. Local soothing dressings only.

SHINGLES (Zoster)

A virus disease, in which groups of blisters similar to herpes appear on the face, limbs or trunk in a pattern corresponding to the distribution of one of the spinal nerves.

SYMPTOMS. Begins with a temperature and pains in the area of a nerve distribution (usually on the chest, where it follows the course of a rib). When the temperature drops, little blisters appear in the painful area. Shingles on the face is dangerous as it can spread from the brow and temples to the eyeball.

TREATMENT. Local soothing dressings and drugs like aspirin or codeine to relieve the pain, which is often severe. Shingles on the head definitely requires medical treatment, in order that the eyes may be protected.

SLEEPING SICKNESS (Encephalitis Lethargica)

Since the First World War various forms of virus disease of the brain have been observed in different countries. This kind of illness has appeared only in this century. The cause is at any rate a virus. In typical cases the illness starts like flu, but is accompanied by extreme sleepiness, which develops into a comatose state. Constipation is a regular symptom of this complaint. The patient falls asleep while standing or eating (he can, however, be aroused at any time and is then completely alert). A temperature is not always present. Usually paralysis of the eye muscles, squinting, etc., occurs.

TREATMENT. This must be left to the doctor. The symptoms always appear to be so alarming that the doctor is invariably called in. The illness is very dangerous, but has become rare in the past decades.

POLIOMYELITIS

Apart from epidemic flu, this is the most dangerous virus disease of our part of the earth. The cause is an exceptionally small virus, which settles in the nerve cells of the spinal cord and the deep parts of the brain. It grows almost exclusively in the anterior horn of the spinal cord (see Nerves and Hormones, Spinal Cord, page 76), which transmits impulses for the movement of voluntary muscles. As the virus grows and these cells become destroyed, paralysis occurs, which is especially dangerous if the upper parts of the spinal cord and the nerve nuclei in the brain are affected. It is in this area of the brain that the centers for the movement of the muscles controlling our breathing are found. In the upper spinal cord are anterior horn nerve cells which supply the breathing muscles themselves.

The illness usually begins with an indeterminate feverish catarrh. There may also be stomach disorders and nose and throat catarrh. At this stage it is not possible to diagnose the complaint. After a short interval a second rise in temperature occurs, accompanied by a sudden outbreak of paralysis, which spreads to its furthest limit in the relatively short time of twenty-four hours. Then the paralysis subsides, leaving various affected parts. It may be a long time before full muscle power is regained after the illness.

Although the epidemics of polio that once were common in the United States are now extremely rare events, the virus still thrives in other parts of the world, particularly in tropical regions. Also, the symptoms of the disease can be deceptive so that an apparently healthy individual actually can be a carrier of polio. Thus, a person planning to travel to an area where the disease may be encountered should receive a booster dose of the immunizing vaccine. Revaccination generally is not recommended for adults who already have been immunized by the live virus vaccine. And, unlike most other live viral vaccine, the oral polio vaccine can be administered safely to women who are pregnant.

Ironically, poliomyelitis has been associated with the development of good health habits in a population. People who live in areas with poor sanitary conditions tend to develop polio infections and develop natural immunity as small children while persons who grow up under the protective umbrella of modern hygiene rules fail to acquire natural immunity in early life and, unless they receive immunity through vaccination, become susceptible to the disease as adults.

INFECTION. In times of epidemic the virus is very widespread, but of every thousand fit people carrying the virus, one at the most becomes paralyzed. The majority of cases (also those with a temperature) pass off unrecognized and even unnoticed. At times like these it is impossible to guarantee effective protection from infection. The virus may reach a person through flies, dust, excreta, etc. The disease may also be contracted through contact with patients or droplet infection (speaking and breathing) from healthy virus-carriers.

INCUBATION. Four to thirty-five days. (Usually ten days at the most.)

IMMUNITY. For life. Artificial immunity for several years can be induced by vaccination against poliomyelitis which virtually eliminates the chances of catching the disease.

SYMPTOMS. Fever and paralysis. Sometimes preceded by muscular weakness and painful muscles, often a stomach upset or nose, throat and bronchial catarrh. Fever may persist a long time. Children comprise four-fifths of all cases.

TREATMENT. The patient must be admitted to a hospital where facilities for the treatment of such cases are available. Every hour counts with polio or even suspected cases. There are nowadays special breathing apparatuses to overcome the dangerous paralysis of the breathing muscles, which is the usual cause of death (10–20 per cent of cases). With the help of these "iron lungs" it is possible in most cases to keep the patients alive until the breathing muscles recover.

Up to now no effective drugs have been found to destroy the germ before it does its damage.

The most important part of the treatment is physiotherapeutic training after the acute illness has subsided. Even after two years, during which period the paralysis may improve spontaneously, orthopedic operations can be performed, in order to make the damaged limbs more usable. This is done by grafting the tendons of healthy muscles to other bones. For example, where calf muscles are not affected, a part of them can be used to enable the patient to lift his foot again, etc.

BEHAVIOR IN TIMES OF EPIDEMIC. If anyone develops a temperature, all physical exertion should be avoided for at least a week. It is best to stay in bed. Overstrain, getting soaked through, operations on tonsils, and vaccination against other diseases after contact with polio will result in a more severe paralysis if the disease be contracted.

PREVENTION. Conquest of poliomyelitis was brought closer to reality with the development in the 1950s of the Salk vaccine, developed by Dr. Jonas Salk, and the licensing in 1962 of the Sabin oral vaccine. The Salk vaccine is of the killed virus type which requires three properly spaced injections to give maximum immunity. The Sabin vaccine, named for Dr. Albert Sabin, uses live attenuated polio viruses. Taken by mouth, the Sabin vaccine simulates a natural silent infection which, besides inducing the development of antibodies in the blood, causes a state of resistance in the intestinal tract to prevent spread of the virus to other members of the population. Immunity is achieved within a week to 10 days after the Sabin vaccine is given, making it an effective means of controlling polio epidemics.

Immunization can be started in children as young as two months of age, using a trivalent (three virus strains) form of the oral vaccine. The doses are repeated at intervals up to the age of 15 to 18 months of age, with an additional dose for children starting primary school. For older children who have not been vaccinated previously, a series of three doses over a period of one year is recommended. Because of the widespread use of polio vaccines in recent years in the United States, it is unlikely that adults will be exposed to the disease. However, they are advised to receive vaccination if they plan to travel to areas of the world where epidemics still are possible.

RABIES

A severe virus disease of the nervous system which can be caused by the bite of infected animals or by exposure to the saliva of an infected animal or a skin abrasion or mucous membrane. Although dogs are chiefly responsible for infecting humans, the virus also can be transmitted by cats, squirrels, bats, skunks, raccoons, and other animals.

INFECTION. Bite of an infected animal. In a fifth of all cases this results in illness. The severity of the wound is not important. Apart from dogs suffering from rabies, the following animals get it with us and are recorded in the list in the order of frequency: cattle, cats, horses, sheep, goats, pigs and foxes.

INCUBATION. Twenty to sixty days, according to the place of the bite, as the virus multiplies slowly along the course of the nerves until it reaches the brain.

SYMPTOMS. In dogs the disease is recognizable by the raging fury which makes them attack and bite animals and people without reason. This is followed by paralysis of the hind legs and lower jaw, and finally the whole body. There is copious secretion of saliva. With people the illness begins with acute depression, which after two or three days develops into a state of extreme nervous excitement. There is painful cramp of the muscles used in swallowing and breathing. The offer of drink provokes terror because the patient is afraid of choking. There is a copious flow of saliva. Some days later exhaustion and paralysis set in. The disease is always fatal if one is not inoculated in time after the bite.

TREATMENT. Inoculation can still be carried out after the bite because of the long incubation period. It must be done as soon as possible.

JAUNDICE (Virus hepatitis)

The most commonly seen form of jaundice is an infectious illness. (Jaundice also occurs from numerous other causes.) Virus hepatitis is a disease of the liver cells, so that bile pigments pass into the blood and stain the skin, turning it yellow.

INFECTION. The disease is transmitted in two ways. The

stools of a patient contain the virus, and so it can be carried by flies if sanitation is imperfect. Another form of the virus is present in some people's blood and is transmitted if a syringe used for giving them an injection is imperfectly sterilized before being used on someone else.

SYMPTOMS. The first indication is usually found in one's appetite, which is reduced. Another symptom is the fact that smokers no longer enjoy a cigarette. In most cases the skin turns definitely yellow and this becomes first apparent in the whites of the eyes. The urine is brown in color.

TREATMENT. Strict bed rest and a low-fat, high-carbohydrate diet may be recommended in some cases, but diet and activity can be adjusted to the condition of the patient. Alcohol consumption should be forbidden during convalescence. Most patients return to normal activity after six to eight weeks.

PREVENTION. Ordinary attention to sanitation and cleanliness. Immune serum globulin injections are available for exposed persons who have not developed symptoms.

WARTS

In warts a virus is found which, when injected into the skin of other people, causes more warts to grow. However, in normal life one does not get warts through becoming infected. The virus always appears to be present.

It is difficult to get rid of warts, and they often recur after treatment. Local application of caustic substances, X-rays and burning off with a hot wire are effective, but there is undoubtedly a strong psychological element in the causation and persistence of warts. It has been suggested that the impressive sight of the X-ray apparatus is the curative factor rather than the rays themselves! Certainly some lay people have a reputation for being able to "charm away" warts or even to "buy" them! It is wrong to scratch or pick off warts, since this makes the virus spread, and fresh warts often grow and may become quite numerous.

LYMPHOGRANULOMA INGUINALE (a venereal disease)

A rare virus disease predominantly contracted through sexual intercourse or other intimate contact. It is especially prevalent in sea-ports, but is also found in large cities where prostitution is prevalent. It has recently become possible, with the help of three new bacteria-killing substances, to effect a speedy recovery.

SYMPTOMS. One to several weeks after having become infected, little blisters appear on the sex organs. These are easily overlooked. After this, inguinal glands swell greatly and sometimes discharge. If not treated, the illness can go on for years. "Lymph accumulations" occur, which can result in the swelling and thickening of the sex organs, and also of the buttocks (elephantiasis).

TREATMENT. The doctor's surest method of diagnosis is to make a painless skin test. The disease is controlled with tetracycline, chloramphenicol, and sulfa drugs.

PREVENTION. Personal protection as for all venereal diseases. One should try to stamp out the disease by treating each case immediately.

TRACHOMA (Egyptian Eye Disease)

One of the most widespread infectious illnesses on this earth. It is one which is found predominantly in warm countries where people are living herded together under very unhygienic conditions. It is passed on through direct contact or by flies and infected articles. The conjunctiva over the eyeballs and the skin of the eyelids gradually become inflamed and discharge pus, and blindness frequently results.

The cause is a very large virus, which can be destroyed by bacteria-killing substances. Up to now the poor countries in the East have not had the necessary medical facilities for overcoming this disease.

FOOT AND MOUTH DISEASE

This is an animal virus disease, which can sometimes be passed on to human beings through direct contact.

YELLOW FEVER

This is a very serious virus disease, which is spread by mosquitoes in tropical countries. It is accompanied by jaundice and is highly dangerous. There is an effective form of
(Cont'd on p. 157)

THE CHEMICAL CURTAIN ((+) = FORMER

Illness	3000 B.C. Quinine	1910 Salvarsan
Malaria	+	
Syphilis		+
Cerebrospinal meningitis		
Streptococcal infections (blood-poisoning, puerperal fever, etc.)		
Pneumonoccal infections (primary pneumonia)		
Dysentery (bacillary)		
Anthrax		
Gas gangrene		
Gonorrhea		
Erysipelas		
Staphylococcal infections		
Diphtheria		
Tetanus		
*Spirochete infections (Jaundice)		
Actinomycosis		
Chancroid		
Scarlet fever		
Trachoma (Virus)		
B. coli infections (urine, gall-bladder)		
Glanders		
Urinary infections by B. proteus and B. pyocyaneus		
Pneumonia from Friedländer's bacillus		
**Bang's disease (Brucellosis)		
Plague		
Tularemia		
Cholera		
Tuberculosis		
#Venereal disease (Virus)		
Typhoid		
Paratyphoid		
Food-poisoning		
Whooping-cough		
Q-fever		
Typhus		
Psittacosis		
*Canicola fever		
*Swamp fever		
Enteritis		

* indicates variations of same disease, leptospirosis

\-\- ** a veterinary disease primarily, but a human form exists

\# treatment is for complications of the disease; the drugs listed are not effective against the virus

REMEDY, ++ = EFFECTIVE REMEDY)

Sulfon-amide	Penicillin	Strepto-mycin	Chloram-phenicol	Tetra-cycline
++				
	++			
++	++			
++	++	++		
(+)	++			++
	++		++	++
	++			++
	++			++
	++			++
	++			
	++	++		++
	++			
	++			
	++			++
++	++			++
++		++		++
++	++			++
++		++		++
++	++			++
	++	++		++
		++	++	++
		++	++	++
		++	++	++
		++	++	++
		++		
		++		++
	++		++	++
	++		++	++
	++		++	
	++			
			++	++
			++	++
++				++
	++			++
	++			++
++		++	++	

vaccination, which everyone going to the tropics must have done.

THE CAUSE OF ILLNESS. BACTERIA

THE CHEMICAL CURTAIN

The victory fanfares of science ring out joyously in its unparalleled campaign against these microscopic enemies of our race. Our scientists and chemists are preparing the same fate for these little invisible enemies that wolves, tigers and lions once suffered at the shot of our guns. Year by year and month by month man's genius is increasing the variety of antibacterial drugs which can be likened to a chemical curtain. These chemicals strike down the invisible enemy in a sick body like a magic bullet. Illnesses which formerly meant long invalidism and possible death, can nowadays be eliminated as easily as one turns off a water-tap.

This can be done more easily with bacteria as they themselves are living creatures and have their own inner physical world with ferments and metabolism and breathing—unlike the viruses, which live and feed on our cells. We can literally poison bacteria and protozoa without harming our own body.

Thousands of years ago clever people in East Asia found the first poison of this kind. It was the bark of the cinchona tree, in which quinine is contained. This is a poison which the human body can stand better than the malaria germ—a one-celled, microscopic creature, which has wrought much havoc among tropical peoples for thousands of years. Alone, the human body is unable to deal with this blood parasite. Now, quinine is poisonous also to humans, but it happens to be much more poisonous, in amounts harmless to us, to the little malaria parasite in the blood. More cannot be expected from a natural substance which was discovered by chance. The quinine in the bark of the quinine tree has nothing to do with malaria. The tree does not contract the disease. The poison is there for other reasons. The fact that it is used by humans is incidental.

Only in our chemical factories have we been able to produce really effective substances for our fight against bacteria—substances which have been specially made and tested for this purpose. Natural substances are only substitutes to be used until we learn how to make something better ourselves.

This thought first occurred to a small, shrewd, exceptionally tough, cigar-smoking Frankfurt chemist, Paul Ehrlich, who, at the beginning of this century, set about making the first chemical "magic bullet" with which to slay bacteria. He was successful. He discovered salvarsan, which kills the microscopic one-celled creatures that cause the venereal disease, syphilis. Then nothing happened for thirty years. The first world war put a stop to further progress.

Then all of a sudden it broke loose like a scientific thunderstorm—new chemical drugs to replace quinine in the treatment of malaria. At the same time came the German sulfonamides. Then Sir Alexander Fleming in England hit upon the idea of using minute fungi which cause mold. This mold, which we have all seen on bread which has been left lying about for a long time, has its own problems with bacteria. Mold and bacteria eat the same food. They get in each other's way and vie with each other in their daily struggle for existence. Yes, and the fungus takes part in this fight with chemical weapons. One special species of fungus squirts penicillin. Now we human beings keep this mold as a "domestic pet" in large tubs in our chemical factories and use it when we need it for our own fight against bacteria.

The idea bore fruit. Over and over again new substances are being discovered in this way, which are more and more sealing the fate of bacteria. According to whatever suits us best, we either use the fungus mold or make our own substitute for it in our retorts, or we invent one on our own. It is quite immaterial. The important thing is to possess a substance which can kill bacteria in our blood without harming our body. With this new step forward another thread has been woven into the "chemical curtain" which protects us from the microbe world.

If one were to record all this in a chart, it would look something like the one shown on pages 155–156.

In their living habits and chemical mechanism bacteria are as different as human beings, crocodiles, birds and rats. It is therefore obvious that one single chemical substance cannot strike at all species of bacteria simultaneously. It does not cure all complaints, but is used in the treatment of definite bacteria illnesses. It is essential to know with which bacteria one is dealing in order to choose the right substance. Otherwise one simply takes a shot in the dark. A newly discovered bacteria-killing substance does not need to be more effective than its predecessors, but it must be able to get at other species of bacteria, which formerly eluded us. This is our aim in weaving the chemical curtain, which protects our life.

It was not possible to name in the chart all the diseases with partly foreign-sounding bacterial names. You may say that the illnesses which I have mentioned still occur, and will go on doing so, despite our chemical weapons. That is true, but in the paragraph on tuberculosis, we shall learn just why it is so difficult in the case of us human beings to overcome bacterial diseases with chemical weapons alone.

And here again we must apply the law of "usually" when dealing with illnesses which are caused by bacteria and one-celled living creatures. These illnesses can usually be overcome with chemotherapeutic substances.

The illnesses usually leave one immune.

Bacteria are destroyed by boiling.

Bacterial diseases, too, can spread in an epidemic, if the conditions surrounding them are favorable. A typical example is diphtheria.

SCARLET FEVER

Predominantly a disease of children, accompanied by a bright scarlet rash.

INFECTION. Mainly by droplet infection while breathing and speaking and also by actually touching the patient. Things that the patient has handled (such as toys) become infectious, as do their articles of clothing.

INCUBATION PERIOD. Two to five days.

EPIDEMICS. These can occur at any time of the year.

IMMUNITY. Lifelong protection after recovery from the disease. Half the population seem to be immune from birth.

SYMPTOMS. The illness begins with a sudden, rapid rise of temperature and shivering. There is difficulty in swallowing, due to an acute sore throat. At the end of the first or at the latest the second day, the rash appears. The spots are first small and separate and then become flame-colored and begin to merge into each other. If pressed with the finger the spots disappear. The area around the mouth remains pale and this is in striking contrast to the fiery red of the cheeks (unlike measles). The rash is specially profuse in the armpits and groin.

The temperature drops at the end of the first week providing there are no complications. The pulse is rapid in proportion to the temperature, but this is not serious. The tongue, which is coated at first, later looks like a strawberry, as it peels. The whole throat is inflamed.

TREATMENT. Most cases can be controlled by a 10-day program of antibiotic injections.

PREVENTION. Isolation of cases until the skin is clear.

DIPHTHERIA

The bacteria themselves hardly penetrate into the body. They invade the tonsils and the mucous membrane of the throat, but are quickly destroyed in the blood. It is the toxins secreted by the bacteria that constitute a danger to the body. They kill and damage the cells of the mucous membrane of the throat, so that the bacteria can feed on their remains. The diphtheria bacilli destroy surface cells with their toxins, but if there is antitoxin in the blood, these mucous membrane cells are also protected. In that case the bacilli may live on them without causing illness. In this way a healthy person is capable of infecting others.

INFECTION. Through droplet infection when speaking, breathing and coughing. Every twentieth healthy person is a diphtheria carrier and can infect susceptible people. The bacteria remain for a long time on objects (toys, dishes, handkerchiefs) and food after being touched with hands which have not been disinfected or carefully washed.

INCUBATION. Two to seven days.

TIMES OF DANGER. Definitely more prevalent in the late autumn.

IMMUNITY. Lifelong after one attack.

SYMPTOMS. Tonsilitis with a steadily rising temperature. The tonsils are coated and this coating usually extends beyond them and looks gray. It gives off a strange sweet odor, which is very noticeable.

TREATMENT. Must stay in bed (as with ordinary tonsilitis). At the slightest suspicion call the doctor. An injection of antitoxin.

The antitoxin is prepared by inoculating small quantities of diphtheria bacilli into horses. This means that the injection given to humans contains horse serum, and may make them become sensitive to horse serum. Hence, whenever a doctor intends to give any injection prepared in a similar way (e.g.

tetanus antitoxin), he first inquires whether the patient has ever had an injection of antitoxin before. If the answer is "yes," the second injection must be given slowly and cautiously, or a reaction (with fever and a rash) may occur.

PREVENTION. Immunization against diphtheria between the age of two and five. In some countries this is compulsory by law. Isolate every patient. Do not let him go back to school for at least four weeks.

ILLNESSES WHICH CAN FOLLOW. The heart muscle and muscles of the eyes and throat are endangered by the bacterial toxins. Paralysis of other nerves can occur, but they usually recover completely. The soft palate in particular often becomes paralyzed temporarily.

WHOOPING-COUGH

Predominantly a disease of children. Dangerous before the age of three.

INFECTION. Through droplet infection when coughing, speaking and breathing.

INCUBATION. One to three weeks.

IMMUNITY. Usually for life.

SYMPTOMS. In very mild cases it is like an ordinary cold, which, however, cannot be cured with ordinary cough medicines. If the illness persists, after eight to fourteen days a horrible kind of coughing spasm ensues. There are lots of short, dry coughs in succession, then a wheezy intake of breath, which is followed by another fit of coughing. Usually this brings on vomiting. When there is a prolonged spasm the child goes blue. The illness can last for months (usually twelve weeks). All this time the patients are infectious. With some children this particular kind of coughing becomes a habit so that they go on doing it for years. This is very alarming for the parents when the children have the slightest chill, and can usually only be eradicated by careful training.

TREATMENT. Bed rest may be unnecessary for older children with a mild case of the disease, but expert nursing care, including hospitalization, may be required for infants. No specific therapy is known but antibiotics may be used to prevent bacterial complications. Mild sedatives are used to aid rest. Small, frequent meals are a part of the therapy. Vomiting and severe coughing gradually decrease with convalescence.

PREVENTION. Vaccination gives useful protection. Avoid contact with children suffering from whooping-cough.

EPIDEMIC MENINGITIS

An epidemic bacterial disease caused by the meningococcus, which enters the body via the throat. This illness was usually fatal (up to 80 per cent of all patients died) prior to the introduction of chemotherapy. Predominantly children and young people up to twenty-five years of age contract this disease.

INFECTION. It spreads from person to person by droplet infection (breathing, speaking and coughing). Healthy adults and children can carry the germ round with them on their tonsils, and thus spread the disease. The bacteria can remain on handkerchiefs and other articles so that they also become a source of infection.

INCUBATION. Two to three days.

IMMUNITY. The disease does not leave one completely immune.

TIMES OF DANGER. Most prevalent in the spring months.

SYMPTOMS. Begins like flu. High fluctuating temperature with headache, shivering fits and perspiration. Usually severe nose and throat catarrh and often violent vomiting. A typical feature is the rigid neck. The neck muscles are cramped and the head is bent backwards. In bad cases the body forms an arch, so that the patient touches the bed only with the back of his head and his buttocks. All arm and leg movements are painful. If not treated in time, hydrocephalus can result. Sometimes the skin shows a rash of small red spots.

TREATMENT. Immediate medical treatment with ampicillin or sulfa drugs usually will kill the germs and cure the disease. But the exact diagnosis and treatment require a spinal puncture for analysis of spinal fluid. (See Nerves and Hormones, page 76.)

PREVENTION. Isolation of patients in times of epidemic. Treat healthy "germ-carriers," who have been in contact with patients, with penicillin.

ILLNESSES WHICH MAY FOLLOW. If treatment is not given in time, there is a danger of blindness, deafness, squint, permanent paralysis, and idiocy.

GONORRHEA

The most common venereal disease. It has not yet been stamped out, as the chronic form in women may go undiagnosed for some time. The vague symptoms of a vaginal discharge are overlooked in the variety of psychosomatic internal complaints of women. The causal organism (gonococcus), like that of epidemic meningitis, cannot live outside the body and dies off very quickly.

INFECTION. Although sexual intercourse is the most common source of infection, nonvenereal infection also is possible, particularly in young children, and in the eyes of adults and infants. The incubation period is 2 to 8 days.

IMMUNITY. Does not exist.

SYMPTOMS. In men, prickling and burning in the front part of the urethra and a discharge, which is at first rather slimy and then becomes green and pus-like. It can spread to the prostate gland if not treated in time. With women the first symptoms are almost negligible, usually only a discharge, and then "dripping" after urination. With the next monthly period the inflammation usually spreads to the womb and Fallopian tubes with a temperature of up to 100 degrees Fahrenheit. In a considerable percentage of cases the rectum also becomes inflamed (painful bowel movements and rectal discharge). The conjunctiva of the eyes can become infected, causing inflammation and a discharge. (For this reason eye-drops are often given to each newborn baby immediately after birth.)

TREATMENT. At the slightest suspicion medical advice must be sought. For uncomplicated cases of gonorrhea, procaine penicillin is injected into two or more sites after oral doses of probenecid; the treatment is the same for men and women. Follow-up examination is recommended after 7 days for men and 7 to 14 days after initial treatment for women. For complicated cases, antibiotics are administered daily for up to two weeks.

PREVENTION. Because of the steady increase of gonococcal resistance to antibiotics, absolute protection with drugs is no longer possible and reinfection is common. It goes without saying that anyone with venereal disease, who has intercourse without knowing that he or she is infected, should inform the partner and send him or her to the doctor as soon as it is discovered. This can be embarrassing, but it should be done as a matter of some importance.

ILLNESSES WHICH MAY FOLLOW. These only occur as a result of negligence, i.e. if the disease has not been treated in time. The most serious consequence with men and women can be sterility due to permanent scarring of the spermatic and "egg" passages.

SOFT SORE (Chancre)

This is also a venereal disease, which is caused by bacteria. It is the so-called third venereal disease.

INFECTION. Through direct contact in sexual intercourse.

INCUBATION. One to three days.

IMMUNITY. Does not exist.

SYMPTOMS. Soft ulcers. The surrounding area is red and painful. The ulcers spread and, if untreated, do not heal for weeks. In the middle they are covered with a greasy, purulent mass. The ulcers are usually to be found on the outer sex organs and in their vicinity. The inguinal glands usually swell and sometimes burst.

TREATMENT. Local hygiene and sulfa drugs or tetracycline for up to 14 days are needed to effect a cure.

TYPHUS

A highly feverish and dangerous infectious disease.

INFECTION. Only through lice that have become infected by persons suffering from the disease. The deloused patient is not infectious.

INCUBATION. Ten to fourteen days.

IMMUNITY. For life after having once had the disease.

SYMPTOMS. Sudden onset with a feeling of chill or shivering and a correspondingly rapid rise in temperature to 103 degrees. Violent pains in the small of the back and limbs. The legs are kept drawn up and the face is bloated. Headaches, giddiness, and a mentally confused condition.

On the third to the sixth day, minute red spots, which are close together and start on the chest and shoulder, spread over the whole body and persist for ten to fourteen days.

TREATMENT. Broad-spectrum antibiotics, such as chloramphenicol or tetracycline, are most effective.

PREVENTION. Delousing with insect-powder (D.D.T.). If travelling to a louse-infested area, it is advisable to be vaccinated.

FOOD-POISONING

A gastrointestinal disorder accompanied by vomiting and diarrhea and which may be caused by a variety of agents including chemical poisons, bacterial infections, and toxic substances produced by microorganisms. Bacteria causing food-poisoning develop in milk, custards, cream-filled pastry, eggs, shellfish, fish, meat, sausages, and some canned vegetables.

Among the various kinds of food-poisoning which are bacterial infections of the intestinal tract there is a real kind of poisoning which occurs when food is contaminated with the bacterium of botulism. This produces a dangerous nerve poison. After eating such food there is vomiting or diarrhea. There is double vision, and then paralysis of the eye muscles occur and one cannot lift one's eyelids, and there is difficulty in swallowing owing to paralysis.

TREATMENT. Bed rest with convenient access to toilet or bedpan, kaolin powder, and drugs to relieve abdominal cramps or sedate the patient. Nothing should be given by mouth as long as vomiting and diarrhea continue. If symptoms persist, call a doctor.

PREVENTION. All canned food which smells or looks suspicious should be rejected. The bacterium can thrive only in the absence of oxygen. This condition is found in the interior of sausages, ham, bacon, and spiced or pickled food and in canned food. The botulism toxin is destroyed by cooking food at 180 degrees Fahrenheit or above for 30 minutes before eating. All bacteria are destroyed by boiling.

TYPHOID

This is an infection conveyed by food.

INFECTION. The source of infection is always the excreta of infected persons. From this the typhoid bacilli get into drinking water, milk, potatoes, lettuces and other vegetables if these are handled by infected persons, or contaminated by flies. All uncooked food is dangerous in times of epidemic.

Three per cent of people who have typhoid do not completely get over the infection. Without showing actual symptoms the bacteria go on living in the gall-bladder. As chronic excretors of typhoid bacilli, these people are very dangerous to their fellow men and are, for instance, forbidden to work in food-shops or stores unless they agree to have their gall-bladders surgically removed.

INCUBATION. Twelve to fourteen days.

IMMUNITY. On the whole, for life if one has had the disease.

TIMES OF DANGER. Midsummer and early autumn, but epidemics can occur at any time of the year if human excreta are used to fertilize vegetables and if typhoid "carriers" (as described above) are employed in dairies.

SYMPTOMS. Gradual onset with a rise of temperature which takes a week to reach its peak (102 degrees Fahrenheit). Usually constipation to start with. Diarrhea and vomiting are rarer. The pulse is slow in proportion to the temperature. What is particularly noticeable about the patient is his mental confusion. The stools are either constipated or thin and bright yellow. In the second week, when the temperature is high, a crop of little red spots appears on the skin. Bronchitis or pneumonia may occur.

TREATMENT. Chloramphenicol destroys the germs and cures the illness in time.

PREVENTION. Inoculation does not always prevent one from contracting the disease, but usually prevents one from dying of typhoid. The use of human excreta as fertilizer should be forbidden and the medical history of food-workers carefully investigated.

PARATYPHOID

This is similiar to typhoid, and due to related bacteria. For infection, symptoms and treatment, see typhoid.

DYSENTERY

An illness characterized by diarrhea, not necessarily with a temperature.

INFECTION. Spread is from the excreta of patients and occurs in the same manner as typhoid.

INCUBATION. Two to seven days.

IMMUNITY. No method of immunization has proved to be satisfactory to date.

TIMES OF DANGER. Danger of epidemics is in the late summer and autumn.

SYMPTOMS. Violent diarrhea (slimy, watery and blood-stained) accompanied by cramp-like pains. Temperature only moderate. Great exhaustion. Neuritis and arthritis rarely occur.

TREATMENT. Replacement of body fluids and salts lost through diarrhea. Ampicillin usually kills the microorganism.

PREVENTION. As for typhoid.

CHOLERA

The severest known form of food-poisoning, which was well known in Europe even fifty years ago. In the Prussian-Austrian war of 1866 the proportion of deaths among the soldiers due to cholera was higher than that due to enemy action. Usually continual vomiting and frequent watery diarrhea take place and the absorption of bacterial toxins from the intestine may quickly lead to death.

INFECTION. The source of infection is always human excreta and spread is as for typhoid. In times of epidemic many healthy people pass out cholera bacilli with their excreta.

TREATMENT. If taken in time, tetracycline antibiotics can destroy the bacteria and reduce the severity of diarrhea. The body fluids and salts lost through diarrhea must be replaced to prevent complications of dehydration and circulatory failure.

PREVENTION. A completely safe water-supply and sanitary drainage. In times of epidemic only boiled water and cooked food (afterwards protected from flies) should be consumed. Inoculation reduces the chance of illness to 1/30 and the chance of death to 1/60 as compared to people who have not been inoculated. People travelling to Asia should be inoculated.

We owe the beginning of our Western standards of hygiene to this fear of cholera. It was because of the epidemics during the last century that the authorities decided to improve sanitation, water-supply and drainage. Thus cholera indirectly saved more lives than it destroyed directly. In this connection

mention must be made of the Bavarian bacteriologist, Pettenkofer, and his assistant, Emmerich, who in 1892, in front of
their colleagues, drank a pure culture of cholera bacteria,
because they did not believe these to be the cause of the disease. Pettenkofer himself became only slightly ill, but Emmerich's condition was serious. Pettenkofer had once had
cholera and was therefore partly immune. It was a senseless
piece of bravado, which might have turned out much worse.

PLAGUE ("The Black Death")

An epidemic infectious disease, which spread across Europe
many times in the Middle Ages, wiping out up to three-
quarters of the population of affected areas. There are two
forms. In bubonic plague there is swelling and ulceration of
the lymphatic glands under the skin. They break down and discharge. Pneumonic plague, caused by inhaling the bacteria,
results in a serious and often fatal pneumonia. The disease still
occurs in the western United States, as well as in Asia, South
America, and parts of Africa and eastern Europe. People
catch the disease from fleas on infected rodents (rats, mice,
rabbits, squirrels). The disease is associated with chills, high
fever, rapid pulse and enlarged lymph nodes.

TREATMENT. The most effective drugs are the tetracyclines,
streptomycin and chloramphenicol.

PREVENTION. Quarantine regulations of the Public Health
Authorities, above all in sea-ports. Vaccination is possible, but
does not guarantee complete protection.

ANIMAL DISEASES *like glanders, anthrax, Malta fever and
tularemia are sometimes passed on to human beings. They
can be cured by the new chemotherapeutic drugs.*

TETANUS

A wound infection due to a bacterium found in the soil in
certain districts. Deep wounds contaminated with soil run the
risk of infection, since the bacteria can multiply only in the
absence of oxygen.

SYMPTOMS. Stiffness starting in the muscles surrounding the
wound, later becoming general. Characteristically the jaw
muscles are involved, so that the mouth cannot be opened.

TREATMENT. The bacteria themselves can be destroyed by

penicillin, but not the toxin, which penetrates into the nerves and nerve cells. For this reason, tetanus antitoxin should be given after any injury causing a penetrating wound.

GAS GANGRENE

This is another wound infection due to bacteria found in soil. It occurs predominantly in war wounds, but it formerly complicated illegal abortion. Around the wounds, gas is produced by the bacteria in the muscles, which swell and crackle when pressed. In the first world war many soldiers died of gas gangrene.

TREATMENT. Antitoxin. The bacteria are destroyed by penicillin G or tetracycline.

SYPHILIS (Lues)

The most severe and treacherous venereal disease. It has a strange history. The first epidemic outbreak occurred in the year 1494, when the French king, Charles VII, had to call off the siege of Naples as so many of his army were laid low by the disease. His army was beaten back by syphilis and brought the disease back to France.

Syphilis was introduced into Europe in 1493 by the returning members of Columbus' expedition. Among the Red Indian tribes of Central America this disease was known by the name of Xiotl, and it apparently appeared there in its more obscure and protracted form. When it first appeared in Europe it was an acute purulent inflammation. The skin was covered with painful ulcers. Today the disease is to be found all over the world. In civilized countries it is almost only contracted through direct contact with the sex organs of an infected person.

SPREAD. Since the discovery of salvarsan in 1910 there has been a marked decrease in the spread of syphilis. Much of this success may be attributed to the increasing enlightenment and frankness with regard to sexual matters. Modesty or shame is a protection only in so far as it prevents extramarital relations. However, once one has become infected, the consequences can be appalling. Fear of discovery and trying to conceal infection from the doctor have nothing to do with modesty. Indeed, it is a moral crime.

In 1910 every tenth patient in ordinary hospitals was infected with syphilis. At that time about 10 per cent of all people had once had syphilis or were still at an infectious stage. In 1932 the figure was only 4 per cent. As we all know, morals were becoming more lax then, so this success was entirely due to the achievements of medical science. Infectious diseases can always be stamped out or checked if one has effective drugs with which to treat the patients, and if one has the opportunity of using them in time. This should never be forgotten.

INFECTION. There are many erroneous views about syphilis. Therefore: it is an infectious disease, the germ of which—the spirochete—can barely exist outside the human body. It can only live for a short time in the outside world, and for that reason it is actually almost only caught through direct infection. The most intimate contact between human bodies takes place in sexual intercourse. The spirochete of syphilis can only penetrate the body when there are skin injuries (small and minute ones). When there is sexual intercourse little abrasions always occur on the sensitive mucous membranes of the male and female sex organs. Of course the mucous membranes of the mouth, lips and the surface of the tonsils can also form an entrance for the germ, but experience has shown us that, under sanitary living conditions, at the most every thousandth case occurs without sexual intercourse (sharing cups, glasses, towels, etc.). It has been proved that syphilis germs can live for forty-five minutes on a moist drinking-glass. On dry ones they die off more quickly.

Apart from these unhygienic forms of becoming infected, one can contract the disease without going through the complete sex act. It is quite sufficient to touch the sex organs with hands or fingers. The use of a condom by men does not necessarily protect them from syphilis as the germs can penetrate the body at other places.

SYMPTOMS. *Primary Stage.* After having been infected, a painless, hard ulcer forms on the genitals and does not heal for weeks. It gradually develops a round, smooth, shiny surface with a sharp edge. The size varies between a pin head and a dime. Several such primary sores may develop at the same time. Ten per cent of all infected people do not get a primary sore. They only become aware of the disease when it has reached the secondary stage, which is five weeks after the appearance of the primary syphilitic ulcer.

Secondary Stage. At this stage different forms of skin eruption occur. Rashes may cover the whole body, or be localized to certain parts such as the upper lip, the soles of the feet, and the palms. Frequently the rash appears on the brow along the hair-line. At this stage the patient is still infectious. These rashes may persist on and off for about two years, although there are periods when they temporarily clear up.

Tertiary Stage (late syphilis). At the earliest some three years later, new, but no longer infectious, ulcers form on the skin and internal organs. If untreated, the nervous system may become involved, and after another ten years, disorders of the mind and degeneration of the spinal cord result. Other organs, too, can become affected at this stage if the disease is not treated. In particular the aorta may be seriously damaged. During the entire duration of the disease, as long as syphilis germs are active in the body (even if they cannot get outside and infect others), the Wassermann reaction and other similar tests on the blood are positive. The disease can always be "confirmed" in the test-tube, even if the infected person is unaware of it, or there is no longer any danger of infection, or the most careful medical examination yields negative results. As long as these blood-tests show a positive result, there is always a danger that the person concerned may develop fresh symptoms unless treated.

It comes as a great shock to some people when a blood-test like this reveals that they are suffering from syphilis. They feel themselves to be innocent, and there is no reason why they should feel guilty. The doctor is not concerned with guilt in the moral sense. All he asks is that they should try hard to recall suspicious symptoms of the sex organs and the skin. One cannot cure an illness if one tries to deny or conceal things; it merely prevents a cure. Syphilis which has remained unrecognized is, moreover, more a sign of relative innocence than past vice. The immoral person with a guilty conscience is more likely to go to the doctor. (See Degeneration of the Spinal Cord and Bad Mode of Living, page 79.)

It is high time we abandoned the harsh words of the last generation of doctors: "Every syphilitic person lies (Omnis syphiliticus mendax)." But concealment of infection remains one of the most serious obstacles in our attempts to stamp out once and for all this disease. With the judicious use of antibiotic drugs, we may be able to achieve this aim.

Congenital Syphilis

If a syphilitic expectant mother is not treated during pregnancy, the disease can be passed on to the unborn child. The child is born, provided there is no miscarriage, with serious syphilitic defects of the skin, bones, and internal organs. Syphilitic babies are about the most infectious things imaginable. Congenital syphilis has nothing to do with "The sins of the fathers shall be visited on the children . . ." Syphilis was unknown to the Old Testament Jews. This prophetic threat of punishment must have referred to quite another illness, if indeed a physical illness was implied. To our way of thinking it is a grievous sin and omission not to have treatment during pregnancy. It is a crime against the child, whose life can be blighted as a result of this negligence. Once organs begin to be destroyed, not even the most perfect bacteria-killing drug can help.

INCUBATION. Ten to thirty-five days.

IMMUNITY. Having the disease prevents one from contracting it again.

TREATMENT. In the early stage the disease can be cured by penicillin injections. Formerly, when salvarsan was used, longer treatment was necessary. According to previous experience syphilis was not considered infectious after four years had elapsed since first becoming infected provided that no symptoms were apparent for two years after treatment. On the basis of present-day experience a shorter limit may be imposed. But this is a matter for the doctor in charge of the case to decide.

PREVENTION. The same as for other venereal diseases (see paragraph on Gonorrhea, page 163). Condoms do not provide safe protection.

The belated consequences of syphilis may usually be prevented if treated in time. At any rate, they have become much rarer since salvarsan was introduced in 1910. We cannot be sure at this point whether penicillin or other drugs can completely cure them. But it is probable. It is possible to prevent unborn babies from becoming infected by treating syphilitic mothers during pregnancy. As 10 per cent of all syphilitic people do not know that they are suffering from the disease, it is the duty of every pregnant mother to undergo a blood-test to establish her freedom from the germ. This should be done even if "she cannot possibly be infected."

MALARIA

This disease is widespread in Southern countries. The germ is a single-celled protozoon which multiplies in the blood. It is carried by mosquitoes. Without the right kind of mosquito and without a mosquito bite there can be no malaria. The mosquito bite, too, is harmless unless there are people suffering from malaria, whose blood can then infect the mosquitoes. Furthermore, when the external temperature at night drops below 60 degrees, the malaria germs are destroyed in the mosquitoes' bodies. Hence the disease does not occur in cold climates. The malaria germs in the human body can be destroyed by chemotherapeutic drugs. The malaria mosquitoes can be killed by D.D.T. Malaria could in fact be wiped out everywhere, if only sufficient money were available. During the war this was done in certain areas. In the battles for the Pacific islands American airplanes sprayed clouds of D.D.T. powder during the fighting and cleared the islands of mosquitoes. Friend and foe alike were scattered with it and thus protected from malaria. But in peace-time also, D.D.T. and antimalarial drugs are performing miracles in the tropics. This success, however, is somewhat counterbalanced by the problems of nutrition and population which have thereby arisen. Countries where the population remained the same for centuries now experience a rapidly growing population as the death rate from malaria dwindles. In Guyana, for example, the population used to be 400,000. Births and deaths counterbalanced one another until 1935, when serious attempts were started to eradicate the threat of malaria. By the 1970s the population of the South American nation had risen to approximately 750,000.

SYMPTOMS. Fever recurring at regular intervals (usually every three days).

TUBERCULOSIS

Tuberculosis is a quite special kind of bacterial infectious disease. The extraordinary thing about it is that the human body can deal with the tubercle bacteria in more than ninety-nine out of a hundred cases without showing any marked symptoms of illness. Probably every adult has imprisoned a few tubercle bacteria in small deposits of calcium salts in the lung or in the lymphatic glands of the abdomen. They cannot harm us from there and we cannot do anything to them.

However, there are people who are unable to encapsulate tubercle bacteria, or who cannot do so adequately, and these people are in danger of contracting T.B. It is impossible to predict who come in this category. These people do not even comprise a fixed percentage of the population. Their number is far more dependent on the amount of tubercle bacilli present in the dust in our apartments, houses and towns. As our living conditions and general standard of hygiene improve, the percentage of people liable to contract T.B. will rapidly drop.

THE CAMPAIGN AGAINST TUBERCULOSIS

The main object of this campaign is to reduce the number of tubercle bacteria around us. First and foremost this costs money. All T.B. patients should undergo medical treatment as soon as possible. People who cough up tubercle bacilli or excrete them in any way should really remain in sanatoria for treatment until all their bacilli are encapsulated in calcium, as happens with other people.

But it is not enough to eliminate and cure infectious T.B. For all the trouble we take, we would never succeed in diagnosing cases so early as to make our air free from tubercle bacilli. But it helps to live under less crowded and more hygienic conditions. If an infectious person lives with five people in one room, he is constantly spreading his germs over five healthy people. If each of the six can sleep in his own room, the swarm of bacilli over the five healthy people at night is considerably diminished. If in addition the sun shines into the room, it helps to kill off tubercle bacilli, which cannot stand sunlight. So an unrecognized T.B. sufferer is far less dangerous in a large, hygienic dwelling, than in a poor, cramped one.

General prosperity and a high standard of living banish T.B. Even wealthy people are endangered as long as others live in poverty. The fate of our health is dependent on the air and dust of our cities.

B.C.G. Vaccination

We can and must do one more thing, and that is to protect ourselves from T.B. This can be done with the help of B.C.G. vaccination, which is usually effective. The cells of the vaccinated person are made ready for action in the event of tubercle bacilli invading the body. They are, as it were, ready to meet the emergency.

This happens to adults at the first contact with a small quantity of tubercle bacilli. These immunize us against their successors. For four weeks following contact our fate lies in the balance. Will our cells succeed in overcoming the infection? Most of us come through without noticing it. But suppose we had not come through? And, even more important, will our children come through? This now is everyone's responsibility. Vaccination against T.B. should be carried out in one's early childhood, otherwise it is pointless. By the time of starting school one child in five has been involuntarily and more drastically vaccinated by life itself, whether it has had an actual T.B. illness or not. It has been vaccinated with highly virulent tubercle bacilli, and not with the harmless B.C.G. vaccine. My advice is: Do not rely upon nature when this is not necessary. People who have been artificially vaccinated (B.C.G. vaccination) are at any rate far less liable to contract T.B. later than those who have not been vaccinated. Should we become infected with tubercle bacilli, whether we become ill or not, depends upon the number of bacilli which attack us and upon our powers of resistance against them at that particular time. Both these things can be changed in our favor.

Is T.B. Hereditary?

Severe illnesses, starvation and hardship can weaken the human body to such an extent that its powers of resistance against T.B. are reduced. There sometimes appears to be an inborn susceptibility, but it has not been proved that extreme susceptibility to T.B. is hereditary. One should realize this if one is faced with the problem of marriage with a tubercular person. Provided that any children are protected from becoming infected, they are in no greater danger than others.

TREATMENT

It would be simple to treat T.B. if it were an ordinary infectious disease. A few streptomycin injections or some isoniazid tablets would be all that was needed. Paradoxically enough, if human beings had no defense against tubercle bacilli, T.B. would have long since been relegated to a place behind the "chemical curtain." Rhesus monkeys, which have no resistance whatever to T.B., can be cured by these drugs because the tubercle bacilli are, as it were, "exposed" in their bodies and are easily reached by bacteria-killing drugs. Unfortunately the human being with T.B. attempts to seal off the bacilli in scar tissue. This partly protects them from the drugs in the blood-stream, which cannot permeate through the scar. The bacilli, however, may break out again subsequently and cause further damage.

Because of this, the curious fact emerges that the rapidly spreading forms of T.B. seen in humans with low resistance are those most amenable to cure by streptomycin and allied drugs. When natural resistance is high, the body's attempts to combat the disease may be completely successful without chemical aid: but if unsuccessful, the reaction serves only to wall off bacilli and protect them from the healing substances administered to the patient. This is why, in so many cases, the cure of tuberculosis is a protracted and long-drawn-out affair.

And so it becomes clear why each individual T.B. case demands special methods of treatment. The treatment is not confined to some such simple formula for success as was once thought possible with venereal disease—i.e., diagnosis, penicillin injection, quick recovery, examination eight days later to check results: finished. With T.B. such confidence could not be expected. The correct treatment of T.B. will always be an independent part of medical science; it will always be a matter for the specialists in lung diseases. Of course it is up to all doctors to diagnose it. And so once again: the earlier it is recognized, the greater one's chances of recovery. In order to attain this end, it is necessary to know about the first symptoms of tuberculous disease.

SYMPTOMS. T.B. is a long-drawn-out pneumonia (inflammation of the lungs). As the original area of infection is very small, the infected person does not notice anything at first. If the body does not succeed in mastering the invading bacteria, a general feeling of malaise may result. A suspicious symptom, and one which should send one to a doctor, is profuse sweating at night, if persistent for a long time. For the same reason, anyone who values his life should not ignore what seems to be a long-drawn-out bout of flu. If a feverish cold hangs on for weeks, it may mean the beginning of T.B. With this goes occasional slight shivering, especially in the evenings, a dry cough, general weakness, sometimes a greater need for sleep.

Severe symptoms such as coughing blood, blood-streaked sputum and loss of weight are so alarming that it is unnecessary to emphasize the need to see a doctor as soon as possible. Starting from the lung (or sometimes from the lymphatic glands of the intestine), the tubercle bacilli can get to any other organ. The symptoms at the portal of entry—usually the lung—may be so slight that the disease may appear in bone, kidney, brain or other organ like a bolt from the blue. It is always a gradual process and is sometimes very difficult for the doctor to diagnose. For instance, T.B. of the bones or joints causes just the same pains and discomfort as rheumatism, or the after-effects of sprains and many similar illnesses.

TREATMENT AND MANAGEMENT. Tuberculosis is not a vanished disease, but its treatment and management have been revolutionized in recent years—so much so that many sanitariums which existed for treatment of tubercular patients have closed their doors, and surgical procedures such as collapse of the lung, which once were common, are now rarely resorted to. This revolution has been brought about by potent new drugs such as isoniazid, streptomycin and PAS. Streptomycin, an antibiotic, was the first "breakthrough" drug for tuberculosis. It was effective in inhibiting tubercle bacilli but, after a period of treatment, patients became resistant to it, or rather the "bugs" did, and were no longer affected by a drug which was lethal to them when they first encountered it. The same tendency to develop resistance applies to other antituberculosis drugs. But, when two or more drugs are given in combinations determined by a physician, benefits last much longer, quite long enough in most cases, to bring tubercular infection under control. As a consequence, the patient's stay in a hospital is commonly reduced to a few weeks as compared to the many months or years of former sanitarium treatment. Nor is it usually thought advisable today for a patient to move to some part of the country reputed to be particularly salubrious for tuberculosis; effective treatment can virtually always be given very near to home.

DEALING WITH TUBERCULOUS PEOPLE

Since T.B. is infectious, caution is required. But patients with T.B. are not necessarily infectious all the time, since they do not all cough up tubercle bacilli. Only really ill patients are "open" cases, i.e. always disseminating their germs. The ideal method would be to segregate permanently all infectious people, but this is not practicable in view of the long duration of the illness. One can only urge them against working in certain occupations while they are infectious. To their own family they are of course responsible and must abide by the doctor's orders. First of all children must be kept away from the patient as much as circumstances permit. The patient must be careful never to spit except into a container of disinfectant. In short, all possible precautions must be taken and the doctor's instructions carefully carried out.

Should one come into contact with open T.B. people, one can console oneself with the thought that, as an adult, one has long since got over one's own T.B. Only if one breathes in quite enormous quantities of tubercle bacteria can anything happen.

SUPPURATIVE (PUS-FORMING) DISEASES

Modern science has greatly increased its defenses against the germs of these diseases, which are extraordinarily sensitive to most chemotherapeutic drugs.

Those dramatic and formerly highly dangerous diseases, which are accompanied by high fever, such as puerperal fever, blood-poisoning and pneumonia, are no longer dangerous if the doctor intervenes in time. Whenever there is fever and rapid spread of bacteria, we can rely on bacteria-killing drugs. It is only necessary for us to recognize the first symptoms in order to start treatment in time.

PNEUMONIA

SYMPTOMS. Sometimes following a severe chill, but often out of the blue. There is a sudden rise of temperature to 100 or 102 degrees Fahrenheit. Often shivering fits, headaches and a sharp pain in the chest, made worse by cough. There is cough, sputum and shortness of breath. Pneumonia may also complicate other diseases such as "flu" and measles.

TREATMENT. Penicillin G; also tetracyclines or erythromycin.

PUERPERAL FEVER

SYMPTOMS. After birth or miscarriage which has taken place under not completely hygienic conditions there is a sudden rise of temperature with shivering fits. The temperature fluctuates and there are shivering fits whenever swarms of bacteria enter the blood-stream. Rapid pulse. Often a rash similar to scarlet fever or small hemorrhages appear on the skin.

BLOOD-POISONING. (Septicemia)

SYMPTOMS. Exactly like puerperal fever, except that the source of infection is not the womb. Possible sources of infection are inflamed tonsils, suppuration in the middle ear, boils, inflammation of the gall-bladder and appendix, and discharging wounds and injuries.

ERYSIPELAS

SYMPTOMS. Begins with shivering fits and rapid rise in temperature. Simultaneously a surface rash and swelling appears, usually on the face, but sometimes on the arms or legs. The skin becomes thick and taut and hot and very red. If the area round the eyes is affected, the lids swell up.

TREATMENT. Penicillin or erythromycin cure the disease. Cold packs and aspirin help relieve discomfort of patient.

IMMUNITY. Does not exist.

RHEUMATIC FEVER

Although this is not a suppurative disease, rheumatic fever is here mentioned because it is due to the same organism that causes tonsillitis and erysipelas, namely, the streptococcus. In some people the late effects of such an infection result in painful and swollen joints and inflammation of the heart. The joints usually recover completely, but in about a quarter of the cases permanent damage is done to the valves which subdivide the heart chambers. These no longer function properly, and as a result the work of the heart is greatly increased and it therefore enlarges and may fail. This is an example of serious and permanent after-effects that may follow an infection with bacteria even after the bacteria themselves have been killed off by an active chemotherapeutic agent.

HOW TO SAFEGUARD AGAINST INFECTION

THE HYGIENIC MODE OF LIFE

Our body is capable of extraordinary powers of resistance and the microscopic enemies of the bacteria world cannot easily harm it. When it works properly it can withstand pretty violent attacks before finally giving away. This does not apply to venereal diseases, where the most robust health is of no avail. Here the only safe protection is chastity, or real marital fidelity. The body must rely on the vigilance of the mind.

But with everything else a well co-ordinated and disciplined body is of the greatest importance. If each of us had one-tenth of a penny in our savings account for each harmful germ disposed of by our body, we should be provided for for the rest of our days.

Our achievement in this respect is really impressive and goes on quietly, day in and day out. But we must not just rely on the body's resistance and make no attempt to avoid bacteria. For that reason we have, over several generations, made a point of observing the rules and demands of general hygiene, and putting them into practice in our daily lives. This is all the more important now that we tend to live crowded together in large cities. Fortunately by now our hygienic habits are an accepted custom, so that we no longer find anything unusual about them.

THE LAVATORY

It goes without saying that we should deposit our excreta where they cannot harm our fellow men. In the large towns harmful human excreta are safely removed by means of a sewage system. In villages and the countryside there is still much to be done in the way of improvement in this respect. Covered privies which keep out flies as far as possible should become an institution in the country. It is not merely a question of absence of smell: there are important scientific reasons for it in connection with prevention of disease.

One of the rules of decent behavior, which, alas, is not always observed by everyone, is that no one should spit in the street. It is not necessary to enrich the dust of our cities with germs from the mucous membranes of our mouths and noses.

THE HANDKERCHIEF

The use of handkerchiefs made of cloth, a common custom for only two hundred years or so, is only of partial value from the point of view of hygiene. This method of blowing one's nose was in itself a great step forward and at the time there were no better materials available for this purpose. But now it is about time we withdrew these "bacteria-spreaders" from current use. It is really quite shocking to contemplate what goes into our handkerchiefs and comes out again. As soon as one develops a cold the handkerchief made of cloth should disappear into the cupboard, no matter how pretty and gaily colored it is. The ideal thing is to use paper tissues, which do not incur great expense, and which can be destroyed after use, for preference by burning. The handkerchief made of cloth should only be used for mopping one's brow!

DO NOT COUGH AND DO NOT SNEEZE

We realize we should not cough or sneeze in other people's faces, but holding a hand before one's face is scarcely more than a pretty gesture. A cloth—and here we must in an emergency resort once more to the handkerchief—constitutes a better filter for the bacteria-carrying stream of drops. One can sometimes prevent oneself from sneezing at an inopportune moment by an effort of will. Yawning is not so dangerous for other people. Here it is quite sufficient to put a hand before the mouth.

The basis of these customs is the protection of our fellow men from infection. During epidemics and in the case of venereal disease these demands of good manners have been strengthened by the law. Actually, with all other infectious diseases there are certain regulations which have to be observed by the doctor.

GENERAL CLEANLINESS

A far-reaching and important means of keeping healthy is cleanliness of hands, body and food. Adequate use of soap affords protection from illness. As the mouth and nose are the two most obvious entrances for germs, it is obvious that in addition to washing the hands before a meal and after going to the lavatory, one should not touch one's mouth and nose unnecessarily. It is not only for esthetic reasons that one does not pick one's nose or bite one's finger-nails.

The normal secretion of gastric juice disposes of considerable quantities of harmful bacteria taken in at meals. Drinking can be more dangerous—in particular cold drinks without food. Drinks pass quickly through the stomach and do not stimulate any secretion of hydrochloric acid. For this reason it is inadvisable to drink unboiled water during the summer in places where the water supply is not absolutely safe.

There is always an element of risk about eating any kind of raw food, but of course one should not overrate the extent of the danger. Neither should one overrate the value of raw food (see Modern Nutrition, Vitamins, page 106). Cooked food is always safer.

It goes without saying that, if one smokes while working, one ought not to rest the cigarette between puffs on something dusty or dirty; but, let's face it, few of us can honestly say we have never sinned in this respect.

Obviously one should avoid using handkerchiefs and tooth-brushes that other people have used. Also you should desist from visiting infectious patients, no matter how dearly you love them.

KISSING

Finally we must remember one more thing. A lot of kissing goes on. When this happens a very extensive exchange of bacteria from the mouth takes place—more than one can inhale when being sneezed at. Nevertheless, grown-ups stand up to it very well. One thing, however, should be made taboo once and for all—the indiscriminate kissing of small children. Although in one's own immediate family circle the usual skin and mouth bacteria are common property, the aunt who comes to visit her nieces and nephews, every four weeks, should be urged by their cautious mother to refrain from smothering the children with kisses. If the aunt must kiss the children, it should be on the cheek.

FINGER-NAILS

In our personal toilet we often make mistakes in hygiene through ignorance or thoughtlessness. Finger-nails and hang-nails should not be pulled or bitten, but cut with a pair of sharp scissors. They can thus be separated from the healthy tissue in such a way as to avoid the danger of inflammation. As well as finger-nails, toe-nails should not be forgotten. With tight-fitting shoes there is a danger of ingrowing toe-nails, which may cause inflammation. Toe-nails should be cut so that they grow toward the middle.

If we itch, we instinctively scratch, but this should be done without infecting the skin with dirty finger-nails. Itching mosquito bites can be relieved with spirits of ammonia. Usually an astringent such as methylated spirit helps to relieve itching.

There are people who pick their teeth, and from the point of view of hygiene there is no objection to using a wooden toothpick to remove scraps of food from between the teeth. On the contrary, they can be cleaned more thoroughly this way than is possible with a tooth-brush, but custom decrees that the practice should not be carried out in public and indiscriminate poking about is injurious to the gums.

EYES AND EARS

The auditory canal is a highly sensitive area and should not be cleaned with sharp objects such as hairpins, etc. The most hygienic way is to wash out the ears with warm water using cotton wool or a soft towel. If there is wax in the ears, some glycerine should be added to the water used to clean them.

Keep your fingers and handkerchiefs away from your eyes when a foreign body has got into them. Try to remove the object by bathing the eye in clear, warm water, and opening and shutting the eye. If this is not successful, the doctor must remove the cause of the trouble.

HEALTHY HOUSING AND KEEPING THE BODY HEALTHY

As well as general hygiene which helps us to avoid any infection, good housing and working conditions and care of the body to keep it fit and sound are very important factors in healthy living. Dry and sunny houses harbor fewer bacteria than damp and dark houses. It is more refreshing to sleep with the windows open than in a damp, close atmosphere, but people who feel the cold very much can do themselves more harm than good by flinging open all the windows. It is not just the oxygen in the air which makes sleeping with open windows advantageous, nor is it the coldness of the air, but the decisive factor is the humidity of the atmosphere, which depends upon the temperature at any particular moment. Some people think that they would suffocate if they slept with their windows shut, but this is not so, for the air can seep through cracks in closed doors and windows quite rapidly.

BATHING

To have a cold bath, winter and summer, is not a particularly good way of cleaning oneself (although it is all right for making oneself spartan). One washes first and foremost in order to clean oneself, and anyone with really dirty hands knows only too well that he must have warm, and not cold, water to get them clean. For those who want to stimulate the skin in the morning they can do far more with a hard brush than with just a cold shower of water.

When taking a hot bath, it is not good to dry oneself immediately without first allowing oneself to cool down gradually. This can be done either by cooling down the shower, or by adding cold water to one's bath-water. Turkish baths, with all that they entail, are apparently very good for the health. They are excellent exercise to keep the walls of our blood-vessels supple. All bodily functions remain more flexible and efficient if we occasionally drive them to the limit of their capacity. But this applies only if we do not always drive them in the same direction. For example, the blood-vessels of the skin should not always be made to feel cold, but alternating hot and cold leaves them supple and elastic.

This interplay between all the various functions of the body is one of the most important principles of good health. The even keel of one's life must sometimes be disturbed; now and again one must get out of breath, or miss a meal and feel hungry, or feel oneself perspiring with heat, or feel the prickling sensation of a cold shower on one's reddened skin.

Firemen have to undergo trial runs, and armies do maneuvers in order to be able to function properly in an emergency. Thus in the same way our body needs exercise, fresh air and sunshine. It is its trial run, which counteracts the stagnating influence of the dreary daily routine and helps, not by an increase in the size of our muscles, which is important, but rather by the interplay between all the bodily functions. It is, of course, obvious that too much exercise no longer represents a trial run. It becomes a really serious emergency, and a man who is exhausted from some sport is running a risk to health. Just as an army on maneuvers does not use live cartridges, so with games everyone should know his limits and bear them in mind.

7. Hereditary Diseases

THE CAUSES OF INTERNAL DISEASES

It may seem surprising that the long chapter about infectious diseases is not all that is required to understand the causes of human ills and what can be done to relieve them. However, there is also the fact that some people are born imperfect and predestined, as it were, to suffer; for hereditary diseases exist. Many congenital illnesses and defects, though, are not hereditary and modern research is putting an end to many of the ills which we used to call inevitable. Sometimes the cause is traced to damage done to the fetus while still in the womb. In the case of mental disorders it is becoming more and more apparent that such illnesses are hereditary to a much smaller extent than we once used to think, and that they are often due to errors in upbringing. Every year relief and prevention of disease becomes a more tangible proposition.

We have learned that the laws of heredity applicable to lower creatures can be applied to human beings only after careful analysis of actual hereditary diseases. Above all, it has been proved that the sterilization laws (such as those which formerly existed in Germany) meant needless hardship to a great many people. There are many hereditary ailments; diabetes is an example of one. But medical science is learning how to use diet, drugs, and other techniques to permit patients with such diseases to have normal, active lives.

The visibly sick represent a diminishingly small percentage of the number of people with a concealed predisposition among the population. If these are excluded from reproducing, the number of living people with a predisposition for disease among the population is virtually undiminished. To put it into figures, if one were to carry out sterilization of the unfit consistently in every generation, a reduction of $1/1,000-1/100,000$ would be achieved, according to the frequency of the illness. To counter this, one must remember that, since the birth of Christ, not many more than sixty generations of human beings have lived. Thus a reduction of at the most 6 per cent in hereditary diseases would be the outcome of 2,000 years of repeated sterilization of sick people—and this is the most favourable estimate—at the worst a 0.06 per cent reduction would be achieved. So it is not worth while passing laws which are going to mean such hardship for many people, simply for the sake of a few possible successes during thousands of years. This would not be applied science, but rather an illusion. Only when we have the necessary knowledge and information at our disposal does our common sense know what is the right thing to do.

CONGENITAL DISEASES CAUSED BY DAMAGE IN THE WOMB

CONGENITAL SYPHILIS

In the chapter on infectious diseases we learned the most important possibilities of damage: some living germs can penetrate the filter of the placenta in the womb and harm the embryo. Congenital syphilis is the best-known form. Syphilis in the mother can be transferred to the child during pregnancy. But it is so easy to avoid this by treating the mother during pregnancy that such cases of prenatal damage occur only very rarely. It could be completely stamped out if a check were kept on all expectant mothers by means of the Wassermann blood-test.

CONGENITAL DEAFNESS DUE TO GERMAN MEASLES

It seems more difficult to avoid congenital deafness and other defects that occur if the mother gets German measles during pregnancy. Unfortunately the illness is not so rare with adults as one might expect with a children's illness. At roughly twenty-year intervals epidemics occur, which may also affect those grown-ups who were not infected during childhood.

INCOMPATIBILITY OF THE PARENTS' BLOOD GROUPS

When a person requires a blood transfusion, his blood group must be determined to see which type of human blood can safely be given. The characteristics which determine a person's blood group are inherited. A test must always be made to ensure that the donor's blood group is compatible with that of the receiver. Some time ago a new kind of blood group (the so-called Rh factor) was discovered, and it was realized that incompatibility could occur between the blood of a mother and that of the child in her womb. This accounted for previously unexplained stillbirths. The child had inherited a blood factor from its father which was not compatible with the mother's. This can happen to about 15 per cent of women.

With the first pregnancy this can never happen, unless the mother's blood has been sensitized by a previous blood transfusion with the wrong Rh blood group. Then the mother's blood develops antibodies, just as against bacteria. In these cases the nourishing blood of the mother destroys that of the unfortunate unborn child during pregnancy. Sensitization of the mother's blood takes place not only as the result of a blood transfusion, but also as a result of the first pregnancy if the father belongs to an incompatible Rh group. Only if the mother produces a large amount of antibody is the child's health endangered. Fortunately, immunization against Rh disease is now possible with an injection of human immune globulin.

8.   Blood Diseases and Cancer

The title of this chapter may well appear strange to many people. You may ask what connection there is between blood diseases and cancer. But normal blood cells as well as the malignant growth of cancer and other growths are first and foremost tissues which continually grow and are replaced. The bone marrow constantly throws out new blood cells into the blood channels, and these cells live and work for about four months, wear out, and are removed. New cells from the marrow replace them. The cells in our blood, in health, represent the results of this rate of formation and the act of destruction of worn-out cells. Blood diseases are first and foremost due to a disordered or accelerated cell growth or cell destruction. Some blood diseases have therefore a cancer-like character.

ANEMIA

If a person receives a large wound and bleeds profusely, he becomes anemic. He becomes very thirsty and makes up his blood volume by drinking water. The blood becomes thinner, that is to say there are less cells per cubic milliliter of blood than in a normal person. There are no longer five millions in the minute measured drop which the doctor counts under the microscope. Correspondingly, the hemoglobin content is reduced. It no longer amounts to 100 per cent. This is the simple anemia of hemorrhage, which occurs immediately after a heavy loss of blood and which everyone can understand. It lasts only a very short time. The bone marrow exerts itself to the utmost and in a few days the harm is repaired and the cells are made up again.

ANEMIA DUE TO LACK OF IRON

However, it is a different matter when a person has a wound which is constantly opening up again, as, for example, a bleeding stomach-ulcer or severely bleeding hemorrhoids. The bone marrow works at high pressure to make good the daily loss of cells. It may succeed in doing so more or less completely, according to the rapidity of bleeding. But hemoglobin is not produced so quickly. The cells become more deficient in it and so less efficient in transporting oxygen. This is because the iron which is lost with the blood cannot be replaced quickly enough. Hemorrhagic anemia is really anemia due to lack of iron. An ordinary diet contains the amount of iron corresponding to ten cubic centimeters of blood. If more is lost, the iron intake must be increased. Then the cell factory in the bone marrow can completely make good very considerable losses in a short time. Its achievement is limited only by the supply of iron.

In cases of long feverish infectious diseases an iron-deficiency anemia occurs. The stocks of iron are adequate but the sick body is unable properly to construct the hemoglobin molecule. Women, during their fertile years, can develop anemia through loss of blood during menstruation.

Of course, exactly the same form of anemia results when complaints of the digestive organs hinder the absorption of iron. For example, this may be the case when there is a lack of hydrochloric acid in the gastric juice. That occurs with some cases of inflammation of the stomach mucous membrane, cancer of the stomach and also after stomach operations.

All anemic people have pale lips. The lack of pigment in the blood is particularly apparent in the mouth and above all in the conjunctiva of the eye. If one pulls down the lid, one is immediately struck by the pale red of the visible small blood-vessels. These people feel weak and tired and have a greater need of sleep. In severe cases there is a tendency to giddiness and fainting.

PERNICIOUS ANEMIA

This is quite a different form of anemia which was formerly invariably fatal. Until 1925, few patients survived longer than three years. This illness and its methods of treatment are an example of the effectiveness of vitamins (page 90). Nowadays no one dies of pernicious anemia. An injection of vitamin B_{12} every few months is sufficient to control the trouble, if the illness has been recognized in time, before damage to the nerves is caused.

These people are unable to utilize a certain substance in food which is metabolized in the liver. They also lack hydrochloric acid in the stomach. Nevertheless, lack of iron plays no part in this. The red pigment is ready for the blood cells in the requisite quantity in the bone marrow, but these cannot be built up in the necessary amount. They are partly too big, partly misshapen, and are all full of hemoglobin.

The complexion of untreated people is a lemon color. There is a yellowish tinge in their pallor. The tongue, too, is usually changed, before they undergo treatment. At the sides the tongue looks red and inflamed and hurts if touched. It is sensitive and burns. Soreness of the tongue is often the first symptom of illness, and is almost always accompanied by indigestion. The mucous membrane of the stomach is no better off than that of the tongue. The stomach fails to secrete a substance necessary for moving protective elements from food into the blood. Quite soon unpleasant sensations become apparent in the limbs, especially in the arms and fingers: feelings of numbness, prickling, tingling, and a cold feeling. This is due to an insufficient supply of oxygen to the nerve cells. The blood is not efficient enough in transporting oxygen because there are not enough cells present. These symptoms are present in all serious cases of anemia. A degeneration of the spinal cord can occur in a small proportion of cases where treatment is inadequate or is given too late.

Pernicious anemia should be recognized and treated as early as possible. If this is done, there is no danger. Formerly one had to rely on very frequent and often painful injections of liver extract in treating this illness. But in recent years we have had pure vitamin B_{12}, which can be injected painlessly and at longer intervals. The injected quantities are incredibly small, for 50 micrograms (50/1,000,000 gram) are enough.

HEMOLYTIC ANEMIA

As well as anemia caused by loss of blood or lack of iron, and pernicious anemia, there are many other forms of this complaint, such as anemia due to poisons, lack of vitamins, and anemia complicating a large number of other illnesses. All these blood diseases are caused by a disturbance of function of the bone marrow. Anemia can also occur as a result of increased destruction of red blood corpuscles. In such cases there is jaundice, as the blood pigment liberated by the destruction of red blood cells by the spleen is turned into bile pigment. These anemias are termed hemolytic (hemo = blood, lytic = dissolving) anemias or hemolytic icterus (*ikteros* = jaundice). In some cases they can be cured if an operation is performed and the spleen removed.

LEUCOCYTOSIS AND LEUKEMIA (Increases of the white blood corpuscles)

The white blood corpuscles are the most independent cells in the human body. That is to say, like one-celled primitive creatures they can move under their own power, and migrate out of the blood-vessels and eat foreign particles such as bacteria. They are a law unto themselves and the number present in the blood-stream is extremely variable. After a meal, for example, the circulating white cells increase by 10-20 per cent. (This is believed to play a part in absorption of fat.) They are released in masses when germs invade the body. Double or three times the normal number then circulate in the blood and carry out the work of defense. As soon as the white blood corpuscles have performed their task, the number again falls.

The increase or decrease of white blood cells is an important finding in numerous illnesses, not only where there is infection. Especially important are the relative amounts of individual species of the cells. This is what the doctor calls a *differential blood count*. Under the microscope 100 white cells are sorted out, and the percentages of individual species of cells are determined. If in an infectious disease many young or immature cells are found, it is a sign that the bone marrow is exerting itself. The cells are mostly formed in the bone marrow as are the red cells.

BONE MARROW PUNCTURE

In some cases it is not sufficient just to examine the cells in the blood. If it appears that their manufacture in the bone marrow has become abnormal, they must be examined in this their place of birth. A specimen of bone marrow must be obtained. This is a completely harmless operation and, if handled properly, is absolutely painless. After numbing the tissues with a local anesthetic, the skin and thin bone of the breast-bone are punctured with a needle and a drop of bone marrow (an almost liquid tissue) sucked up. This is spread out on a small glass slide and examined under the microscope, just like a drop of blood from one's finger or ear lobe.

LEUKEMIA

This is something quite different from a leucocytosis and is not only an increase of cells in the blood, but a wild, uncontrollable growth in the bone marrow. This may go on for years relatively harmlessly, but can, however, take place at a tremendous speed. The white cells no longer grow in the way required by the body; they run wild and spread and refuse to be checked. They occupy the entire bone marrow and, in severe cases, settle in other parts of the body as well, where they form new places of growth and go on growing until the formation of red cells is completely suppressed. Their activities eventually destroy life. They lose their ordinary shape and useful abilities in the process. They are a body tissue which has gone wild—a sort of cancer. Their development can be followed more closely than is possible with ordinary cancer, since every drop of blood gives the doctor information. For that reason one can say with greater certainty how great the danger is, unlike cancer of the internal organs.

SYMPTOMS. There is little point in describing the first symptoms of these illnesses in such a way as to make them comprehensible to the layman—and it is indeed scarcely possible to do so. There are at least twenty-five different complaints, which can be distinguished from one another only by blood-tests. Only these tests can give information concerning the patient's fate. One of the most frequent early symptoms of leukemia is a feeling of tension in the upper left abdomen. The spleen, which is situated there, is trying desperately to master the cell masses and increases considerably in size. Very often there is an increased tendency to bleed—little spots under the skin, nose-bleeds, bleeding gums, etc. With most forms the lymphatic glands on the neck and in other parts of the body swell and form palpable masses. Sometimes there is fever.

TREATMENT. There are various methods of checking and suppressing this wild growth of cells. There are drugs which interfere with the production of the white blood cells in the bone marrow. One of these drugs is a close chemical relation of mustard gas. If injected carefully, and due attention is paid to the blood picture, leukemia can be checked for a time. Another drug, urethane, has a similar action. X-ray treatment of the entire body can also check leukemia. Research on drugs of this kind is continuing, but up to now there is not one which can completely cure the disease. One has to use them all in succession, as soon as one loses its effect on the patient. By utilizing these various methods to the best advantage the life of the patient can be prolonged for years, except in very severe cases. Every doctor calls in a specialist if he feels the task to be beyond his own capacity. These doctors are known as hematologists and are specialists in blood diseases.

APLASTIC ANEMIA

There is also the opposite of leukemia and it can become equally dangerous, as there may be complete failure of the bone marrow. This may result from certain poisons, sensitivity to certain drugs and, in rare cases, for no apparent cause. The dangerous thing about it is not so much the lack of red cells, but the shortage of white cells, without the help of which the body's defense against infection breaks down. Then even an ordinary attack of tonsillitis becomes serious because of the lack of resistance.

If the cause is removable—for instance, sensitivity to a drug whose use can be stopped—there may be spontaneous recovery. But in many cases it is necessary to give whole blood transfusions to prolong life until the bone marrow is able to resume its normal function.

BLEEDING DISEASES (HEMOPHILIA)

All of you will have heard with a faint shudder of the hereditary blood disease which has played such a tragic role in some European royal families. It is a hereditary disease which can only occur in the male members of the affected families. The condition is transmitted by the females, who themselves remain perfectly healthy. The factor transmitting the disease is linked to the chromosome that determines the sex in the unborn child. Usually women who transmit this disease have 50 per cent entirely healthy children, 25 per cent healthy girls, who can nevertheless transmit the disease like their mother, and 25 per cent sick sons. As has already been said, we must apply the law of "usually" here. Certain women may produce completely healthy children or, on the other hand, all sick sons, and daughters capable of transmitting the disease. One can assess the percentage of healthy and sick children with reasonable accuracy only after taking a census of thousands of births. Affected males lack one important factor from the complicated clotting system of the blood. Thus it happens that their blood does not clot when shed. Even the most trivial injury is sufficient. A slight knock on the elbow or elsewhere on the body is sufficient to cause rupture of the smallest blood-vessels. Immediately blood pours into the tissues so that taut, painful, blue and green swellings result. The torn blood-vessel is not plugged by a clot as quickly as is usually the case and so even a nose-bleed is dangerous. Extracting teeth becomes a highly risky operation. Although transfusion of normal whole blood relieves the condition, many patients can be treated by additions of fresh normal plasma to their blood or by injections of antihemophilic factor (AHF).

THROMBOPENIA (Lack of blood platelets)

There are other bleeding diseases which are not hereditary. One of these is a bone marrow defect resulting in a disorder in the formation of blood platelets. These are minute bodies which circulate in the blood in fairly large quantities, and contain substances which when released set in motion the mechanism of clotting whenever blood is shed. The blood platelets are called thrombocytes (*thrombos* = clotting; *kytos* = container). Hence the name thrombopenia (*penia* = lack, poverty).

One can recognize the condition by purple spots which appear on the skin after the slightest injury and above all by little specks of blood on the skin when the blood-stream in the arm is temporarily interrupted by means of a tourniquet.

OTHER BLEEDING DISEASES

Disorders of the complicated clotting mechanism of the blood with its many substances can occur for other reasons, but are rare. As nearly all the clotting substances are produced in the liver, the mechanism is likely to be affected in disease of the liver. However, the liver complaint must be at a considerably advanced stage before bleeding becomes serious. By careful and exact examination it is very often possible to detect an increased tendency towards bleeding in liver disease.

A serious deficiency of vitamin C also manifests itself in an increased tendency toward bleeding (scurvy). This is not a disorder of clotting, but an increased fragility of the smallest blood-vessels. They easily break at the slightest contact, as, for instance, during chewing, or brushing one's teeth, when the gums are somewhat roughly treated. It is easy to overcome the trouble, not only by vitamin C itself, but also by similar vitamin-like substances which are known as rutin.

Many erroneous beliefs and superstitions exist concerning cancer, both as regards causation and cure. Unfortunately these may sometimes result in serious harm. There have been occasional items in the press featuring so-called cures for cancer devised by unqualified laymen. Such publications may, tragically enough, undermine the patient's confidence in his doctor's advice. It must often happen that patients hesitate when advised to undergo operation as the only hope of cure, simply because they have been misled by incorrect information. Often this raising of false hopes leads to death by neglect of proper treatment. Let us therefore consider carefully the nature of cancer and the effective methods of treatment.

WHAT IS CANCER?

Cancer starts as a change occurring in some of the cells in an organ, so that they run wild, degenerate and no longer carry out their natural functions. They begin to multiply of their own accord and at the expense of their fellow-cells. They grow out of all proportion to the actual needs of the body and attack and invade other tissues.

Not every growth (or tumor) is a cancer in the medical sense. No one would regard a wart as a cancer, but it is obviously a little independent growth. There are two sorts of growths—benign and malignant (or cancerous). By a benign growth we mean those which are not dangerous and which do not invade or destroy neighboring tissues. An example of this type of growth is the *fibroid,* a tumor of the womb which is quite common in women over thirty. This grows as a self-contained mass without invading the wall of the womb. Of course, even benign growths may cause trouble if they become very large or if their size makes them press on adjacent organs and cause pain. Another example is the tumors consisting of fat cells ("lipomas"), which often occur under the skin. They need removal only for cosmetic reasons. The surest way of distinguishing harmless from malignant growths is to cut away a small portion (known as taking a biopsy) and examine this under the microscope.

MALIGNANT GROWTHS (Cancer)

Unlike the tumors described above, the malignant growths have two characteristics. As they grow they destroy the adjacent normal structures; and small numbers of cells break off from the main mass to be carried by the blood-stream to other parts of the body. These secondary deposits behave in each new locality in exactly the same way as the primary growth from which they originated.

TREATMENT OF CANCER BY OPERATION

In view of what is known about cancer it is obvious that the disease is cured only if the degenerate cells can be completely removed. If the disease is diagnosed in time and the first cancer cut out, the patient is cured. The actual danger is not so much the operation as the possibility that single cells may have already passed into other organs. For that reason it is sometimes necessary to remove the nearest lymphatic gland as well (e.g., in the armpit when an operation for cancer of the breast is performed). On account of the danger of spread, every operation on a cancer must also remove a good margin of healthy surrounding tissue, since if the cancer were cut into, the cells would get into the blood and form deposits elsewhere.

X-RAY TREATMENT

Cancer cells can be destroyed also by X-rays or radioactive chemicals such as radium, though this form of treatment is usually reserved for growths which by their nature are difficult to remove. Unfortunately X-rays also destroy ordinary healthy tissue, though cancer cells are much more susceptible than these to X-ray damage (all actively growing cells are more easily damaged than mature cells). The problem is therefore to protect the adjacent healthy tissue from the rays. With growths near the surface this is easy, but with deep internal growths the problem is more complicated. One technique is to focus the X-rays on the site of the tumor and then to continually rotate the patient around the X-ray tube (or the tube around the patient) during treatment. By this means the tumor receives the full dose, while the skin and intervening structures are only partially irradiated.

Minute amounts of radium can be enclosed in little hollow metal tubes (radium needles) which can then be inserted directly into an accessible growth.

DRUGS

No drug in the usual sense of the word has any curative effect on cancer. However, in two particular forms, life can be prolonged and symptoms relieved by the use of sex hormones. These two are cancer of the prostate gland in the male and of the breast in the female. Cancer of the prostate can be held in check by doses of female sex hormones or estrogens. Many patients who have had such treatment have now lived more than five years. Formerly the longest recorded survival was nine months. In addition, pain, discomfort and difficulty with urination are relieved. Such results are not, however, seen in all patients, and this is even more so with breast cancer. In this condition, hormone treatment may occasionally help a patient in whom the condition is too advanced for surgery, but in many cases it has no effect. It cannot replace operation or X-ray treatment when these are possible.

Everyone should realize five important points about the incidence of cancer:

(1) Cancer is not hereditary.

(2) Cancer is not generally infectious, even though some kinds apparently are transmitted by viruses.

(3) Cancer is not incurable.

(4) Cancer generally is not caused by our present mode of life, although some individual cases of cancer can be traced to certain lifestyles, such as to the use of tobacco.

(5) Cancer today is no greater threat to mankind than it was 50 or 1,000 years ago. The fact that there are more cases of cancer is simply because more people live to be over 40 than formerly, and methods for detecting cancer now are

better. On the positive side, your chances of recovery from cancer have never been greater than they are today.

All misunderstandings which exist about cancer are based on ignorance of the law of "usually," which we have come up against over and over again in this book, and which has proved to be indispensable to us in our real understanding of illness.

The knowledge contained in these five points is the best antidote to alarming and misleading information about cancer. It is the best and only remedy for dispelling fear. A person who knows enough about cancer is better protected than any other. For, only if he comes to the doctor in time, can he be cured, and that is why we have devoted a whole detailed chapter to the prevention of cancer.

WHAT CAN ONE DO ABOUT CANCER?

Prognosis

One of the most difficult questions of tact and conscience for a doctor is to decide just how much to tell a cancer patient and his relatives about the nature and seriousness of the case. He should not raise any false hopes and, on the other hand, he must not destroy the patient's courage and will to live by painting too grim a picture. It is only when all hope of improvement has gone that suffering becomes intolerable.

This problem demands complete understanding of human nature and skill on the part of the doctor, for there are scarcely ever two patients in the same situation to whom he can use the same words. In the case of cancer his words usually carry more weight than at other times, and it is on them that the happiness and grief of a whole family rest. Considering that any such person may need an exceptional measure of perception, sympathy and understanding, how much more difficult is our task in this book, where we are endeavoring to enlighten a vast and unknown public on such vital matters. We think that we may prevent untold suffering if we give healthy people an adequate knowledge of the first symptoms of malignant growths.

Only if the cancer patient undergoes medical treatment in time is there really any hope of a cure, since all methods of cancer treatment which have stood the test of critical scientific investigation are based on the destruction of the malignant growing tissue. It is obvious that this can be achieved only if the malignant growth has not yet already spread to essential organs and if its colonies have not been formed in numerous parts of the body (via the lymphatics and the blood-stream). These conditions are found only when the disease is in its earliest stage. Even the best doctors and the most complete Health Service of a country can succeed in their battle against cancer only if cancer patients come to them when they are still reasonably fit. Thus the idea of enlightening the public about the first symptoms of different forms of cancer seems appropriate, as the patient's help must be enlisted in this matter.

FEAR OF CANCER

While it is natural and reasonable to fear cancer, there is an equally unnatural and unreasonable fear with which we have to contend, and that is "cancerophobia"—the unfounded and senseless fear of cancer. There are people who are obsessed by such an unreasonable fear of cancer that they can no longer enjoy life. They imagine themselves to be incurably ill and beyond hope, when they are, in fact, perfectly healthy and even the closest medical examination fails to show the slightest suspicion of cancer. Of course this senseless fear of illness can be found with a thousand other "imaginary" ailments. Most of us are acquainted with the sort of person who is always suffering from a different ailment and keeps going from doctor to doctor; one moment his liver is affected, then it is the gallbladder, and finally the kidneys, etc. But that is something quite different from this mysterious, mental symptom of cancerophobia—this senseless fear of cancer.

One must go further if one wants to make this mysterious dread of cancer comprehensible. In what way does cancer differ from the other diseases which we know? Firstly, most laymen believe that it is incurable, that a person who gets cancer is beyond hope of recovery and that medical science is powerless. We shall soon see that this is not altogether correct. But this idea that cancer is incurable is very widespread and helps to lay the foundation for a psychological symptom such as the unreasonable dread of cancer.

The second point in which cancer differs from other diseases is that its cause is unknown. People do not know how they get it, but believe that the doctor's diagnosis of cancer is tantamount to a death-sentence. Another point of difference between cancer and other diseases is that it originates within the body whereas other diseases such as infections or injuries come from without.

All these peculiarities contrive to make cancer an uncanny disease, and one which we may rightly fear. Every normal person experiences a feeling of apprehension, a certain degree of fear at the thought of cancer. But that is not cancerophobia, which can spoil a person's happiness and ruthlessly intrude upon his enjoyment and his peace of mind. We must learn to distinguish clearly between these two things—the mental illness, cancerophobia, and the normal feeling of apprehension at the thought of cancer.

This distinction may perhaps best be illustrated by the following example: Imagine that a mentally stable person with some feeling of apprehension at the thought of cancer is clearly and intelligently enlightened on the subject—as we have endeavored to do here. He will learn that cancer is not incurable if discovered in time. He will also learn that cancer is not hereditary, even if it occurs more frequently in some families than others. He will see clearly that one cannot contract cancer through infection. He will also learn more about research workers' views on the origin of this strange disease. In short, he will know more after reading this chapter and the disease will have lost something of its uncanniness for him. His apprehension will be less, because his knowledge is greater.

But with another person—one with a tendency to cancerophobia—there is the danger that the opposite effect may result. He will pore over the account of the first symptoms of cancer of the various organs and devour its contents, and his conviction that he is suffering from cancer will be strengthened, even though his doctor has told him that this is not the case. Every little feeling of discomfort and ailment will be regarded as a symptom of cancer. In short—after reading the chapter on cancer his cancerophobia will be greater.

There may be deeply rooted psychological causes for the development of cancerophobia. In some cases it may be unconsciously based on fear of retribution for some past misdeed (actual or imagined). In others it may be engendered by experience of cancer in a relative or friend. Such deep fears cannot always be allayed by logical argument even when the person consciously accepts the logic.

This is not to suggest that someone is suffering from cancerophobia just because, having read the description of early symptoms, he goes to see his doctor only to be told that his fears are unfounded. The last thing one would wish to do would be to deter anyone from seeking medical advice for fear of being considered neurotic. But the sensible person will always be relieved to discover that his worries are without foundation.

CANCER IS NOT A SCOURGE OF CIVILIZATION

A great many people hold the view that cancer is a disease of civilized countries and that the defects of our Western civilization are responsible for its increasing prevalence. If one takes a brief look at the statistics relating to causes of death in the past decades, there is apparently much to support this view. From year to year there is an increase in the percentage of deaths from cancer.

One might really be tempted to attribute this increase to defects in our civilization or other harmful effects of our own ever-increasing technical progress. However, careful analysis shows it to be otherwise. In point of fact our improved standards of hygiene and our own advance in medical science, which are the direct outcome of our technical progress, are responsible for the average span of human life becoming considerably longer. This of course means that the proportion of older people in the population has become greater; and cancer is a disease which occurs mainly among older age groups.

While only about five of every 100,000 people under thirty die of cancer, between one and two hundred people aged from thirty to sixty and 650–850 people of seventy die from this cause every year. Among even older people the figures are 1,000–1,200. So it is understandable that even a slight increase in the older age groups among the population can considerably influence the frequency and number of deaths from cancer. If one were to calculate the number of deaths which would occur if there had been no change in the age groups of the population, one would see that the risk of cancer is actually decreasing. The reason for this has not yet been accounted for. Perhaps the progress of our civilization and our improved diet and hygiene have resulted in a decline of carcinogenic stimuli and substances.

Cancer seems to have become more common because modern medical science has checked and practically eradicated all other fatal diseases which formerly carried off many young people. Nowadays many old people, who in former centuries would have died in youth, survive to the age when cancer is more common.

It is a fatalistic thought with which we are faced when we realize that, in spite of all our scientific efforts and work, instead of perfect health, one serious disease of old age stares us in the face. One's reaction is to cry out, 'How can we protect ourselves from this inexorable fate?' The question could be answered only if we really knew how all the various forms of cancer originated. Only then could we say, 'Do this, don't do that, and avoid doing anything likely to induce cancer.' But in these matters only a small amount of the necessary knowledge has resulted from our research work.

CARCINOGENIC SUBSTANCES (Substances known to produce cancer)

Tar Products

Tar has been shown to contain substances which cause cancer if repeatedly painted on the skin of animals in the laboratory. But this has no significance for the ordinary person.

Soot

It has been known for a long time that chimney-sweeps used to have an increased liability to develop cancer of the testicles. This was due to the irritation produced around these organs by repeated contact with soot which had worked its way in through their clothes. Once this was realized and attention drawn to it, it was found that attention to clothing and scrupulous cleanliness abolished this increased risk.

Aniline

A similar risk was formerly incurred by workers in aniline factories. They tended to get cancer of the bladder. This substance, which entered their bodies either via the skin or was inhaled, was excreted in the urine and probably remained for a long time in a fairly concentrated form in the bladder. This danger too has been removed by changes in production methods. The danger exists only if one works for at least two years with aniline or similar substances (see chapter on Poisons, page 129).

Another example of the ill effects caused by carcinogenic substances, which seems rather curious, is worth mentioning. It has been found that, in hot climates, cancer of the penis is much rarer among those religious groups which practise circumcision. One could deduce from this that any lack of cleanliness on the part of a non-circumcised person would result in accumulation of secretion (smegma) under the fore-skin of the penis, and it is possible that by the breakdown of this smegma, carcinogenic substances are formed. So one can see that general hygiene and cleanliness can serve in some small measure to prevent such a disease as cancer.

Radium

The ill effects of irradiation have made cancer of the lung an occupational disease in certain radium (and uranium) mines in one part of Germany. The ores from which these radioactive substances are won emanate rays which constitute a constant irritation to the lung tissue. Chronic irritation of this kind over a period of many years is conducive to the formation of cancer cells. It seems strange that in the process of gaining one of our most powerful weapons for treating cancer—radium—people run the risk of getting the disease. In civilized countries it is of course taken for granted that the strictest precautions are taken to safeguard uranium workers and for this reason they are only allowed to work in uranium mines for a few years. In this way one can reduce the degree of irritation to the lungs sufficiently to remove all danger.

X-rays

It is not only workers in uranium mines who run the risk of getting cancer as a result of being constantly exposed to radiation, but also all other people engaged in work with similar substances. X-rays also possess the power to produce cancer, and when they were first used, a number of pioneer research workers died of X-ray cancer. Nowadays we have learned to protect ourselves by means of lead screens, lead aprons, etc., so that this danger appears to have been removed and all that is necessary is proper supervision and training of the staff to see that these precautions are carried out.

Sunlight

It must be realized that not only radioactive rays and X-rays can cause cancer as a result of chronic irritation of the tissues, but that sun rays, which are normally so beneficial to us, can, if too intensive, be dangerous. Exposure to sunlight has an effect on the skin that resembles chronic exposure to X-rays. Farmers, sailors, sportsmen and sun worshippers are among groups with a higher than average incidence of skin cancer. Fair-skinned persons, particularly blond or red-haired individuals, are most susceptible and should learn to avoid overexposure to sunlight.

One hardly need mention that the sunlight in temperate regions is not sufficiently powerful to cause cancer. We need not be afraid of the sun. If we occasionally suffer from sunburn at the beginning of the summer, it is painful and causes us sleepless nights, but it is not conducive to cancer.

Asbestos

There is increasing evidence that asbestos fibers may be a contributing factor in lung cancers. The tiny fibers, only a millionth of an inch in diameter, are used in automobiles, textiles, and in building materials. Clouds of the fibers may be in the air in urban areas, and such fibers are easily breathed into the lungs. Workers, as well as their families, exposed to asbestos have a much higher rate of lung cancer than those not exposed.

False Alarms: Tarred Roads and Exhaust Fumes

There are unproven scientific theories and surmises which have unfortunately been given undue prominence in the press. One of these theories which has been voiced by some doctors, although it has never been proved and indeed probably never will be, is that by the use of asphalt and, above all, tar on our roads, the entire population is being constantly brought into contact with carcinogenic substances. People have tried to attribute the apparent increase in cancer of the lung in civilized countries to this factor, and statistics have even been produced to prove that in the countryside, away from tarred streets and the exhaust fumes of cars, cancer of the lung is rare.

Now it is very valuable for scientists to devote a great deal of time and thought to these problems and publish their own views on the subject in order to stimulate scientific discussion. But it shows lack of responsibility to alarm the public, before there is any evidence to substantiate their claims; and we can only repeat emphatically—we are nowhere near any proof that there is any connection between tarred roads, exhaust fumes from cars, and cancer of the lung.

Smokers and Cancer

Although the exact cause is unknown, there is a strong statistical relationship between cigarette smoking and lung cancer. The incidence of lung cancer among heavy cigarette smokers is about 20 times that of non-smokers. The occurrence is more common among men but is rapidly increasing in women. The evidence has been convincing enough to warrant an advisory from the U.S. Surgeon General in 1964 that "Cigarette smoking is a health hazard." The elevated death rates have been associated almost entirely with cigarette smoking rather than cigar and pipe smoking.

Fear Is Always Wrong

Thus we have observed what is known of precautions against cancer. As one can see, there is not much to be done, and this will remain so until science can tell us exactly how cancer or the different forms of cancer come about. In the meantime there is very little we can do to safeguard ourselves from the disease. One feels almost tempted to say, "Eat, drink and be merry, for tomorrow we die—and to hell with cancer." This is another way of saying that one must believe in one's good health and good fortune, and not spoil one's life with senseless worry and anxiety.

Perhaps future research will show us that a person who is jolly and free from anxiety can derive from his mental strength physical reserves for his body's defense. There may perhaps be justification for the theory that in all our bodies and among all the billions of cells, single cancer cells are formed from time to time in the course of a dividing process. This theory, which research workers seriously believe in and indeed have good cause for doing so, would mean that we all get a cancer cell some time in our life. And since not everyone by a long way gets cancer, we might deduce further that most people's bodies are able to cope with those cancer cells, by developing forces which nip the single cancer cells in the bud.

How Can I Protect Myself from Death from Cancer?

Now we have reached the stage when we can stop our fruitless efforts to answer the question "How can I protect myself from cancer?" We know that we can find many more practical answers to the question, "How can I protect myself from death from cancer?" The most general answer, and one which cannot be repeated often enough is: "By giving the doctor the chance of diagnosing the disease as soon as possible, should I have the misfortune to get it." That is the first and most important rule and it is the only thing that science really has to offer us—the earliest detection of cancer and the earliest complete removal of the growth-cells either by operation or ray treatment.

Believe me, all the doctors in the world would triumphantly proclaim the fact if there were any other effective means of combating cancer.

Nothing can cure cancer except the removal or destruction of the cancer tissue. *There is no other remedy for cancer.* All non-professional claims to this effect are dangerous falsehoods, which endanger human lives, because they make people with cancer less willing to undergo an immediate operation or irradiation treatment.

Drugs at best limit the growth of the cancer. But cancer cannot be cured by drugs.

Propaganda which is designed by non-medical people to attribute such powers to certain drugs is the greatest menace which threatens us in our task of fighting cancer.

But forgetting these hard words of condemnation, which only apply to what has happened up to the present day, we must conclude, from the few indications of the possibility of future cancer remedies, the following: One can say almost with certainty that a drug to cure all forms of cancer will never be discovered. If our future research gives us drugs to cure cancer, there will presumably be substances which will only be effective with certain forms of cancer. It is true that these surmises cannot be proved, but nevertheless we would not like to oust them at this juncture, as they lend weight to the warning which we again urge you to heed in all seriousness: "When there is cancer the only hope is to remove the growth-cells at the earliest possible moment."

EIGHTY PER CENT OF CANCER PATIENTS ARE CURED

If a person suffering from cancer goes to the doctor early enough, he is not incurable.

Of a hundred women who come for treatment while they are in the first stages of cancer of the womb, eighty leave the hospital cured and can then say of themselves, "I had cancer."

With present-day knowledge among our population, this percentage of people with cancer who undergo early treatment unfortunately only amounts to 10 per cent. Those who do not wish to die of cancer must know enough about the disease to be able to be counted among this category of people who are operated on while they are in the first stages of cancer, so that they, too, can say afterward, "I had cancer." Only in this way is it possible for us with our present-day facilities to make cancer curable on a large-scale—i.e. when not only 10 per cent, but all people with cancer, are operated on in time.

HOW TO GUARD ONE'S HEALTH

Careful, but not over-anxious observation of one's own body can protect one from dying of cancer, just as it prevents one's condition from deteriorating in any illness, or from spreading illness.

Never let your own flesh and blood be a matter of indifference to you, even when your looks begin to fade and you lose interest in the way your body functions. You still want to go on living. In other words: Don't go to the doctor with the idea, "Doctor, I think I've got cancer." But go preferably once too often if you notice a little lump on or beneath the skin, which you do not understand and which does not disappear, or if you have symptoms which do not seem to right themselves: things which you have not experienced before, such as a constantly recurring pain in one's stomach, a persistent cough, in fact any symptom which does not clear up of its own accord.

It would be wrong to say that, "In order to protect oneself from dying of cancer one should, for example, have a thorough overhaul every two months." The doctor has no magic cancer detector and can only start a systematic search when there is some indication of cancer such as pains or little lumps in the skin.

These symptoms can be discovered by a person who knows and watches his own body, for nothing is more sensitive than the nervous system, which runs across our body, sending its signals to our mind in the form of pains or other uncomfortable sensations. Unfortunately this signal system can let us down, and, for example, transmit faulty messages. For instance, pains from the gall-bladder can be felt in the right shoulder. Some people have such a sensitive nervous system that the minor organic disorders which are an everyday occurrence are registered as major pains and disorders. Their nervous system makes, as it were, mountains out of molehills. They have such a variety of pains and disorders that the whole warning apparatus is thrown out of gear. Thirdly, areas can be affected which are not supplied with pain nerves, and, as it were, remain silent.

With all these necessary reservations a healthy balanced person can rely on his body to give him warning about cancer.

THE AGE AT WHICH ONE IS LIKELY TO GET CANCER

There is some justification for counting cancer among the diseases of old age, although it is necessary here to modify somewhat the term "disease of old age." The age at which one is likely to get cancer is not seventy, but, according to most cancer research workers, there is an appreciable tendency for men to get it after forty-five and women after thirty-five. Cancer is possible before these ages, but it is very rare. So men and women should start observing their bodies more carefully from forty-five and thirty-five onwards for the purpose of detecting symptoms of cancer.

What does this observation entail? The following table shows us how often the various organs in both sexes are affected by cancer.

The frequency with which cancer occurs in the various organs of the body. The figures show the percentage of cancer of individual organs in proportion to the entire number of cases of cancer.

	Skin	Womb	Breast	Lung	Digestive Tract	Prostate	Other Organs
Woman	13	15	23	3	21	—	25
Man	23	—	—	18	21	10	28

CANCER OF THE STOMACH

We can see from this table that cancer of the stomach is the most common form of cancer with both sexes. Now, stomach ailments are very common. Cancer of the stomach can at first give rise to all kinds of minor stomach trouble, such as occur with inflammation of the mucous membrane, ulcers, etc. It is, however, unforgivable if a middle-aged person ignores constant indigestion over a period of weeks, without allowing himself to be medically examined. A stomach upset usually gets better, as we all know, in eight to fourteen days at the longest. All symptoms of stomach trouble which persist for a long time—i.e., frequent belching with an unpleasant taste, pains after or during a meal, or when hungry, heartburn, nausea, vomiting, loss of appetite, and a feeling of fullness after a meal—all these must be regarded as potential symptoms and should make one go to the doctor after fourteen days or three weeks at the latest. Even then, the chances are fifty or a hundred to one that it is a harmless stomach ailment. If, however, it is accompanied by loss of weight and a dry, yellow skin, one should not delay a visit to the doctor. Even then it need not necessarily be cancer, but the danger that it might be is much greater.

CANCER OF THE WOMB

With this form of cancer the first symptoms are just as difficult for the layman to distinguish from other harmless ailments, as with cancer of the stomach. Therefore my advice is once again, "When there are suspicious symptoms, it is better to go to the doctor once too often than too seldom."

It is especially essential for a woman to be medically examined if, after the menopause, bleeding occurs, however slight. But a woman also should be examined by a doctor if, in her pre-menopausal years, bleeding is noticed after sexual intercourse, or after lifting heavy objects or straining at the stool. Usually, this bleeding is not very severe and may not last very long and the loss of blood may be slight.

There is a simple and painless method of determining the presence of cancer of the womb even before the more serious symptoms such as bleeding appear. A few of the cells that are naturally shed by the cervix, at the opening of the womb, are collected by the doctor and studied under a microscope. This procedure, called the Pap smear or Pap test, was developed by Dr. George Papanicolaou to detect cancer of the womb five or more years before other symptoms occur. If cancer cells are detected by the Pap test, the woman has a better than 80 percent chance of recovery. For that reason, all adult women should receive a Pap test at least once a year.

For women who for various reasons cannot be examined by a doctor with facilities for examining cells of the cervix, there are do-it-yourself kits available with instructions for obtaining samples. The self-administered sample is then mailed to a laboratory for microscopic examination.

CANCER OF THE BREAST

Women who are at the age when cancer is likely can do more to protect themselves in the case of cancer of the breast. The first symptom is always a small hard lump—painless at first—in the female breast. These lumps or knots can be rec-

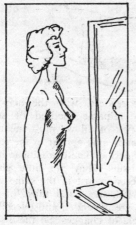

Fig. 31

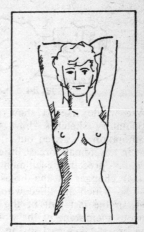

Fig. 32

ognized by the doctor in the course of a general examination only by careful and systematic feeling all through the breast tissue.

In recent years, in the course of a large-scale campaign of

enlightenment in the U.S.A., gynecologists have made an educational film for the purpose of enlightening the public on the subject of cancer of the breast. Special importance was attached to the demonstration of the correct method of examining one's own breast.

Women were advised to "knead through" the breasts point by point every two months. Such repeated examinations tend to develop an instinctive feeling for one's own body and one feels all areas, as it were, from two sides. First the sensory nerves of the fingers register the area which has been "kneaded through," and then the sensory and pain nerves of the area itself register the process once again. Naturally one can detect small changes in one's own body better than a doctor who examines many patients each day.

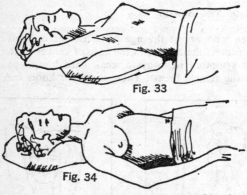

Fig. 33

Fig. 34

We would like to show our readers, with the help of explanatory sketches, how this valuable method of self-examination is carried out. But first of all we must mention that in any female breast little lumps may appear in the fourteen days preceding each monthly period. These are due to hormonal changes in the breast tissue. They are little gland nodules which are filled with secretion just in the same way that, in the last half of the period, the gland tubes of the mucous membrane of the womb are distended and overfilled. The breast takes part in this cycle of changes. So these self-examinations should be carried out in the first few days following a period, in order to avoid unnecessary mistakes. At the same time it must be realized that, apart from these temporary lumps of hormonal origin, not every knot or lump discovered need necessarily be an indication of cancer. It is the doctor's job to make this decision. If he cannot decide just by feel alone whether it is a harmless or a malignant growth, he may advise its removal so that the diagnosis can be made with certainty by the microscope.

The first examination starts with a careful inspection of the breast in a good light in front of a mirror (of course the upper half of the body should be unclothed). This is done first with the arms by the side and then with them raised behind the head (see Figures 31 and 32). One must keep a careful look-out for little contractions of the skin, changes in the nipples, any asymmetry of the breasts and any protuberances under the skin.

For the second examination one lies down flat with a small pillow or cushion pushed under one's shoulders (see Figures 33 and 34). *Figure 33:* Correct position for examining the breast oneself. A pillow has been pushed under the shoulder in order that the pectoral gland sits properly in the thorax. *Figure 34:* Faulty position for examining the breast oneself. If the shoulders lie flat on the support, the breasts fall sideways.

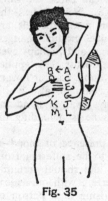

Fig. 35

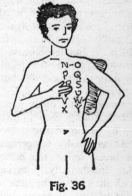

Fig. 36

First the inner side of the left breast is carefully felt with the right hand (as shown in Figure 35). The left arm should be placed under the head. One after another the fingers are pressed down flat, working their way downward from above, bit by bit, so that the whole breast on the inner side is felt. The hand must always follow the direction indicated with arrows in Figure 35—from breast level to the middle of the body. Then changing the position of one's arm the outer half of the breast is examined in the same way, starting at the bottom and working up to the collar-bone (see Figure 36).

It is the opposite direction of the one which is taken when examining the inner side. Then the same procedure is carried out with the left hand for the right breast.

So one can do a great deal to protect one's life by occasionally carrying out these examinations from the thirties onwards. But it is unwise to repeat them too often, not because one can do any harm, but because one may be inclined to get panicky about cancer.

We know from experience that an early cancer grows so slowly that a period of two months between examinations is quite adequate. If anyone feels impelled to do so more frequently after having read these lines, she should reason with herself as to whether she is suffering from cancerophobia.

CANCER OF THE BOWEL

With cancer of the bowel the same problem exists as has already been described in this chapter with cancer of the stomach. Many other harmless illnesses can cause the same symptoms as cancer in the early stages. Nevertheless the general rule applies again: if a person whose bowels are normally regular in their functioning notices gradual changes, which are not temporary, but always recur and perhaps even get worse, he should definitely go to the doctor. This applies not only to the elderly, but also to the young. Cancer is very unusual in young people, but other illnesses are also worth treatment! The older person must always bear in mind the fact that with such intestinal symptoms he is defending his life by going to the doctor.

An especially dangerous sign is the presence of blood in the feces, unless the person is known to be suffering from piles. Incidentally, piles can be treated and should certainly be dealt with as they can seriously interfere with our enjoyment of life. Persistent constipation, arising in a person of previously regular habits, is another sign which should make him go to a doctor. The opposite—loose stools or diarrhea which go on for a long time should not be passed off lightly without consulting a doctor. Alternating constipation and diarrhea must be regarded as especially suspicious.

Persistent abdominal pains, especially when cramp-like in nature, should, of course, never be ignored. Should they be accompanied by weakness, loss of weight, loss of appetite, nausea and vomiting, one would presumably consult a doctor immediately without special advice. It should be mentioned that the chances of cure with cancer of the bowel are better than with other forms of cancer, because complete operative removal is often possible.

CANCER OF THE ESOPHAGUS

Malignant growths of the esophagus, which are commoner in men than women, can first be recognized by difficulty with swallowing. Pain on swallowing which occurs deep in the chest should definitely make older people go to the doctor. Similarly, a repeated sense of pressure behind the breast bone when swallowing large and hard mouthfuls must be regarded as suspicious. Another symptom not to be ignored is the occasional regurgitation of a mouthful of food. Of course these symptoms may be due to other causes, but only a doctor can differentiate between this and other illnesses, and he should carry out a medical examination at the earliest possible opportunity.

CANCER OF THE LUNG

The early symptoms of cancer of the lung may resemble the symptoms of other, less harmful diseases, just as we saw with malignant growths elsewhere. But with cancer of the lung this may be particularly difficult as the disease may be preceded by chronic bronchitis over a period of years, in which case the first symptoms of cancer are obscured by cough and shortness of breath due to the bronchitis. It is, of course, difficult for the doctor in charge of the case to observe this new turn. But one should never ignore a persistent cough when there are no obvious signs of infection or fever-ishness accompanying it. If, in addition, there are traces of blood in the sputum, it is criminal folly not to go to the doctor. If you have a cough which persists for more than four weeks, you must seek medical advice.

LATE SYMPTOMS

The following symptoms apply to cancer in an advanced stage: wasting away with a yellow, lackluster appearance, loss of weight, fatigue, subdued mood, extreme loss of appetite, lack of interest in life. Such symptoms would obviously make a person go to a doctor, but they are no longer the early symptoms, which offer the best chance of cure. Things should never be allowed to get to this stage. But even these late features may be due to diseases other than cancer and only expert medical opinion can determine their cause.

Cancer is not incurable if diagnosed in time, but the only reliable treatments require complete removal or destruction of the malignant growth through surgery, radiation, or chemotherapy. Whoever shrinks from these accepted treatments for cancer is signing his own death-warrant.

9.   Hormones and Endocrine Disorders

The discovery of hormones was a revolutionary event in the history of medical science. Now for the first time it was possible to intervene directly in the body's functioning. Illnesses were discovered which had been caused by faulty functioning of the hormone-producing gland. On page 89 the table shows us what happens when there is too much or too little of certain hormones.

HORMONES AND OBESITY

People often speak of glandular disorders when some form of obesity is meant—the strange story that one gets fat in spite of not eating excessively. It is a fact that there are people who put on flesh despite appearing to eat no more than their thin friends. Even though they may not eat to obvious excess, they do in fact eat more than is necessary to meet the body's demands for energy. That is very little, as one can see in the section on "What should fat people eat?". It is beyond question that overeating plays a decisive part in the disorder of obesity. But there may also be a fault in the secretion of growth hormone by the pituitary, so that it is, as it were, concentrated on the building up of fat. All food consumed in excess of absolute energy requirements is laid down in fat instead of just being burned up, as with most people. The "thermostat," so to speak, is set at too low a level. Young women are sometimes affected by this after the birth of their first child. Overeating during pregnancy lays the foundation-stone for obesity (for pregnancy diet see page 311). Beyond a shadow of doubt the first link in the chain of causes of obesity (disorder of the pituitary) is to be found in the mind. Gluttony and a love of sweets originate in the mind and in the last resort in one's childhood experiences and upbringing.

PREGNANCY

Pregnancy brings about a fundamental hormonal change. For many women, there is a feeling that their physical and mental powers are at their highest level during pregnancy. And in pregnancy, they have achieved an important goal.

But with the complexities of life today, this salutary effect of pregnancy can be turned into a harmful one. The vitality of young womanhood may not return after pregnancy. The sex glands may not function as expected and she may lose some of the sparkling, seductive vitality which was an important ingredient in the early days of her marriage. However, the problem may be related to attitude as much as to hormones.

The upbringing of many young girls with an emphasis on "getting married off" is fundamentally to blame for this sad state of affairs. When marriage has been the prime object, married love may cease with the first child. The young woman may become fat and indolent. There is a gradual loss of interest in sustaining a loving relationship. On the other hand, in a marriage where happiness is the ideal, a woman can have both children and a full and satisfied sex life. With proper diet and exercise, most mothers can retain the weight and figure they had before they became pregnant. This rule holds true through repeated pregnancies as can be observed in magazine and newspaper photographs and television appearances of actresses, professional women, and other notables who have been able to maintain their youthful glamour while also playing active roles as mothers of one or more children.

CHANGE OF LIFE (Menopause)

A second difficult time in the life of a woman is the menopause. Often this is wrongly thought to be the end of one's sexual life. Certainly the full flow of sexual hormones declines at this period. Certainly it means that one cannot have any more children. But it does not mean and must never mean no more love. That is the danger that destroys the sustaining tension in the mind, nerves and hormones. It is then that one becomes fat, to a large extent because one lets oneself go over food and tries to substitute sweets for love. Most longings, regrets and sorrow for something that one is missing can easily turn into hunger, with a craving for little tidbits, such as our mothers used to give us as an expression of their love. These are deep and simple reflexes which dominate our emotional life. Our hormones obey them implicitly.

DIFFERENT FORMS OF OBESITY

Only in rare cases can pituitary hormones be used in treatment of obesity. The treatment of obesity remains first and foremost a question of diet, particulars of which are to be found in the section on "What should fat people eat?" on page 117. There are, however, forms of obesity which occur when other ductless glands no longer function. If, for example, a woman is sterilized by X-rays or by an operation for the removal of her ovaries, fat accumulates, especially in the upper part of the thighs, in the skin of the abdomen and in her breasts. Male eunuchs—men who, as a result of injury or illness, lose their testicles—also become fat.

When there is overfunctioning of the pituitary gland stimulating the adrenal cortex, or when there is overfunctioning of the adrenal cortex itself, obesity also results. This is known as Cushing's syndrome, and there are fat deposits, especially on the face, throat and neck. The limbs remain slim.

When there is underproduction of thyroid hormone the body increases in size, especially the face. This, however, is not fat, but a mucoid swelling of the tissues under the skin.

This is known as myxedema and can easily be treated with thyroid gland hormone.

Increased production of insulin by the pancreas (the rarely occurring opposite of diabetes) may also result in obesity. Unless there are clear indications of endocrine disease, treatment must be based first and foremost on diet, and, in order to carry this out strictly, the patient must be convinced of the connection between overeating and obesity.

The opposite of obesity is rarer. There is a severe form of emaciation which occurs with another disorder of the pituitary. People suffering from this can eat enormous quantities without putting on an ounce of fat. In its severest form (Simmonds' disease) death can result. Also, with excess production of thyroid hormone, people get thin in spite of the fact that they eat a lot.

Naturally chronic disorders of the appetite (gastritis in heavy drinkers, for example) can make one thin. There are also disorders of appetite which are purely mental in origin and which are probably the most common cause of thinness.

But the influence of hormones on the body is not confined to determining its size and shape. The size of the body is determined during the normal period of growth by the growth hormone of the pituitary. If this growth hormone suddenly runs wild at a later age because of a pituitary tumor a disease called acromegaly (*akros* = extreme; *megas* = great) results. Then the hands, feet, nose, chin, ears and tongue grow larger.

DIABETES MELLITUS

For some reason which has yet to be explained, insulin production by the islet cells of the pancreas is insufficient in some people. The result is diabetes.

A complete or relative lack of insulin in the blood prevents the storage of glucose in the cells of the liver; the blood and tissues are flooded with glucose. This is harmful, as more fuel is given to the cells than they can use. The presence of the correct amount of insulin promotes the burning of sugar by the cells. Thus, despite the excessive supply of glucose, the cells suffer from a deficiency because they cannot make proper use of it. As a result fat becomes the body's main fuel, and, from this, acid remains are left which are poisonous in excess. The excess of glucose is passed out through the kidney and is lost. The extra glucose passed via the kidney requires an increased amount of water for its excretion. This loss of water in the urine makes one constantly thirsty.

For this reason a constant feeling of thirst and an increased output of urine are often the first symptoms which make one pay a visit to the doctor. Another symptom of the disease is loss of weight.

Insulin Treatment

It is easy for the doctor to diagnose diabetes. There are simple chemical methods of testing for the presence of glucose in urine. However, the treatment calls for great skill, for the deficiency of insulin varies in individual cases. This will naturally depend upon the amount of food taken each day. The patient is therefore put on a fixed diet and the amount of insulin gradually increased. The insulin is prepared from the pancreatic glands of animals. To determine the correct amount, sugar passed out in the urine must be measured every day. Where necessary the blood-sugar is measured as well, which calls for an efficient chemical laboratory.

The diabetic patient's metabolism is put right by careful adjustment of the quantity of insulin given. Insulin has to be injected as it is destroyed by the digestive juices of the stomach if taken by mouth. The patient must learn to inject himself under the skin of his upper thigh with specified quantities of insulin each day. He must also learn to work out correctly the carbohydrate content of his food, for if he alters his intake of carbohydrate, it upsets his doctor's adjustment of insulin. If he eats too much carbohydrate his blood will be flooded with sugar, and if eats too little the injected insulin will reduce the sugar in the blood to such an extent that the brain no longer functions properly and a condition of confusion and unconsciousness results. He must know that, at the first symptom of insulin overdosage like this, he must immediately eat a lump or a spoonful of sugar (preferably glucose).

The diabetic patient should also know that his body needs more insulin than usual when he has a temperature. Therefore, if he gets any form of fever his doctor may prescribe more insulin (10–20 per cent more than the normal daily amount), but of course he must not reduce the amount of carbohydrate in his food. If the appetite is affected, he can substitute four level teaspoonfuls of sugar in a drink for every slice of bread of his prescribed diet.

New "diabetes pills" which can be swallowed like an ordinary tablet can replace the need for insulin injections in some very mild cases of diabetes, or reduce the size of the insulin dose, but very careful medical supervision is, of course, required.

The correct treatment of diabetes depends greatly on the cooperation of the patient himself. The better he learns to make use of the diet charts given him by his doctor, and the better he learns to understand his body's insulin requirements, the greater his freedom with regard to his diet and the better his body cells can be protected from too much sugar, or from the opposite—insulin coma. Unfortunately many patients, who at times display high intelligence, are never able to master completely this art of self-treatment. Such people are for the most part undisciplined eaters. They easily make the mistake of indulging a sudden craving. If they give way to their inclinations, they eat at very irregular hours. The disobedience of some diabetic patients can go so far that quite incomprehensible and well-nigh suicidal neglect of diet regulations occurs. In such cases psychiatry may reveal the patient's wish to revert to a hospital atmosphere, where a bevy of doctors and nurses administer solicitously to his needs.

Actually the daily requirement of insulin is influenced by emotional disturbances, mental conflicts and excitement. Conditions of excitement, because of the increased adrenaline output (see page 84), demand more insulin. But also deep-seated mental conflicts, especially those which are connected with fear about the anxieties and burdens of life itself, make the diabetes worse and increase the demand for insulin.

DISORDERS OF THE THYROID GLAND

In ancient Rome it was customary after marriage to feel the young woman's neck soon after the wedding night, in order to see whether the thyroid gland was swollen. It was believed that from this one could tell whether the marriage had been happily consummated. Thus the thyroid gland has long been associated with physical exertions involving excitement. One might almost define the thyroid gland hormone as the hormone of mental and physical "sustained effort." Just as the sympathetic nervous system and the secretion of the adrenals increase the efficiency of the cells in times of acute excitement, fright or rage, so the hormone of the thyroid does for similar, but more sustained emotional conditions. The quantity in which the hormone is produced is dependent upon a pituitary hormone, which stimulates the thyroid gland. This is also influenced by mental processes.

There is an illness resulting from overproduction of thyroid hormone which in Germany is called Basedow's disease. It is known as Graves' disease in England and America, and under other names in other countries, according to their patriotic feelings! It is best to call it thyrotoxicosis (toxic = poisonous). There is excessive thyroid secretion out of all proportion to the normal demands of the body. As a result there is greatly increased consumption of glucose by the cells and the patient loses weight in spite of a good appetite. The sufferers also become nervous and highly emotional and in mild cases it is difficult to tell the disease from purely psychological disorders.

The causes for overproduction of thyroid hormone are but rarely found in the thyroid tissue itself. This, as a rule, simply responds to stimulation by the thyroid stimulating hormone (T.S.H.) released from the anterior pituitary. The thyroid stimulating activity of the pituitary gland is highly interdependent on mental and emotional processes as well as on changes in the hormonal secretion levels of the sex glands. The pituitary gland in this way makes the thyroid a highly adaptable organ. It thus reacts in normal functioning bodies as a means of adapting to sustained emotional and physical effort. The causes for detrimental over-stimulation of the thyroid therefore have to be found among a variety of mental, emotional and physical factors. It is especially noteworthy that times of hormonal changes in the body, i.e. pregnancy, puberty and menopause, account for slightly but measurably raised thyroid activity. It seems quite possible that, in these circumstances, the iodine supplied with the normal diet can become insufficient. This happens because, with increased thyroid activity, the iodine-containing thyroid hormone is produced and broken down at a faster rate. During metabolism of the iodine from the broken-down hormone naturally greater quantities are lost in the urine. It is, therefore, of considerable importance, especially during pregnancy, to increase the intake of foodstuffs rich in iodine (seafish). Otherwise any shortage in iodine is likely to cause enlargement of the thyroid, as so often happens in the development of simple goiters during and after pregnancy, at puberty, and during the change of life in women. Simple goiter is definitely a different disease from thyrotoxicosis. Its development is largely dependent on iodine shortage in the diet. As a rule these simple goiters are much larger than the thyroid swellings accompanying genuine thyrotoxicosis.

In advanced cases the disorder is easily recognizable. The internal "fire" is manifested by the feverish, moist skin, by the wide-open, protruding eyes, the racing pulse, the jumpiness and nervousness, and a tendency to dissolve into tears at the slightest thing, and by the trembling hands. The thyroid gland is usually somewhat swollen and soft. (Thyroid swellings are called goiters.) The disease sometimes starts suddenly as the result of a shock.

There are several methods of treatment, including surgery, drugs and radioiodine therapy. Surgical removal of much of the thyroid gland usually returns the patient to normal health.

Among the various chemical substances that can be used to prevent hormone formation in the thyroid gland are derivatives of thiouracil and methimazole. Adrenergic blocking agents also may be used to suppress symptoms. But doctors frequently resort to surgery when drug therapy is unsatisfactory.

In doubtful cases the diagnosis of thyrotoxicosis may be made by measuring the patient's basal metabolic rate. This is done by recording the quantity of oxygen consumed during quiet breathing in the fasting state while lying down. Clearly, if there be increased cell metabolism, the oxygen requirements will be greater than those of a normal person. The extra amount is recorded as a percentage: thus a thyrotoxic patient's basal metabolic rate may be expressed as, for example, "+ 40 per cent."

In recent years very advanced techniques for studying thyroid function have been developed by means of the application of radioactive iodine. By administering a "tracer" dose the rate of absorption of iodine in the thyroid (thyroid uptake), and especially the rate of turnover of inorganic iodine into thyroid hormone by the thyroid, can be studied by measuring the radioactive iodine collected by the thyroid and emitted from that circulating in the blood-stream. These methods of assessment of thyroid function have greatly advanced our knowledge during the last decades and allow much more accurate diagnosis of the variable forms of thyroid disturbances.

Radioiodine can be used not only to determine the degree and type of thyroid disturbance, but also, in appropriate large doses, it can effectively be used for partial destruction of over-functioning thyroid tissue. The intensified radiation in these cases destroys the thyroid tissue slowly in the course of some weeks, resulting in the same state of affairs as an operation.

There are cases where the thyroid does not secrete enough hormone. When there is a deficiency of iodine in food and drinking water, as is the case in the so-called "goiter districts," the thyroid gland lacks the basic substances necessary for the production of its hormone. It cannot fulfill the tasks required of it by the pituitary, and in its vain efforts to do so, it swells up considerably, and the result is a goiter. It is not an over-functioning of the thyroid gland, but is, on the contrary, a symptom of insufficient hormone production. The person becomes indolent, his eyes become sunken, and his skin turns dry and puffy. The basal metabolism is lowered. These symptoms are known as myxedema and can easily be cured by taking thyroid extract regularly.

If myxedema occurs in childhood or when there is a congenital disorder of the thyroid gland, this indolence, which is part of the hormonal disorder, becomes such that idiocy results. It is like a miracle to watch for the first time the rapid rise in intelligence of these idiot children when they are given thyroid gland treatment. The cause of these defects of intelligence due to failure of the thyroid gland can easily be recognized. With all other forms of idiocy, thyroid extract is useless and, in too large quantities, always detrimental to one's health. Thyroid gland hormone preparations, indeed all hormones, are drugs which may only be taken if prescribed by the doctor. They have strong effects, which can be a boon only if used at the right time and with exact knowledge and understanding of the illness.

DISORDERS OF THE SEX HORMONES

Two important changes in a woman's life are puberty and menopause ("change of life"). Both are based on changes in the production of sex hormones. These crises are dependent on the conditions prevailing at the time. Neither puberty nor menopause constitutes an emotional or mental "thunderstorm" with naïve, sensuous races. They regard them as imperceptible changes, which are met with knowledge and understanding. It can be the same with us, too. But the fact is that most of our thirteen-year-olds are suddenly confronted with strange internal forces which they cannot understand. Some young people are not mentally prepared for the sudden increase in sex hormones. Unless enlightened, they do not understand what is happening to them. From within suddenly come new and imperious urges, the existence of which may have been denied and concealed by their parents and teachers for twelve years or so. This did not arise while the amount of sex hormones in the blood was small, but with their sudden violent increase, combined with the beginning of sexual maturity, the whole inner emotional balance is upset.

The adolescent begins to be greatly attracted to the other sex—with a longing for union, having children, and an inner struggle between continence and a desire for sexual experience.

MENSTRUATION

Women are subjected to fluctuating emotional cycles by their sex hormones. In the first half of the average 28-day menstrual cycle, estrogen hormones dominate the female reproductive physiology as the lining of the womb, the endometrium, is prepared to receive a fertilized ovum. During the second half, progesterone hormones which are essential to finally condition the endometrium and maintain a pregnancy, if it should occur, are secreted in greater abundance. Because these hormones also affect other bodily functions in the woman, the phases of the menstrual cycle frequently are marked by apparent changes in personality.

For many years the emotional changes in women during the different phases of the menstrual cycle were thought to be merely psychological or "psychosomatic" in nature. Doctors who have studied emotional fluctuations in women have reported that 80 percent of the crimes of violence committed by women occur during the progesterone phase of the cycle. After the start of menstruation, many women are at the opposite extreme of activity and complain of feeling not up to par.

It would be simple enough to attribute to such variations in temperament psychological reasons. But doctors have found more likely physiological changes that can account for the personality changes that seem to appear in some women during different phases of the menstrual cycle. A woman might seem indolent during her menstrual period because of a loss of hemoglobin during the bleeding phase; the effect would be like the symptoms of iron-deficiency anemia. But during the progesterone phase, the hormone would act upon the kidneys to alter the balance of chemicals normally retained or excreted by the body. One result of this effect is that water would become accumulated in the tissues of the body, including the tissues of the brain and nervous system, producing headaches, irritability, and a general condition sometimes referred to as premenstrual tension. In addition, there might be more obvious physical symptoms of water-logged tissues such as a swelling of the ankles.

Coincidentally, the symptoms of premenstrual tension tend to vanish within a day or so before the beginning of a menstrual period. And many women who suffer from the symptoms of premenstrual stress find relief by taking a mild analgesic like aspirin for headaches. Other drugs might be prescribed as needed by the doctor, including sedatives or tranquilizers, as well as diuretics which can reduce fluid accumulation in the body tissues. By consulting a doctor, therefore, a modern woman subjected to extreme emotional fluctuations during her menstrual cycles can obtain some control over the physiological causes of manifestations that formerly were thought to be merely psychological in nature.

Any woman who experiences unusual symptoms during a menstrual cycle should, of course, consult her doctor. The new or unusual symptoms suggesting a visit to the doctor might be a heavy menstrual flow if the woman ordinarily has a small flow, or if she experiences a small flow when usually she has a heavy flow. Or if the pattern of cramps or other types of discomfort suddenly changes for no apparent reason. For example, the cramps may be accompanied by a backache. Such changes in menstrual effects can indicate an abnormal condition that requires medical treatment.

Any unusual variation in the length of the menstrual cycle also may indicate a possible abnormal condition. An unusual variation would be a cycle that changes rather abruptly from 28 days to 23 days or 33 days. Although we usually state that the average menstrual cycle lasts 28 days from the first day of menstruation until the first day of the next menstruation, about one-third of all adult women have a normal menstrual cycle that is several days shorter or longer than the average. And it is considered quite normal for an adolescent girl to have a cycle of 33 or 34 days while an older woman may have a cycle that is shorter than average. But the changes from longer to shorter cycles should be gradual, over a period of some years. And it is the rather sudden change in length of menstrual cycle that would warrant a visit to the doctor.

And although alterations in normal menstrual activity can be traced frequently to organic causes, psychological stresses also can influence menstrual variations. It has been shown that the pituitary gland, which controls the secretion of sex hormones, receives signals from the hypothalamus portion of the brain.

HYPERSEXUALITY

One's capacity for love in the physical sense is not entirely connected with the amount of formed sex hormones. What is sometimes known as hypersexuality (over-sexed) frequently is due to mental inhibitions in connection with one's ability to gratify one's desire. As a result, many individuals who seek gratification of sexual urges in abnormal ways appear "insatiable." Such behavior as sadism or masochism (a combination of sexual desire with inflicting or receiving pain) seldom is connected with the amount or quality of sex hormones in an individual. Although some people believe the amount or quality of sex hormones determine homosexual behavior, homosexuality actually is a matter of mental attitudes; both men and women have male and female sex hormones, even though they are distributed differently, and some sex hormones are formed in the adrenal glands.

As we have said, abnormal sex behavior may bear the stamp of "insatiability" since it does not afford gratification of one's own natural urges. The mental development of these people during childhood is such that normal gratification of the sex instinct is no longer possible. The act of sex leaves them unsatisfied and they constantly strive after new ways of complete gratification, but never succeed in this.

FRIGIDITY AND PROMISCUITY

Frigidity in women also may represent a form of abnormal behavior when the normal sex function has been diverted so far from its normal goal that it surfaces in other mental forms. An example from classical literature is the quarrelsome, scolding woman Xanthippe as described by the Greek philosopher Socrates. Another mental form of escape for a

or mental. Menopausal disorders are an illness and are not something "normal," to be accepted as part of getting old. Nevertheless, this idea is widespread and the sense of change cannot always be overcome unaided. Some must be helped by sex hormones while others may enjoy some degree of sex life into their seventies or eighties without such help.

THE WOMAN BETWEEN FORTY AND FIFTY

With women menopausal symptoms are well known: between forty and fifty, inexplicable hot flushes occur with a temporary reddening of the face; irritability, sudden outbreaks of perspiration, palpitations, stomach and bladder disorders. The monthly periods may still occur when these symptoms manifest themselves, but they are usually irregular. Any rise in blood-pressure is usually temporary, but many cases of high blood-pressure are not discovered until this time as the patients had slight symptoms only and did not go to the doctor about them. Some women with no children have been known to suffer more at the menopause than those with many children. There is a tendency to depression and despondency, which, in rare cases, may lead to insanity. Insomnia is common, and also a growing inner restlessness.

By the use of sex hormones the unpleasant symptoms accompanying the change of life can be greatly alleviated, if not completely cured. But actually one is only postponing the mental-physical problem. By the artificial administration of sex hormones one restores the sex condition of youth. The monthly periods start again, even though there is no longer any ability to conceive. This is in no way "unnatural" or harmful, but is simply a repetition of an organic change in the mucous membrane of the womb, which took place every four weeks as a result of the influence of precisely the same substance produced naturally by the body. The female sex hormone used for this is estrogen, which can be prescribed by the doctor under various trade names. These are artificially produced chemical substances, which have exactly the same effect. There are, however, mental disorders associated with the change of life which cannot be treated with hormone preparations. They are independent of the physical adjustments of the menopause and are precipitated by the increasing awareness that "the gate has closed behind them."

The Change of Life In men

This is far less noticeable than with women, whose new stage of life is marked by the cessation of their monthly periods. With men, on the other hand, there is a general decline in powers, which is seldom accompanied by such nervous symptoms as excitement and hot flushes as experienced by women. In this condition men feel a decline in their mental powers and efficiency and their optimism changes to an attitude of pessimism—in serious cases a deep and dangerous melancholia results. Nobody can say how widespread these symptoms are and to what extent the whole vitality and efficiency of a race is affected, especially in those countries where the population consists mostly of old and aging people.

Thus occasionally the symptoms are serious enough to permit a comparison with the female climacteric—the basis of which is, as we know, the lack of female sex hormones. And here, too, we find that we are dealing with an illness due to hormone deficiency. By giving treatment with testosterone —the male sex hormone—we can succeed with a few injections in even rescuing people from the mental hospital and restoring them to their families.

Testosterone is not a universal rejuvenator of men, as some promoters of the hormone like to boast. It does not help to rid us of bald pates, wrinkles, and paunches. In fact, its use has been associated with an increased risk of prostatic cancer. But it helps some regain mental vitality. And a great deal depends on this vitality—even life and death. Proof of this was given by a large number of sick old men, who had had slight accidents, and did not show the slightest inclination to get up again, wasting away miserably. In the experience of their doctors, they were simply waiting for death. Some of them were given testosterone and others were not treated in this way. Most of those given the medicine recovered, but the others did not.

Enlargement of the Prostate

This is a common symptom in aging men. The prostate surrounds the urinary tract below the bladder. When it is enlarged, urinating becomes difficult. The urine does not come out in a full stream, but drips slowly and, in serious cases, only when the bladder is over-full and is under great pressure, and even then often after a wait of some minutes. In many cases an operation is necessary. Aging men should not regard this as a normal disorder of old age: it is an illness, which definitely requires treatment. The longer one lets it drag on, the higher the risks of the operation. If the retention of urine persists for some time owing to an enlarged prostate gland, there is always the danger of inflammation, which may spread to the kidneys.

10.   Nervous-Functional Disorders

PSYCHOSOMATIC MEDICINE

It is scarcely possible to understand an illness properly without knowing its nervous and mental implications. Every organ of the body and the interplay between the various organs are dependent on the brain, without which they could not function properly. For this reason mental changes can usually be detected in all internal illnesses. Because this natural connection between the mental and physical process in internal illnesses was previously neglected by medical science, modern medical research is devoting itself more and more to this branch of medicine. Psychosomatic medicine is practiced in all countries of the earth. Psychosomatic illnesses, such as disorders of the thyroid gland, some heart ailments, stomach ulcers, asthma, etc., are, in the last resort, mental disorders, in which, unlike hysteria, psychoneuroses (illnesses caused by mental inhibitions) and the more serious mental illnesses, physical suffering takes the place of mental suffering. Usually a mental-nervous disorder starts off the illness, which later, through resulting damage to cells and organs, takes on a physical character. For example, in asthma the recurrent mental-nervous constriction of the small bronchioles, the breathlessness and the choking cough can cause the little vesicles of the lungs to burst. In the course of years this results in an incurable disease of the lung called emphysema.

In cases of psychosomatic illness the mental affliction is hidden and deceives both doctor and patient with regard to the true nature of the illness. This is partly because there is less stigma attached to illnesses of this kind than to those of the mind, which have been surrounded with an aura of disgrace ever since primitive days, when superstition was rife. This moral condemnation of a certain class of diseases of the mind, where the bodily functions remain quite unimpaired, is so deep-rooted that psychosomatic treatment is extraordinarily difficult. If an asthma patient is advised to go to a nerve specialist or psychotherapist, he usually feels offended. He considers this equivalent to telling him he is insane, and for him that is much worse than to be told that he is suffering from a severe disease. With mental patients, however, the disturbance is only to be found in the place of its origin—in the mind. With psychosomatic patients it is the organs which have "gone mad." The mental illness has spread to the body.

And so we nowadays regard certain illnesses as diseases of the mind which are concealed behind physical disorders and pain.

AFFLICTIONS OF THE MIND

Among these are those special cases which manifest themselves only or predominantly in mental disorders. It is not physical defects, but the patient's mental condition, which renders him unfit for normal life. With serious forms of mental illness one can be just as incapacitated as someone suffering from articular rheumatism with completely stiff joints. The patient who, although healthy in body, is incarcerated in an asylum is just as much cut off from life as the one who is doomed to the sick-bed with rigid limbs. In milder forms work and a normal life are possible up to a point.

The greater part of all mental disorders is not due to hereditary causes, as research during the past years has shown more and more clearly. Most of these illnesses originate during the long and difficult years of growth and mental adjustment to life and the conditions around one. They represent a failure in this task of adjustment, the purpose of which is to achieve the best possible balance between the inner world and outer world. The body's requirements and its private urges and impulses must be brought into harmony with the outside world and its opportunities. This is not innate, but has to be learned step by step by every child, just in the same way that it has to learn to walk, speak, etc. Diseases of the mind are more likely to result from environment than from heredity.

IDIOCY, FEEBLE-MINDEDNESS AND STUPIDITY

One might say, "The Gods themselves struggle in vain against Stupidity," without thinking that stupidity, too, is an illness due to defects or disorders in intelligence. There are medical terms for the different degrees of defects of intelligence and almost all of these are known to laymen as terms of abuse. The severest form of low intelligence is idiocy. A less severe form is imbecility, sufferers from which are just about able to mix with other people and can perform some kinds of repetitive work. Those classed as morons form the transition between imbeciles and people of normal intelligence. More recently, the term mental retardation has been accepted to describe the three or four percent of our population who, "because of arrested or imperfect development of intelligence, are incapable of competing on equal terms with normal individuals or of managing personal affairs with ordinary prudence."

Such intelligence defects as these may be due to a number of prenatal causes; they may be congenital (see the section on "Congenital Diseases caused by Damage in the Womb," page 187). Then they are the result of a damaged brain tissue, which does not function in a completely normal way. The simplest way for the layman to recognize them is to visualize an impaired intelligence. These patients have difficulty in learning and cling tenaciously to the little knowledge they have so laboriously acquired. They fall for the most stupid practical joke six times in one day. However, if they are teased too much in this way, they tend to become fundamentally suspicious and at times refuse to be helped to overcome the difficulties which learning and life present for them.

There are other symptoms of mental illness, which to all outward appearances are the same as those due to intelligence defects. Almost everyone has experienced the awful reaction of fear in an examination, when one sits there idiotically—one's mind a complete blank. An overwhelming mental inhibition can temporarily paralyze an otherwise normal person's intelligence. This mental vacuum during emergencies may exist as a permanent condition, as a subgroup of psychoneurotic illnesses. It is often very difficult for a doctor to distinguish between this seeming feeble-mindedness and genuine feeble-mindedness. However, close observation of the patient usually reveals a glimmer of intelligence. Those who are feeble-minded as a result of inhibition can in some ways show remarkable precision of thought and action. They are "cunning," as, for example, in pilfering snacks from the refrigerator and covering up their tracks. In such cases they are even able to use their mental defectiveness as a camouflage, and for that reason they are often beaten as children, which only makes the illness fundamentally worse. Beating makes no one more intelligent, but rather more deceitful. One learns to camouflage oneself better.

Mentally Defective Children

For this reason it is of paramount importance for parents who believe they have a mentally defective child, first to consult an experienced specialist before resigning themselves to the fact. It is not so necessary for them *to tell the doctor about the symptoms of mental defectiveness which they have observed, but rather to report all indications of a partially preserved intelligence.* In this way they can considerably simplify the doctor's work and receive quicker and better help themselves. They must observe the child and inform the doctor when it has grasped something particularly quickly. Such children usually behave badly and do things one does not like to tell others about, i.e. stealing, telling lies, and making excuses, deliberate deception about going to sleep, etc. If possible, treatment should be started before the child goes to school. The sooner apparent feeble-mindedness, which can gradually get worse, is recognized, the greater the chances of cure. It is a psychotherapist's job, since kindergarten teachers and schoolteachers are insufficiently trained to be able to deal adequately with such cases.

HYSTERIA

Of all mental illnesses hysteria is the most easily cured. Psychotherapy gained its first fundamental experiences with it fifty years ago. Real hysteria is always connected with movement and perception. It is an illness on the frontier between the mental inner world and the outer world and can occur in an extraordinary number of different guises. There is an hysterical blindness, in which the patient cannot see, even though the eyes are normal, the retina is healthy and the optic nerves are sound. There are hysterical forms of paralysis, when one cannot move a certain limb, even though the nerve routes and muscles are intact. It is this mental process of "switching off" which is the fundamental characteristic of hysteria. It is the illness of repression, the illness of "one cannot be what one is not allowed to be." The patients keep unpleasant thoughts (above all, inadmissible urges) within themselves below consciousness. They "repress" experiences, and especially sexual desires and feelings, which they cannot themselves accept. Of course they only succeed in this up to a point. Their repression has to have an outlet, and with hysteria it usually takes the form of inappropriate movement or expressions of emotion. The patients laugh unrestrainedly on certain occasions, when others would be more inclined to weep. They get inexplicable spasms of weeping. In short, they behave in a conspicuously "hysterical" manner. All other people react to their behavior with an instinctive irritability, and it is this feeling of irritability which gives the layman the best clue that it is hysteria. One feels like throwing a bucket of cold water over the offender's head, or kicking him, or punishing him in some way. But of course all that sort of thing is not only not going to cure the patient, but will in fact make him worse. The "normal" person, however, feels only a desire for revenge and is not so much concerned with curative measures.

Hysteria is frequently associated with repressed sexuality. For that reason it was most widespread among women at the turn of the century. In the meantime conditions and circumstances have changed and society acknowledges, almost without reservation, the right of every adult of either sex to sexual satisfaction in married life. Even extramarital relations, which were formerly frowned upon and regarded as something quite beyond the pale, are now generally condoned.

The only successful method of treatment for hysteria is psychotherapy.

In order to prevent hysteria parents should adopt a sensible attitude in all matters relating to sex. It is unforgivable to threaten children with severe punishment for being "curious about sex," as though sex did not exist. It is always parents or those responsible for the children's upbringing who lay the foundation for sexual repression in the three-, four- or five-year-old child. The patient himself cannot be blamed for his illness. He is quite innocent. He has learned to behave like that. He is trying to live according to the principle of "one cannot be what one is not allowed to be."

PSYCHONEUROSES

It is not entirely easy to classify properly the various forms of mental illness. They are not caused by bacteria, which can be grown in test-tubes and identified. Even illnesses caused by living germs are not always easily differentiated on the strength of external symptoms. For example, there are a number of different kinds of inflammation of the lung, each of which demands a different method of treatment. This depends entirely on the bacteria responsible. In the same way it is impossible to classify mental illnesses on the strength of their external symptoms. With a disorder like hysteria, not only repression and distorted emotional outbursts are involved. Hysteria has come to be counted as belonging to a subgroup of psychoneuroses. (The name [*psyche* = soul, *neuron* = nerve, and so, nerve illness] is outmoded and is not entirely descriptive.) These are disorders which can virtually be cured by psychotherapeutic methods as we know them today. The patients are not so far withdrawn that they are impervious to the doctor's voice. They remain in contact with the real world and have avoided creating their own insane world, in which they could live in "happy" detachment, even though cut off from the actual pleasures of our world. Different symptoms are found in these people, characteristic of different forms of psychoneurosis.

OBSESSIONAL NEUROSIS

In speaking of neuroses, one means forms of psycho-neuroses other than typical hysteria. In one form certain obsessions manifest themselves which are prompted by an inner compulsion. The obsession may take the form of con-pulsive washing. Such people feel compelled to go out and wash their hands hundreds of times a day, without really knowing why. There are sometimes repetitive acts, as when a patient has to do the same thing over and over again, such as putting on and buttoning up his trousers. A counting obsession is also common, i.e. counting telegraph poles when passing them in a train, or steps when going up them, or letters when reading. Normal people sometimes make a practice of this counting mechanism when they cannot sleep; it prevents disquieting thoughts from penetrating consciousness. With obsessional neurotics the obsessional act serves the same purpose. The obsessional neurotic is hampered by self-imposed restrictions and exaggerated moral scruples and cannot overcome these compulsory restrictions himself. He cannot obey the command of his will to fight and defeat his "inhibitions."

Almost all cases of impotence are due to neurotic causes. It is these mental inhibitions—these "inner cage-bars"—which deny the patient his own pleasure. It is, so to speak, a morbid form of qualms of conscience, which directly affects the nervous mechanism. Neurosis is the illness of an over-trained conscience. Anything that meets with even the slightest inner disapproval becomes magnified to an all-pervading and crippling conscience-taboo. The smallest details of one's upbringing, even though long since forgotten and often of no consequence, become insuperable "conscience obsessions." The person is virtually unable to move without coming up against qualms of conscience. This morbid state of mind has of course nothing to do with a religious conscience, since it makes demands which appear utterly ridiculous to an adult and his moral code, and yet the patient is nevertheless unable to overcome this. These people often commit crimes for the mere purpose of being punished by the law, and the judge affords them a certain relief from their inexplicable inner guilt. They are criminals who become so because they feel the need for punishment.

One might say that the neurotic's upbringing has been too effective. They have too great and too rigid and inflexible a conscience. For example, in impotent people the warmth of sexual excitement becomes isolated from the actual experience. It is actually often too intense excitement which brings about a premature ejaculation. Nevertheless, this is a symptom of impotence, the switching off of an emotion due to an incomprehensible unconscious fear, similar to pangs of conscience.

Psychoneuroses cannot be successfully treated without the help of psychotherapy. Misleading names for the various forms of psychoneurosis are psychoasthenia (mental weakness); psychopathy (mental suffering); neurasthenia (nerve weakness). They convey to us nothing definite.

To prevent psychoneuroses a sensible upbringing from early childhood is necessary. There is hardly anything more dangerous than to train a child to be too obedient and docile. No adult is able to understand all a child's motives and nothing is more detrimental than to break a child's will as a matter of principle. A well-known cause of neurosis is an over-rigid training in cleanliness, by which we mean any training attempted before the child is nine months old. (Without any compulsion or supervision children instinctively become clean, although not until they are four years old, which is too late and therefore also detrimental. For details, see pages 351 ff.)

It is also dangerous to threaten children with severe punishment for "playing about with themselves" (i.e. their sex organs), for this can also lead to impotence and much unhappiness later in life. One must be particularly careful not to use such expressions as, "Then the doctor will have to come and cut it off"; "A wicked man will cut your nose (or finger) off." Remarks like these are always found to be the actual cause of a severe "castration complex." Formerly it was believed that this complex originated within the child itself as a necessary part of its development. But nowadays we know that it is due in every case to remarks or behavior of this sort on the part of adults. The "castration complex" is not innate and is not an inevitable symptom in a child's development. It is dependent on the environment in which the child grows up. Their inner obedience has rendered them unfit for life. That is one road which the neurotic can take.

The Neglected Child (Delinquency)

The other possibility is to cast all conscience to the winds and simply ignore its twinges. This is what happens to the neglected child, who has grown up in such a hard world that he cannot accept the demands of morality and reason without becoming bogged down in a morass of neurotic inhibitions. However, he is never completely successful in his attempt to "go to the dogs." For there remains a crude and, for the untrained layman, completely incomprehensible discrepancy between uninhibited stealing on the one hand, and an over-strict conscience on the other—for example, in money matters with one's friends. There invariably remain vestiges of an over-strict conscience.

The neurotic does not only repress past experiences and

emotional stimuli. His main weapon in the fight against his "inner cage-bars" is the switching off of emotions. Experiences and perceptions become divorced from their context.

PSYCHOSES (Mental illnesses)

Psychoneuroses merge into more serious mental illnesses. These serious mental illnesses are technically known as schizophrenia (split personality) and manic depressive psychosis (fluctuating between over-excitement and melancholia). Both illnesses are not actually hereditary, although a tendency to them in some families is quite understandable, when one considers the fact that the methods of upbringing and the attitude of the grown-ups towards the small child remain strangely unchanged throughout generations. It is family atmosphere that is conducive to the development of the illness. One is not compelled to regard it as an hereditary predisposition. This is actually unlikely for the reason that almost a hundred years of careful research has failed to find any changes in the patient's brain which might be expected with an inherited defect.

Schizophrenia

In schizophrenia the patient has not been able to make mental contact with reality, or he has withdrawn again from this contact with reality. He lives in an inner dream-world, which sometimes appears as a sharply defined illusion. Normal people can best visualize this illness by thinking of an inventor or professor who is completely obsessed with his own ideas and becomes more and more alienated from daily life until he lives entirely in his own inner world. He then no longer has the mental energy to carry out the simplest tasks in daily life. With this alienation from reality his thought also becomes confused and he is untouched by the experiences of reality. Reason no longer has any place in such a person's imagination. Finally this free and unbridled imagination becomes so powerful that it swamps even ordinary perceptions. The patient "sees," for example, a person walking about on the ceiling. This is called an hallucination. When it is something seen, it is a visual hallucination. If voices or noises are heard, which is more common, it is an auditory hallucination. All perceptions can take on a hallucinatory character.

Manic-depressive Psychosis

These patients have phases when they are "keyed up" beyond measure and are overflowing with life and vitality and an urge for activity. When it reaches such a pitch that thoughts and ideas follow one another in such rapid succession that they can no longer be expressed coherently, one talks of mania. A never-ceasing spate of words pours down on all who are within earshot and no thought is completely or fully expressed, let alone put into practice. Probably everybody knows such trying and garrulous talkers among normal people, and they can often be gay and entertaining at parties if their eloquence is allied with scintillating wit. In some professions it is necessary for a person to have this kind of disposition to a mild degree, but in cases of real illness there is no rhyme or reason in the patient's incessant volubility.

In the disease this manic phase is almost always followed by deep melancholia—depression, which persists for a long time. Every healthy person experiences such emotions at times of normal mourning, or when one has a guilty conscience and is full of self-reproach. In these patients, however, the guilt feelings in the depression-phase swamp all other mental impulses. There are morbid feelings of guilt which originate in the subconscious. Depressive psychosis is the peak of mental inhibition. The sick subconscious conscience drives the patient to suicide in a kind of self-punishment. This danger is greater here than in any other kind of mental illness.

Shock Treatment

If one considers these various examples of mental illness, one can see that even definite insanity can be characterized by an exaggeration of normal characteristics and idiosyncrasies. It is the same brain which each of us carries in his skull.

But the difficulties which treatment of such illnesses presents are quite a different matter. The withdrawal from the world, the abandonment and denial of reality, can be so extreme that the patient, incarcerated in his own imaginary world, is deaf to all calls from the world of real people. For this reason present-day psychotherapeutic methods of treatment are successful only in rare cases, although experimental treatment which has been carried out in many places for research reasons has shown encouraging results. We may be sure that in a few years' time this problem, too, will be solved. In the meantime, however, we must content ourselves with more primitive methods, i.e. drugs or shock treatment, which have the effect of a "trial death" on the patients. Just as a "normal" person often comes to a full appreciation of life and the world and all its beauty when he is faced with death, these "shocks" forcibly restore the patient's contact with reality. The illness does not actually disappear, but the patient learns to behave more unobtrusively. He has the feeling that his brain has been shaken up and a new layer of thoughts and emotions covers the still sick layer of his soul.

LEUCOTOMY

Another method of dealing with mental illness is to cut into the brain. By means of an operation it is possible to separate almost completely the frontmost part of the brain from the rest. The connections in the inside of the brain are simply cut through with a knife. The patients learn to build up a new, if somewhat limited personality out of the remaining part of the brain. They have less imagination and are therefore less likely to get mentally ill. Of course, an operation such as this is bound to impair one's efficiency and one can never afterwards be a full and complete personality.

THE MENTAL HOSPITAL

There is a second serious problem to be faced in treating cases of severe mental illness, and that is a danger to the community. For example, with schizophrenic patients, whose inner world cannot be approached from outside, unpredictable and unforeseeable impulses towards violence may suddenly overcome them. This has nothing to do with provocation beyond endurance by other people, for situations in which a person would have the greatest difficulty in controlling an impulse to strike another person down or to shoot him would in most cases leave the schizophrenic patient absolutely cold. It is not that he is less self-controlled than others, but that he is driven in an unpredictable way and by some strange compulsion to crimes of violence. For this reason it is unavoidable, in the interests of public safety, that such patients should be removed to a mental hospital.

The Legal Side

This often involves difficult legal situations, since our law is still predominantly concerned with punitive rather than preventive measures. Strictly speaking a person can only be removed to a mental hospital after having committed a punishable offense and not as a protective measure. On the other hand, civil law must safeguard the freedom of the individual against abuse. It is often so difficult for a doctor to determine whether a mental patient might possibly turn violent, that our legislation cannot rely on this without running the risk of abusing this freedom of the individual. However, in most cases the legal problem is solved in a different way.

A seriously deranged patient is generally not capable of leading a normal life or of supporting himself or his family. For this reason his relations are obliged to put him under protection, as he is otherwise liable to cause himself and them economic and material harm. This procedure necessitates an application to a court. On the strength of this application the patient's mental state is always checked by an expert summoned for the purpose and this generally entails a period of observation in a mental hospital. A medical certificate or the patient's voluntary consent is necessary before the patient can be sent to a mental hospital for observation.

However, if the patient suddenly turns violent, he can, of course, be removed by his relatives and the doctor in charge of the case—with the help of the police if necessary—to a mental hospital (as is the case with any other illness) without first going through legal proceedings. The necessary legal measures are carried out subsequently in such cases.

EPILEPSY

Epilepsy can occur as a result of a brain injury due to an accident or a war wound. It can be recognized by recurrent sudden attacks during which the patients twitch convulsively and fall unconscious to the ground. In severe attacks, the patients foam at the mouth and lose bowel and bladder control. Another way of recognizing the attacks is that patients bite their tongues. In some cases of epilepsy, an irritation may begin in a small area of diseased brain tissue and spread to the whole brain. However, in many epileptics the illness can not be traced to a specific brain injury. It develops in them for reasons which are not clearly understood, either in childhood or puberty.

Epileptics are highly irritable and may fly into a rage over trivialities. (Incidentally this is characteristic of almost all people with brain injuries.) In many cases the frequently recurring attacks have a harmful effect on the brain itself and in the course of the illness some patients get more and more dull and, in serious cases, become imbecile. Epilepsy often occurs with schizophrenia. Many patients have hallucinations and hear voices, etc. It is important that the family and friends of an epilepsy patient avoid an overly protective attitude toward him. Studies have shown that epileptics who are physically and mentally active, and otherwise well-adjusted have fewer seizures.

It is impossible to predict the outcome of epilepsy. Some become completely cured and no longer need treatment. The attacks may disappear for years and decades. Many epileptics lose none of their mental efficiency, despite attacks. These attacks themselves may disappear temporarily or permanently or be replaced by minor mental symptoms, i.e. a sudden fit of complete "absent-mindedness," which occurs with lightning swiftness and is only temporary, or an inexplicable and strange mood of depression, which is also of short duration. Annoyance may bring on or aggravate an attack.

Heavy drinking also aggravates the attacks and, in serious cases, causes damage to the brain, which brings on epilepsy. Cocaine always brings on attacks with epileptics.

Epilepsy tends to run in families. It may be congenital.

In treating epilepsy one tries to suppress the patient's excitement and with it the attacks by means of sedatives.

SUICIDE

Mental illnesses not only render one unfit for life, but often end in suicide. Neurotic depressive patients are especially liable to commit suicide during periods of deep depression. It is an expression of their deep melancholic mood and morbid guilt feelings. It is quite useless to try to reason with them and refute their morbid and senseless self-accusations with the logical proof of their impossibility. This does not usually afford the patient any relief; he becomes more entangled than ever as he feels himself to be unworthy of the confidence of the one who tries to comfort him. Whoever tries to counter the patient's guilt and sin mania with the natural arguments of the layman, increases the danger of suicide. The logic of reason is unacceptable to patients suffering from mania and any well-meant attempts to comfort them heightens their feelings of guilt.

In schizophrenia, also, there is a risk of suicide. As one might expect from the nature of the illness, the chain of thoughts and emotions leading up to this act of self-destruction cannot generally be appreciated by an observer. The patients can work out and execute the suicide plan in the most ingenious way. Unusual kinds of suicide are typical, especially those where the body is completely destroyed, i.e., jumping into a turbine, throwing oneself under a train, etc.

In a psychoneurosis, the illness of inhibition, the danger of suicide occurs only if the patient is in a depressed condition.

Accidents

The suicide attempts on the part of neurotics may appear to be accidents. In these accidents conflicting emotional impulses bring about a scarcely comprehensible carelessness, or a failure of one's presence of mind. Only a very small proportion of all accidents are completely unavoidable. Those involved are almost always unconsciously responsible for causing the accident.

For example, 5 per cent of all motorists cause 33 per cent of all car accidents. Thus this small group of accident-prone people are involved in ten times as many accidents as a comparable number of remaining drivers. Large business concerns have investigated this. A long-distance trucking business was able to reduce the number of accidents to one-fifth by transferring all drivers who had had more than two accidents to other jobs. Slippery roads or failure of the vehicle are less decisive than the failure of the driver. It is absurd to make a legal issue out of this human failure, unless of course there is proof of driving while under the influence of drink or with undue negligence.

These accidents may, in fact, be a concealed form of attempted suicide. However, they usually have a less serious character in that a mere broken bone is sufficient to satisfy the patient's subconscious desire for self-punishment. They are thus similar to the suicidal attempts of hysterical people, which are usually arranged in such a way that they are discovered and averted in time. Hysterical people who commit suicide, almost always only die because they are discovered too late, or because they are ignorant as to what constitutes a fatal dose of poison, etc. Such suicide attempts have an unconsciously demonstrative and dramatic character. Hysterical people do not attempt suicide because they themselves do not wish to go on living, but rather to show others that they cannot go on living. Naturally this attitude annoys people. But it is without doubt an illness and a morbid outlook and is the expression of arrested development on the part of a person whose emotions and attitude to life have remained unchanged since he was four or five years old.

Prevention of Suicide

It is of course the bounden duty of all relatives and onlookers to prevent all suicidal attempts on the part of mentally sick persons, even if they cannot bear these people on account of their morbid mental qualities. Any suicide attempt is a definite reason for taking the person concerned to a nerve specialist, preferably a psychiatrist, since it is almost always symptomatic of mental affliction, even though this may not appear so on the surface. A suicide attempt is as much the symptom of illness as a stroke or a dangerously high fever, and requires examination and treatment. The prospects of improvement and cure are no worse with this illness than with any other.

"NERVES"

"My nerves are on edge." How often do we hear that said. "Nerves" is a completely wrong and useless expression. It is not the nerves that are sick, which is quite a different matter. For example, the nerves are diseased in poliomyelitis or tetanus infection. With ordinary "nervous over-excitability" the patient exhibits morbid excitability due to mental causes and not to the nerves themselves. It is a symptom of a mental disorder—of a constant inner tension such as is experienced termporarily by everyone before an examination, a performance on the stage, or before the starting-signal in a race. Especially in sporting events this is the expression of the "switching on" of the stimulation of the sympathetic nervous system and the adrenals, which are needed for extra effort. On the other hand, whenever there is undue mental excitement, superfluous muscular excitement appears to be switched on as well, as though mental concentration were possible only when linked to physical tension, as was originally the case in the early days of primitive man. Whereever mental concentration was necessary, one automatically found oneself compelled to exert oneself physically, whether this was in a battle of defense or hunting. For this reason we still feel the need for "distracting" muscular movement when doing brainwork. Some people stride up and down the room while they are thinking. Others nibble their pens. A large percentage smoke too much, which involves activity of the hand and lip muscles.

The need for such distraction becomes greater the more difficult those inner obstacles which have to be overcome are. Tiredness is one of these obstacles. We shall see later, when dealing with the complaint of tiredness, how much lack of zeal or interest in a job can be a contributory cause of getting tired quickly (see page 279).

"Nerves" and Being Overworked

Therefore there is some connection between "nerves" and the fear of the demands made on one. It is like a prolonged state of suspense and fear experienced before an examination. As such it may well be symptomatic of overwork and its cause may be the discrepancy between the ability of the person concerned and the work required of him. It is immaterial whether these excessive demands are made by others or whether he himself is attempting too much. A decisive factor is the resistance of part of his personality against what he is required to do.

However, real "overwork" is only very rarely the sole cause of "nerves." Nervous fear nearly always has inner neurotic causes. These are based on an emotional conflict which one refuses to recognize and which has been pushed aside by one's consciousness. All situations which create a temporary state of fear and suspense with palpitations, etc., can cause "nervousness," i.e. the half-hoped-for, half-dreaded meeting with someone with whom one is in love; or being entrusted with a job for which one had ambitiously hoped and yet which one believes to be beyond one's capacity. In fact, all situations where it is a question of having to do something and not feeling quite up to it. Graves' disease (thyrotoxicosis) is based on similar emotional conflicts. The hormone of the thyroid, which is passed out in increased quantity, is a substance which increases "sympathetic" efficiency in a sustained way similar to the short-term action of excitement in the sympathetic nervous system (see page 222).

Treatment

The treatment of "nerves" rests mostly with the patient himself. He must realize in time that he just cannot go on like that. He must not drag on for weeks, letting the symptoms get worse, but must realize the absolute necessity of relaxation, even if this means economic disadvantage. Nothing is more wrong than to make unavailing efforts of will-power and to drive oneself to work when one is mentally breaking down. This heightens the "nervousness," makes the breakdown worse, and prolongs the illness. Symptoms like this should no more be ignored than tonsillitis or tuberculosis.

If one waits too long, the illness has physical repercussions, e.g. heart trouble. The treatment of these costs more time, money and labor than it would if one were to combat one's nervousness in time by real relaxation in the form of a proper holiday right away from one's accustomed surroundings. One should not only get away from one's profession, but also from one's whole family. In many cases the latter is more important than the first. So it must be a real holiday, away from everything that is part and parcel of one's daily life. Of course it is completely wrong to go somewhere where a new atmosphere of tension prevails. Complete mental peace and an attempt to come to terms with oneself are absolutely necessary, at least at the beginning of this period of recuperation. In the second half of the holiday it is in most cases conducive to recovery to try to regain confidence and joy in one's own efficiency by indulging in sporting activities or games requiring mental skill. Thus innumerable later "physical" ailments and disorders can be avoided by relaxing sensibly like this at the first symptoms of increasing "nerves."

If this simple expedient fails, the cause may be more deepseated than a case of a person whose capacity is unable to meet the demands of the outside world. Then the nervousness is symptomatic of a neurosis, which cannot be removed by drugs or a period of recuperation. "Nature cures" are also completely useless. There is only one possibility of a cure, and that is psychotherapy.

ILLNESSES WHICH ORIGINATE
IN THE MIND

According to our present views there is no illness in which the central nervous activity of our brain, including the life of our mind, does not play a very important part. One can deduce from this, therefore, that with every illness bodily activity is influenced by the mind, as has already been pointed out over and over again in various chapters of this book. So by now one ought to have an idea what this means. There are, however, a number of illnesses which come about, as it were, without external cause, and these form the majority of those complaints for which medical science has not been able to find any cause. These are the illnesses that are known as psychosomatic illnesses (see page 232).

This actually is a misnomer, as all illnesses of human beings are psychosomatic. But it is used to indicate that some illnesses with physical symptoms have their origin in the mind. With these illnesses the mind has affected the interplay and function of various organs. We have seen an example of this kind with disorders of the thyroid gland (see page 222).

HIGH BLOOD-PRESSURE

The medical name for this complaint is hypertension (*hyper* = over, and tension is derived from *tendere*, to stretch). The section on "The Inner Workings of the Heart and Kidneys" gives details about raised blood-pressure (page 56) and how it starts.

High blood-pressure can also accompany kidney diseases or, in rare cases, over-functioning of the adrenals.

However, raised blood-pressure itself is a different matter. It is something that happens in every normal person when he flies into a rage or is in the grip of similar emotional excitement. Then his blood-pressure rises. This is part of the normal functioning of people and animals. High blood-pressure as an illness is a permanent, not a temporary, mental tension of this kind. To illustrate this let us call it an illness of perpetual anger, this rage being denied an outlet (e.g. some violent act) by the person's "inner cage-bars." This rage or anger is not admitted to consciousness by the person and for that reason takes on a permanence maintained by nervous and hormonal factors, instead of vanishing in one sudden outburst and returning to a healthy balanced state. In the early stages of the illness the blood-pressure is subject to marked fluctuation. There are quite normal days which may be followed by a week of high blood-pressure, according to the circumstances of daily life and character development of the person.

Personality Profile

The typical character picture of high blood-pressure is a conciliatory, particularly amiable and obliging personality, who laughingly puts up with all insults, slights or provocation.

As children they were mostly particularly unruly, until at some stage in their development they experienced a sudden change of temperament and became more subdued. Exaggerated self-control is characteristic of these people. They take themselves too much in hand, either because they are naturally violent or bad-tempered and so always getting into trouble, or because their profession demands great self-control. One of the most dangerous professions for this is that of a housewife if the marriage and family life are not completely harmonious. With our present-day conditions of life this illness is more common in women than in men. The conditions of Western civilization are particularly conducive to high blood-pressure. Race and predisposition are of secondary importance.

Patients with high blood-pressure are for the most part employed in subordinate positions and professions. They are usually too modest about their intrinsic ability and are too timid or shy to assert themselves. They are inhibited in sexual relations. Many men are impotent or suffer from premature ejaculation during the act of sex. Women frequently are frigid. Many men with high blood-pressure take alcohol, which helps them to overcome their crippling shyness. For the same reason they frequently break out of marriage or a solitary existence and have extramarital sexual relations of an irresponsible nature. A tendency to drink and sexual immorality do not cause high blood-pressure. You do not get the illness because you drink, but rather you drink because of the nature of the illness. People with high blood-pressure are extremely punctual and reliable workers. They fulfill all tasks given to them, even if they break down. They are also willing to work overtime to please their superiors and only grumble in secret, although this they do almost the whole time. They adopt a somewhat domineering and despotic attitude toward their spouses.

Prevention

Everyone who is threatened with high blood-pressure can do a great deal to prevent it. He can take stock of his own behavior and attitude and perhaps do away with his exaggerated self-control, however convenient and desirable it may appear to his fellow men. Above all one should under all circumstances avoid bringing up children to be too docile and obedient. This only renders them unfit for normal life and paves the way for high blood-pressure and other illnesses. A person has to get on in life, and he learns how to do this in his relationship to his parents in the first years of his life.

About every tenth person over forty years of age suffers from high blood-pressure. Approximately one-fourth of all people over the age of fifty die as a result of high blood-pressure; that is to say, high blood-pressure causes more deaths than cancer. For this reason parents should occasionally sacrifice their principles when bringing up children, since the foundation of this later fatal illness is laid down in the child's early years when his character starts to develop. Life itself compels us to restrain our aggressive urges and impulses sufficiently and a child should not be punished or threatened every time it shows its own will-power or personality. High blood-pressure is a serious business.

If an adult feels he is being taken advantage of in his profession and he is unable to stand up for himself, or if such a person cannot achieve his aim in his profession because he feels himself to be inadequate and lacks the necessary courage to set about things, he should give up all thought of material advantage and change to an occupation in which things are easier for him.

Treatment

Drugs and physical treatment are among remedies employed in the control of high blood-pressure. While some patients benefit from a low-sodium, or salt-free, diet, recent studies suggest that modern medications are generally more effective and provide a simpler means of controlling blood pressure because nearly all canned, frozen, and otherwise packaged foods today contain sodium. There are exceptions, however, such as high-blood pressure patients with kidney disease, who require low-sodium diets. Some patients also find relief through transcendental meditation or similar methods of relaxation. Obesity is another consideration; more than half the people with high blood pressure are overweight. Of course, in high blood-pressure improvements occur on their own. Careful observation has shown that there has always been a change in the patient's circumstances when this is the case. Similar effects can be achieved temporarily by intensive treatment with drugs. Confidence in the doctor in charge of the case plays a decisive part in the patient's improvement and this salutary effect of trusting one's doctor can be reinforced by sedatives. But the patient must not lose heart when he suffers a relapse. It is a good thing for a patient to understand the basis of psychosomatic illnesses, as he can then learn to anticipate dangerous situations and avoid them.

The Consequences

In the beginning the blood-pressure fluctuates between normal and high, and the rise in pressure is based entirely on constriction of the small arteries of the body, and this has mental and nervous causes. As time goes on, this leads to stiffening of the walls of these little vessels—so-called hardening of the arteries. Then the vessel walls can no longer relax when the nervous strain disappears. At this juncture it is scarcely possible to get the blood-pressure down completely. Naturally the heart has to work harder in permanently raised blood-pressure. It is always being called upon to exert itself to the utmost. Its walls develop like the muscles of a heavy athlete in training, above all, the walls of the left ventricle. The heart then looks like the silhouette of a duck in an X-ray photograph. This state goes on for many years, but eventually the heart will fail. Although healthy in itself, it can no longer fulfill its task on account of the constant high pressure with which it has to cope. It breaks down, and when climbing stairs the patient gets short of breath and at night has to get up three or four times to pass water. Failure will occur earlier when there is a rheumatic heart ailment as well as high blood-pressure, as is sometimes the case. Then the heart has to maintain its high-pressure work with leaking valves as well.

Far more often than rheumatic valvular disease, high blood-pressure is combined with disease of the coronary vessels. Increased work of the heart muscle demands a greater blood supply. Approximately one-third of all patients with diseased coronary vessels are suffering also from high blood-pressure. The dreaded outcome of this illness is death from heart failure.

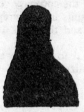
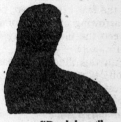

X-ray of normal heart.   Fig. 37   *"Duck-heart" X-ray.*

The next commonest cause of disability in high blood-pressure is a stroke. In this, generally because of particularly high blood-pressure, a vessel in the brain bursts. The effects of the stroke vary according to the position of the damaged artery. Usually paralysis on one side of the body results. At the beginning there is unconsciousness. The face is either pale or bluish and the breathing is stertorous. Death may take place after some hours or days of unconsciousness, if the bleeding has destroyed vital parts of the brain. Milder strokes are, however, followed by recovery. Strokes occur most often in spring and autumn.

Another serious outcome of high blood-pressure is a kidney disease. This develops slowly over a period of many years till death finally occurs as a result of the kidney's breakdown.

NARROWING OF THE CORONARY VESSELS
(Coronary Insufficiency)

Narrowing of the coronary vessels may be part of general constriction of the arteries in a case of high blood-pressure. But it also occurs as an illness on its own, with its own characteristic mental and nervous causes. In the beginning there is usually only temporary constriction of these vital arteries. The exact reason for the distribution of the pain, which radiates to the inner side of the left arm, and the "tightness of the chest" (angina pectoris) which goes with it, is not known. All that is known is that stimulation of the parasympathetic nerves causes the coronary vessels to contract and that of the sympathetic nerves dilates them (see section on Nerves and Hormones: sympathetic and parasympathetic nerves, page 82). It is known also that the pain produces fear and that in turn the fear causes more constriction of the coronary vessels.

Narrowing of the coronary vessels results in a discrepancy between the blood supply of the heart and the work of the heart muscle.

With this illness it is easier than usual to describe a personality type which is also plainly recognizable to the layman interested in psychology.

Personality Profile

Such people are generally industrious, ambitious personalities, who show great self-control and perseverance. They go all out for success and achievement and plan their lives and careers. They are almost always highly successful in their profession and are particularly suited for academic work. They generally become doctors, clergymen, lawyers and senior officials in positions of responsibility. They tend to assume responsibility. They are hard workers and may take stimulants, like coffee and cigarettes, in order to be able to keep at work longer. They appear to be model husbands (and fathers), but nevertheless they often fail to find proper sexual satisfaction in their marital relations, in common with people suffering from high blood-pressure.

Prevention

It is difficult to recommend a mode of behavior that might prevent this illness since the character of the patients represents a widespread educational ideal in our Western civilization. One can only say that it is dangerous to neglect the softer, more tender and emotional side of human nature. Incessant overwork with a constant eye on the future is not compatible with healthy living. Unfortunately such patients usually ignore the doctor's advice to work less, to relax more and to shoulder less responsibility until it is too late and the temporary cramp of the coronary vessels has turned into a genuine rigid constriction, endangering the patient's life.

Perhaps some patients can be helped by a warning to love their wives more and refrain from excesses; to have sexual intercourse only with the loved person and to rid himself of the feeling that only with a stranger can he really "let himself go." Heart failure during a sexual embrace has been known to occur.

Coronary disease is predominantly a masculine complaint. However, there are indications that it is increasing among women.

Professional setbacks, slights and other restrictions of one's own powers of authority set up dangerous emotional conflicts which bring on the symptoms in sufferers from this complaint.

Treatment

It is vital to stop every attack with drugs prescribed by the doctor. Trinitroglycerine and similar substances are used; these take effect in a matter of seconds and dilate the coronary vessels. The greatest difficulty lies in the characteristic ruthlessness of these patients with regard to their own body. When each severe and painful attack (chest and left arm, sometimes also the right arm) with its frightful feeling of fear is over, they again forget the doctor's warning to relax and take it easy in their job. It is one of the few illnesses in which heavy smoking may endanger life. Nicotine constricts the coronary vessels, even in healthy people. Therefore there must be no slackness about forbidding smoking in this illness.

The condition of poor blood supply of the heart muscle due to constriction of the coronary vessels can be recognized on an electrocardiogram (ECG) (see page 55).

DISORDERS OF HEART RHYTHM AND EFFORT SYNDROME

This includes attacks of palpitation and heart-fluttering (paroxysmal tachycardia), fits of giddiness from fluctuations in the blood-pressure or slackening of the muscles of the vessel walls in various areas of the body, and temporary breathlessness. Usually there are slight pains in the area of the heart. These symptoms do not indicate any damage to the heart itself, but a functional disorder based purely on faulty guiding of the work of the heart and circulation by the nervous system. Often such patients have in their youth had mild symptoms, which are the forerunners of the various forms of the illness. But they occur also as a result of genuine injury to the heart. Thus a severe infectious disease like diphtheria or typhoid can poison the heart.

In such cases the electrocardiogram is sometimes a valuable means of diagnosis. Generally, however, normal heart tracings are found, or, what is even worse, errors are made on the strength of insignificant changes. Above all, the patients themselves overrate this method of examination to their own detriment. They say, "The infallible machine has recorded my illness in black and white. I am suffering from heart trouble." Nothing is more dangerous for these patients than anxiety about their heart. They also tend to react to their symptoms of illness with despondency and fear. Concealed anxiety, the reasons for which they just will not admit, does more than anything else to bring on this illness.

These feelings change the action of the heart. One has the palpitations of fear. The blood-vessel walls slacken. The bloodstream and blood-pressure can no longer be regulated quickly enough and in the right way to the necessary amount. When climbing stairs the heart and circulation do not adapt well to the extra exertion. This is termed the "effort syndrome."

Also, however, in actual heart disease, an accompanying heart neurosis (neuro-circulatory asthenia) makes the patient feel worse.

Disorders of rhythm may determine in heart patients whether the feet and legs will swell, or whether breathing will become difficult even when lying down. This happens independently of whether the heart valves are more or less leaky. A heart can make up for extraordinarily severe damage to its valves, but it can also fail to do so. This "decompensation"— filling of the tissues with water, blue lips, and breathlessness —is not always due to a breakdown of the heart, but also to its steering by the nerves. In this case it is not the servant, the good heart, which is at fault, but the master, the guiding nerves. Of course, the results are exactly like failure of the heart itself—for example, when damaged by poisons, or by bacteria in an infectious disease, when the heart really does break down.

Personality Profile of Patients with a Heart Neurosis

According to the law of "usually," people suffering from heart neurosis, with whom we are going to deal in this paragraph, show typical mental characteristics; they are friendly and obliging and are well liked. If they feel unsure of themselves, they change erratically between shyness and timidity and blatant showing off of themselves and their abilities. They anxiously avoid open hostility towards others. They dislike being alone, but even with intimate friends they are usually inhibited and depressed. On the other hand, they may be noisy and gay in company. In sexual matters they are usually insufficiently informed and are frequently revolted by and afraid of sex. Women are shy with their husbands and children and tend to exaggerate the significance of family rows. In work they are somewhat unreliable, but with the necessary supervision they are capable of doing valuable work. Their emotional side tends generally to be somewhat exaggerated.

Such patients often have had strange fears and phobias with regard to dogs, horses, trains, etc., in their childhood. These often persist in a concealed form in later life. They are nearly always afraid of suffocating in closed rooms or in crowds—for instance, in the cinema. They always sleep with their windows open and overdo hygienic precautions. With some this fear of being shut in amounts to claustrophobia. To a large extent these patients show timidity and an over-vivid imagination. They are generally very heavy smokers and drink a lot of coffee. They may become actors and like to perform in public. The illness is brought on by a gradually increasing sense of failure in life and is often precipitated by a wrong move or disappointment in one's private life, in relation to one's family and friends.

Prevention

It is not easy to make any recommendations here. One should not feel completely reassured when a doctor says of a child that it has no heart defect, but only neurosis of the heart. That is every bit as serious. The little word "only" must be eradicated at all events. It is a matter of complete indifference to us whether or not the pathologist is likely to find visible changes when he does an autopsy. The important thing is that the heart and circulation should function properly during one's lifetime. It is all the same to a person if his organs are diseased or just do not function properly because of mental-nervous reasons. It is still an illness, even if drugs cannot cure it. Anyone who allows himself to be put off with the statement that "it is only a question of nerves," will go on being ill.

If such a person could achieve a cure by will-power and determination, he would never have become ill in the first place. But he cannot master his unconscious fears without knowledge of their cause—and, in serious cases, without the help of psychotherapy. In order to understand this, one must read again the paragraph on the fear of cancer (page 200). We are only human, and all the more so when we are ill. Without a mind our organs are dead pieces of flesh. Out-of-date medical science of past decades behaved as though it did not realize this. It got us into the way of saying, "It is only nerves. For shame, one isn't so feeble as to have anything like that." Thus the illness remained untreated. Is it surprising that nowadays we are horrified at the increase in illnesses of this kind? If these illnesses are not treated, they must become more prevalent.

We should at least adopt preventive measures with children. Childish fears are a neurotic symptom and are not normal. They can often be removed after a few sessions with a child psychologist; often a recommended change in one's family habits is sufficient. At least one spares the patient a life of fear and the danger of heart and circulatory complaints. And it is just with heart neuroses that well-nigh miraculous successes can often be achieved, even with adults, after a few sessions with a skilled psychotherapist. Usually a long period of psychotherapeutic treatment is not necessary.

DIGITALIS IN HEART DISEASE

Wherever damage to the heart muscle is established, be it inflammatory, rheumatic or from some other cause, digitalis preparations (from the foxglove plant) are useful. The heart muscle—and only the sick heart muscle—becomes stronger. If digitalis does not help, other drugs must be used. Digitalis is one of our most valuable drugs.

A sick heart which is being treated with digitalis needs it for years. It is not a harmful substance, even though it would be possible to kill a person with large quantities of it. (For that matter spinach, if eaten by the ton, could poison someone, since it contains oxalic acid. Nevertheless, the idea that one should not eat spinach because it is poisonous in large quantities has never occurred to anyone.) Digitalis in ordinary dosage is not poisonous.

ATTACKS OF PALPITATION

These are best dealt with in the simple way described on page 58.

But reading these paragraphs still does not tell you all about heart disease. You must also read the chapters dealing with the function and construction of a healthy body and mind.

MIGRAINE

This is a form of headache, which occurs in repeated attacks. The pain may be one-sided. Generally the attacks are preceded by mild disturbances of sight or speech. During an attack the patients shun the light and feel sick, sometimes vomiting. After the attack is over they experience a pronounced feeling of heightened well-being, which is characteristic. The attacks come quite suddenly and may be over in a few minutes.

Migraine pains are caused by dilation and stretching of blood-vessels inside the skull, and occur as a normal effect of stimulation of the sympathetic nervous system. As a result of close observation of attacks of migraine in the course of psychotherapeutic treatment, it has been established that this faulty stimulation of sympathetic nerves is due to the fact that anger and annoyance experienced by the sufferers are immediately suppressed. The rage is bottled up before it even has time to send up the blood-pressure. When it is possible to understand this anger and to give vent to one's feelings, the pain may quickly go.

Unfortunately one cannot describe clearly the personality types among migraine sufferers, although the following characteristics are found either in a concealed or open form: lack of humor, intellectual ambition, reticence and a tendency to be domineering, as well as to take offense easily, irritability and signs of envy.

The attacks can be terminated by a drug, which is known

as ergotamine. In many cases two or three simple consultations with a doctor versed in psychotherapy may stave off attacks to a large extent. In such a case the circumstances which bring on the attack must be recognized and the connection made clear to the patient. Changes in mode of life, profession, holiday pursuits, friendships and affairs of the heart are the "drugs" prescribed by the doctor during these consultations.

RHEUMATIC HEART DISEASE

The reader has already learned about one side of rheumatic illnesses in the chapter on "Infectious Diseases" (see page 180). It is something like a slow blood-poisoning, which goes on for years. The bacteria have the peculiarity of producing no immunity. On the contrary, the sick person becomes more susceptible to them through the illness. The hormones of the adrenal gland (cortisone) have proved to be an effective remedy. The body manufactures these hormones itself and can produce them in any quantity. Infection and bacteria do not play the decisive part in the illness. What is more important is the correct working of the endocrine glands connected with the mental and nervous processes in the brain and vegetative nervous system.

The two danger-points at which rheumatism attacks are the heart and the joints. In the heart, the muscle itself can become affected or only the important valves. The latter is the most common form of rheumatic heart disease. The damage is not shown in the electrocardiogram. Only the doctor's ear can detect the change by the murmur caused by the blood as it flows through the damaged valves.

An X-ray photograph of the heart does not show the change immediately. Only after a long time can a change in the shape of the heart be recognized. The heart gets large, just as do the muscles of an athlete as a result of training. It must do this to maintain the necessary circulation in spite of leaky valves. The enlargement of the heart affects only the parts where there is greatest wear and tear. In most cases the heart compensates sufficiently by this enlargement so that many patients do not notice anything wrong provided they do not try to perform very heavy work or set sporting records. The heart's ability to make up valvular damage borders on the miraculous.

Unfortunately we do not allow our heart to get on by itself with its difficulties. We usually drive it hard—quite unwittingly and innocently, of course—because of a heart neurosis. A remark by the doctor when informing his patient of the result of a routine examination may precipitate this. It is dangerous to know about a valvular defect without being properly informed as to its real meaning. It does not mean that one must think incessantly of one's "sick" heart and that one should behave like an invalid. Valvular disease which the heart muscle has overcome by "training" and enlargement does not make one only half fit. That results only when the muscle cannot compensate.

The real danger of a valvular heart defect is the fear of suffering from heart trouble. Anyone who avoids this—and he can do so with a clear conscience!—and all other nervous fears, is doing his heart and himself the best service. An example of the mental danger of nervous anxiety about a sick heart—and one which nearly had a tragic ending—is given on page 81.

Personality Profile

Rheumatic heart diseases are more common in women than men. The mental characteristics of the patients are similar to those with heart neuroses. They are popular because they feel a great need to please and often possess a childlike naïve charm. They are sociable and amiable and are good company. They are less shy than people with rhythm disorders. The neurotic traits are the same in both groups (fear of suffocation, nervousness, nightmares). They admire people of whom they are afraid or who treat them badly. A tendency to self-abnegation and "playing the martyr" is apparent. Rheumatic heart disease usually does not occur alone but together with symptoms as are described in the paragraph on disorders of the heart rhythm. Correspondingly the mental behavior of the patients in both groups is very similar.

Treatment

The valvular heart defect can be corrected in many cases by surgical means that substitute man-made valve parts of plastic and metal for damaged natural tissues. Drugs may be needed frequently to protect against further infections.

Sick-Visiting

By knowing and understanding this, friends and relations can do a great deal for the patient's recovery and aid the drugs which he is given. As far as possible, do not sympathize too much with him when visiting, but help him to tackle his mental problems and worries. So much can be done when the patient feels that he can unburden himself to a kind, sympathetic person. This is better than trying to spare his feelings by evading the issue or not talking about the matter. By "not stirring things up" one does in point of fact stir up a great deal more in the patient. If one visits the patient and does not discuss matters which, although dreaded by him, he had hoped to talk about, one leaves him alone with his worries. Deep down inside he feels himself to be an outcast. With kindness and sympathy one can do a great deal towards the recovery of friends with heart trouble.

RHEUMATOID ARTHRITIS

Everyone has probably heard of this. In past years it was just called "rheumatism." The rheumatic damage affects the joints, which swell painfully, and the condition can last a long time. The exact cause is unknown and although there is no evidence that the disease is directly related to rheumatic heart disease, some of the tissue damage effects of both ailments are similar. Emotional factors usually are involved in both diseases. And by understanding the differences in the mental behavior of people, one can understand why the seat of illness in the body may differ, i.e., heart or joints.

Mental Foundations

Research has shown that articular rheumatism, which is also more common among women than men, belongs to the "illnesses of bottled-up anger." It has mental sources similar to high blood-pressure and migraine. It is also an illness of the sympathetic nervous system. The mental behavior of the patients is similar to that of sufferers from hysteria. Naturally this is not apparent to the layman, since the illness takes place in the body and not as an obvious disorder of the mind.

With articular rheumatism, too, we find an irritable character, which tends to be hostile to any form of domination. What is extremely typical is a servile desire to dominate others by sacrificing oneself for them. The patients show great restraint with regard to all their emotions. Women who later get rheumatism tend to indulge in boyish games out of doors in youth. People with a tendency towards rheumatism nearly always marry indulgent and very often physically handicapped partners. Towards their children they are exacting and at the same time over-concerned. They do a great deal for their children, but there again it is a dictatorial kind of advice and help which they proffer, and they sacrifice themselves for the children in order to dominate them. These patients are not very popular. They may be shy and childlike. There is some evidence, because of hormonal involvement, of a link between arthritis and sexual activity. Symptoms in women, for example, disappear during pregnancy. However, an apparent lack of interest in sex by many arthritic patients may be due to the pain and discomfort experienced in sexual activity.

Situations which Precipitate the Illness

These may be all kinds of events in which it is not possible to find an outlet for bottled-up anger, for instance in the form of servile tyranny. That can happen when a husband is unfaithful to his wife, thus escaping from the servile, domineering love. It can also be the birth of a child, since looking after an infant involves only service and no compulsion. It can be a death in the family, when a relation who has been dominated in this self-sacrificing way is taken from one. So one sees that it is an inner significance rather than an external occurrence. A nervous and heightened muscular tension always comes about as a result of the chronic excitement, and is followed by the rheumatic damage to the joints.

Treatment and Mental Prevention

In articular rheumatism there are peculiarities of character which cannot be removed by simple advice or a few sessions with a psychotherapist. As far as character is concerned, these people have managed to get through life relatively well. In order to eradicate the mental causes of the illness they usually need a long course of psychotherapeutic treatment. Mothers or fathers with rheumatism (heart as well as joints) and high blood-pressure would do well to control their own over-fussiness with regard to their children, as far as is possible. Over-protection coupled with strictness conduces the "rheumatic character."

The chances of success with medical treatment are most satisfactory if the patient sees a doctor when the first symptoms appear. Analgesic and anti-inflammatory drugs, exercise to maintain joint flexibility, and adequate bed rest, as well as emotional rest, form the basis of therapy.

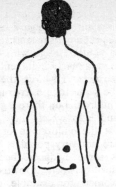

Fig. 38
Sciatica.

SCIATICA

As well as rheumatism of the heart and joints there is also a rheumatism of the nerves, most commonly the sciatic nerve. The pain may extend from the lower back to the ankle. Most common causes of the sciatica pain are arthritis of the spine or a ruptured ("slipped") spinal disc, but it also may be caused by poor body posture. Treatment may include heat applications, muscle relaxing drugs, and bed rest. But the problem should be treated by a doctor because permanent damage to the nerve could result from improper treatment.

DISEASES OF THE BLOOD-VESSELS

There are a number of illnesses which begin insidiously and in which temporary or permanent obstruction of the arteries in the arms and legs occurs. Just as the heart can become sick and altered, so can the blood-vessels of the circulation. Generally the final obstruction of the arteries is preceded by temporary constriction as a result of nervous stimuli. This goes on for a long time, but it does not cause a rise in blood-pressure as usually only individual areas are affected. The consequences of this closing of vessels are grave for the tissues supplied by the affected arteries. These tissues are destroyed because of lack of food and oxygen. Fingers or toes become numb and dry up. They may have to be amputated if gangrene sets in (as the result of infection). Obstruction of the vessels is very painful. It manifests itself in the early stages by cramp in the calves or arms, which occurs after a long spell of walking or handiwork. On resting, the pains subside since the resting muscle needs less glucose and oxygen than the working one.

Blood-vessel disorders also affect the veins. Almost everybody knows someone with this illness, usually called varicose veins. "Varicose veins" in the rectum are known as hemorrhoids. These are particularly unpleasant as they tear and bleed if one's motions are hard. Hemorrhoids can bleed so profusely and frequently that formation of new blood in the bone marrow cannot make good the loss, and anemia results.

A consequence of varicose veins is ulceration of the feet or legs, which does not heal up and from which many old people suffer.

The treatment of all these complaints must be started as soon as possible. Drugs that help dilate blood vessels, such as tolazoline and derivates of the vitamin nicotinic acid, give considerable improvement. Use of tobacco must be stopped because it constricts the vessels.

PHLEBITIS (Inflammation of the veins) AND THROMBOSES

In diseases of veins (varicose veins and the like) painful inflammation of the vein walls plays an important part. The blood may clot inside the vessel when the vein wall is damaged by inflammation. This greatly interferes with the return of blood from the limb (generally a leg) to the heart. The foot swells just as it does when the heart is not working adequately. The doctor can easily distinguish between the two kinds of swelling in the legs as he can feel an enlarged liver if the heart is not functioning properly. It is swollen just like the feet. In inflammation of the veins with blood-clotting (thrombophlebitis) there is a risk that a portion of the clot will break off and get carried along with the blood-stream through the heart and into the lung vessels, where it gets stuck. That is called an embolism and can result in death. Generally, however, only a small part of one side of the lung is cut off from its blood supply by the embolus and heals up without undue ill-effects. Vein thromboses of this sort often occur after surgical operations, and also after childbirth, if the patient is compelled to lie still for a long time.

With varicose veins one need not go to bed, but can walk about during the daytime provided the legs are firmly bandaged.

Asthma

Asthma consists of attacks in which the finer bronchi are constricted and in spasm. This causes great difficulty in breathing. In particular expiration becomes difficult. The wheezing noise made when breathing can be heard without a stethoscope. Typical asthma attacks do not last long, but they should always be treated by drugs. In asthma patients the nervous mechanism has, as it were, gone awry and reacts to the slightest stimuli in the air which they inhale. These patients are over-sensitive to such substances as pollen, cat's hair, feathers and flour dust. There is hardly anything which has not provoked asthma in some patients. They are over-sensitive to them. This over-sensitivity to certain substances which results in such violent body reactions is known as allergy.

Emphysema of the Lungs

If asthma persists for a long time, the numerous attacks over a period of years, with spasms of coughing, cause the lung alveoli to burst. It is in these that the exchange of oxygen between air and blood takes place. The result is called emphysema (over-inflated lung), in which there is reduced efficiency in exchanging gases. In addition, mucus collects in the lung alveoli which have become much larger owing to rupture of adjacent walls. Coughing does not completely get rid of this, and inhaled bacteria grow in it and give rise to bronchitis and a persistent cough. Lung tissue which is irritated by this inflammation can then set off the asthma reaction over and over again.

Mental-Nervous Processes

Constriction of the bronchi in both sick and healthy people is brought about by the parasympathetic nerves. As has already been described, our emotional life is involved in this nervous system. However, one cannot describe a typical asthma personality. The background becomes apparent only when the deeper parts of the person's personality are examined. Superficially, as a normal knowledge of human nature can show us, widely different types of character occur in asthma, but underneath, psychoanalytical research in recent years has revealed the complaint to be an "illness of longing." Invariably it is a phobia of separation from one's natural mother or (later) a "mother-substitute." This "mother substitute" need not be a female person. It can be something connected with fate—something indefinite, so that when the need arises for independent action the longing can have the effect of a "separation trauma." The attack of asthma is in fact a return to the suppressed sobbing of children, who are told not to cry when they wish to do so.

People with a deeper insight into human nature will have noticed that asthma patients are not quite adult in their relationship with their mothers. They have never quite been able to dissolve the "tie to mother" which we all experience in the course of our development. On looking at the matter more closely one finds that these people were usually expected to exercise self-control in emotional matters at too early a stage in their childhood, with the result that they reacted to this seeming rebuff on the part of the mother by clinging all the more closely to her. In cases where psychotherapy has removed this impediment of childhood and the sick person has matured mentally, the over-sensitivity to certain substances does not vanish, as test inoculations on the skin with the substances in question still show. However, these substances no longer bring on any attacks of asthma.

Prevention

To prevent asthma, it is a good thing when bringing up children never to forbid them to cry and not to encourage them to be independent too soon. In this way one impedes their development since they all have the natural urge to try out and learn everything as far as their abilities permit. It is all a question of the right moment. If a child is forced to be independent too soon, it clings to its parents all the more and often remains unduly dependent all its life.

Treatment

In treating asthma there are numerous possibilities for the doctor to choose from, according to the circumstances of the individual case. The most important thing is to arrest each attack with drugs as soon as it begins. That is fundamentally simple. One need only give a drug which equalizes the faulty balance between stimulation of the parasympathetic and sympathetic nerves. The only difficulty is to decide which of the numerous drugs will be most effective in any given patient. If need be the doctor and patient must co-operate and try several drugs in succession until the most effective one is found. It is useless to keep changing one's doctor if he is not successful straight away. If you go off at once to another doctor, he has to start again from scratch and so it takes much longer for the patient to get the right drug. One thing, however, should not be overlooked when an asthma patient is choosing a doctor. Since this illness is to a great extent of psychological origin, the effect of the doctor's personality on the patient is of particularly great importance. He must have a doctor in whom he has confidence as a person. As a type the doctor must appeal to the patient.

In chronic asthma, various drugs are available to the doctor, such as prednisone, aminophylline, and, for infective cases, antibiotics. Breathing exercises, good nutrition and avoidance of fatigue are helpful. Patients also may benefit from changes in climate and changes in professional or domestic circumstances. In a great many cases success can be achieved with a short spell of psychotherapeutic treatment, above all in the early stage and during adolescence. In other cases lengthy psychotherapeutic treatment is necessary.

HAY FEVER, HAY ASTHMA, SPRING CATARRH

These are all allergic illnesses where certain pollen substances from blossom (usually flowering grasses) constitute the allergy. For that reason they are seasonal illnesses, which generally reach their peak in June. The mental and nervous foundations are the same as with asthma. Nowadays there are extremely effective drugs which prevent these attacks. They are called "antihistamines." Histamines is the actual substance produced by the body during an attack of allergy and it causes the urticarial spots on the skin, or the excess nasal secretion in hay fever or in an ordinary cold. The antihistamine substances (for example, Benadryl), prevent the irritation produced by histamine from taking effect. People who suffer from a running nose at certain times of the day or on certain occasions can prevent this embarrassing state of affairs by taking some tablets of an antihistamine drug, but they must go on taking it always.

Nettle-Rash (Urticaria)

Like asthma, this is an allergic and at the same time psychosomatic illness. The allergy substances are usually contained in food. The most common are strawberries and crab meat. Some hours after eating food containing such substances, large red itching spots appear on the skin. Treatment is by antihistamine tablets. In addition one tries to find out by tests which foodstuffs bring on the attack and therefore should be avoided. Urticaria can also be caused by direct skin stimuli (touching stinging nettles brings it on in everyone), or even by inhaling substances (the scent of primroses).

Stomach Ulcers

The formation of ulcers in the stomach or duodenum is a sort of inflammation of the mucous membrane and causes exactly the same symptoms. There is no difference in treatment whether the X-ray photograph reveals an ulcer or not. The only difference here is that the ulcer breaks down from time to time over years or decades. There is a danger that the ulcer may get so deep that the stomach or duodenum will perforate. This is dangerous and requires immediate operation. Severe bleeding may occur from the ulcer and this can be recognized by black feces or by vomiting of blood. (*N.B.* Spinach and red wine can make the feces black in a healthy person.) A bleeding stomach ulcer urgently requires medical treatment.

With this illness—regardless of whether an actual ulcer can be seen or not—pain occurs after meals. According to the circumstances of the individual case the interval between the taking of food and the appearance of the complaints varies in duration. There is often vomiting. As regards diet, full particulars can be found in the chapter on nutrition in the paragraph dealing with people suffering from a weak stomach (page 109). Ulcer patients may have had a weak stomach from early youth. Even when they are free of pain they generally find that not all food agrees with them.

Mental-Nervous Foundations

When a patient has an ulcer there is overstimulation of the parasympathetic part of the autonomic nervous system. This can be controlled by the use of belladonna, scopolamine, and similar drugs. Examination usually reveals the presence of excess hydrochloric acid in the stomach juice. The stomachs of these patients behave as though they were always having to digest something or as though they were just offered a tasty serving of meat. They go on secreting at night and between meals when healthy stomachs are at rest. The causes underlying this are largely psychogenic and have been recognized as such by psychoanalytical research in recent years.

Personality Types

In ulcer cases, too, it is difficult to sketch a definite type of character as it is a matter of a deep-seated, repressed tension of longing, which is replaced on the surface by its very opposite. In the section on "Hunger and Love: the Mind and Its Influence on the Stomach" on page 75, the connection between the nerve stimuli and such "higher emotions" is explained.

The patients either deny themselves (for reasons of pride) the gratification of their secret desire to be petted and made a fuss of, or they encounter opposition all around because of their excessive demands in this respect. Deep down inside themselves they long to give themselves to others and to be as dependent on them as an infant is on its mother's breast. The majority come to terms with these "unseemly urges" in such a way that they become, on the contrary, particularly responsible and are tireless in caring for their family; they never rest and even take more distant relations under their wing. They usually accomplish much and are particularly fond of choosing professions where they can continually hustle around and be active. Then there is a group of patients in whom the exact opposite applies. They try to be as dependent as possible and are unreasonable in their demands on their relations in respect to care and attention. When it becomes necessary to wean themselves of this habit and they repress their desires, increased activity of the stomach mucous membrane results. In the overactive patients the deep-seated tensions have the same effect on the stomach, especially when they need to exert themselves and concentrate particularly hard on their activities, i.e. when their pride has driven them particularly far from their secret "soft core." Outside and inside counter-balance each other. The stronger the deep-seated longing becomes, the greater the compulsion to be active, and vice versa. Before the First World War the illness was found predominantly among women. Now it is the other way around.

Treatment

Having described the psychological aspect, it is possible to understand a well-known medical experience, namely, that four weeks of hospital care—quite independent of drugs and diet—will cure a stomach ulcer. It is not the drugs and special kind of food, but the fact that the patient can let himself be cared for by others and indeed fully appreciates his right to do so. This releases his deep "tension of longing" and causes the constant nervous over-excitement of the stomach to stop. In the past fifty years ulcer patients have been treated, according to the prevailing theories of the time, with varying diet —sometimes rich in proteins, sometimes the opposite, sometimes rich in fat and sometimes with little fat, and several other variations. In most cases the ulcers could no longer be detected in the X-ray picture after four weeks. Almost every year new drugs for the treatment of stomach ulcers are brought on to the market. They are all amazingly effective as long as the doctor in charge of the case is convinced of their efficacy. The effect may vary according to which doctor runs the department and gives the treatment. As soon as a drug for stomach ulcers is tried out on numerous patients under perfect experimental conditions, that is to say, when doctor and patients are not told who are receiving the new substance and who are not, there are no differences. All that remains is the "Magic of Medicine"—the fact that the doctor is treating and caring for the patient, and it is this which cures the patient. Research before this was realized was bound to go wrong because it ignored the decisive psychological factor in stomach ulcers. Nowadays all this is changing, especially as psychotherapeutic treatment is extremely effective for stomach ulcer.

Prevention

All people with a weak stomach, who have a tendency to ulcers, should try to strike a happy medium in their private lives to counterbalance the strain and competition found in professional life. They must always let themselves be cared for and petted by another person. They must allow others to assume responsibility in some matters, whether these people be wives, husbands, or friends. They must appreciate the loving care which has gone into the preparation of their meals and they must take sufficient time to enjoy them in peace. A good table is something for which they should thank providence. There is always time for eating, and the time spent on treating and curing stomach ulcers is much longer than the time needed to eat and digest one's meals properly.

CONSTIPATION

Thousands of people are, year in, year out, greatly concerned about the state of their bowels. Many are often seriously worried if they are irregular in this respect—people who are otherwise the personification of self-assurance and placidity. So let us state the facts. It is normal to have a bowel movement once a day. There are, however, quite a number of people following an equally "normal" frequency of once in two or three days. The amount varies according to the composition of the food and the water content of the excreta. Meat does not leave much waste matter; whole wheat bread and cabbage leave a lot, and milk and cheese leave practically none. There is no cause for alarm if one's stools are small, provided one is more or less regular. If one has not had elimination for some days, one should not expect to pass a larger quantity the next time this happens. The excreta becomes concentrated in the large intestine. Water is absorbed, so that the quantity gets smaller. Don't let this worry you. Nothing will be left behind. One need not be afraid of that if every one does not have a stool for a week. Of course all this applies only to people who have "always" had trouble with their bowels. People who are otherwise regular in this respect should regard any irregularity as a symptom of illness and go to a doctor.

The thing one should never do when constipated (this applies to people who have a tendency toward this) is to wait anxiously for one's bowels to be opened. If one nervously awaits "the call of nature" each day, one simply inhibits it. Conscious thought will interfere with nerve processes that function best automatically, and which one does not notice until the body gives a signal. (Then one should not hesitate to obey. People who habitually suppress it will eventually suffer from constipation.) For this reason going to stool becomes such a habit with most normal people that "the call of nature" comes at the same time each day. The internal clock strikes when the time has come. It is a simple nerve reflex which works to the hour. People who persist in interfering with this fine web of nerve connections must not be surprised if it lets them down.

Mental-Nervous Causes

The intestinal function of evacuation is influenced by the involuntary parasympathetic nervous system. This is part of one's unconscious nervous functions, which work best when one is emotionally and physically relaxed. In people who are always in a hurry and live at top pressure, the nerve processes are inhibited. For that reason people with high blood-pressure, rheumatism and migraine generally have trouble with their bowels.

In our early youth our excreta were a kind of favor—a present to our mother—the first form of payment, as it were. She did not want the bother of washing diapers, and rewarded and praised us if we did her the favor of producing our stool at the appropriate time and place. This was really the first possibility we had of fulfilling our obligations toward others and in this way this unsavory business has become so much a part of our emotional life, strange as that may seem.

Naturally this works the other way round. Our feelings affect the functioning of our intestine. People who are loath to give anything away are also constipated in the physical sense. Suspiciousness is a trait which has an adverse effect on the bowels. Three-quarters of all people who suffer from a mental disease of suspicion called paranoia (persecution mania) are chronically constipated. The same applies to pessimistic people, and sufferers from depression. Thus constipation may be the symptom of a severe mental disorder. However, it is not the only symptom in such cases. As always, the mental conditions conducive to chronic constipation may be found in the patient himself or in his relations to his environment. It can be one's own meanness, as it were, but it can also be lack of generosity on the part of a loved one. Dependents who believe they are getting a raw deal may become constipated in this devious way. "If you don't give me anything, I won't give you anything," is the line they adopt.

Treatment

It helps if the sufferer avoids becoming a prey to the idea
that he is ill. Naturally chronic constipation is a disorder,
but it is not an illness, to be remedied with cathartics and
enemas. It can always be overcome and the simplest way to
set about this is to give up being worried and really do something about it. This can best be done by oneself. You have only
to restore the automatic nerve reflex and get it to work once
more. This may take somewhat longer than in children. At
the age of thirty our nerve routes are slower than at the age
of two. Getting the reflex which controls the opening of our
bowels to work again entails a definite plan, which must be
adhered to.

(1) After careful consideration a definite time of the day should
be chosen when one is most likely to be free and undisturbed.
This may either be in the mornings (remember, on Sundays
one gets up later!) or in the lunch break or in the evenings
(this is difficult if one's hours of work vary). The time of day
is immaterial; what matters is that it should be always the
same.
(2) At the chosen hour one regularly pays a visit to the toilet.
On principle one should allow oneself half an hour for this.
There is no harm in taking a newspaper or book. (It is considerably more polite than reading at the breakfast table!) With
some people four weeks of this drill is sufficient to restore the
bowel reflex to proper working order. Should this fail, medicine must be taken to expedite matters.
(3) Continue with the first two points, but take a laxative
which you know will be effective. Vegetable laxatives or similar laxatives are good. People with hemorrhoids must use a
suitable ointment or suppository to relieve the pain when their
bowels are opened. This is part of the preparation for the
session fixed for the appointed time. You should prepare for
the first session with a large dose of a really effective laxative.
This is repeated for three consecutive days. Then you gradually reduce the quantity of the laxative over the course of
four weeks. You go on reducing the quantity until the bowel
reflex works by itself without the aid of medicines. Then you
stick rigidly to the regular habit and hour (timing yourself
to the minute).

Before doing all this you should read once more the
example of a conditioned drug reflex in the section on the elec-

trocardiogram, page 55. There one can see the amazing effectiveness of such reflexes. A dog's reflexes can even be trained to simulate a heart disease. In the case of a healthy functioning the training is of course fundamentally much simpler.

Nutrition

In addition to training one's bowel reflex to work at a definite time of day, one must make sure that one's diet contains adequate roughage. The intestine moves more quickly and vigorously if it contains some indigestible residue. Being full gives it exercise. Indigestible matter of this sort is contained in whole wheat bread, the coarser varieties of vegetables and in plant foods, which contain little fat; above all in vegetables like lettuce, radishes, etc. Meat and milk are unfortunately not so advantageous. Milk should only be taken in a sour form like yogurt, and meat only together with green vegetables. Potatoes contain little waste matter and do not make up for the meat, which is also deficient in waste matter. Meals containing a lot of fat are always bad since fat does not leave any waste matter.

CHRONIC TENDENCY TOWARD DIARRHEA AND INFLAMMATION OF THE INTESTINE (COLITIS)

There is also the opposite of constipation, as probably everyone knows from personal experience of an "upset stomach." This usually lasts only one to two days, However, there are people who always suffer from "loose" stools and have to go to the toilet several times a day. This occurs also as a symptom in other illnesses; for example, patients suffering from Graves' disease are afflicted in this way. It is, however, generally the mental-nervous counterpart to habitual constipation. This chronic tendency to diarrhea is usually combined with damage to the intestinal mucous membrane, which comes about in a similar way to inflammation of the stomach mucous membrane and stomach ulcers. With it, too, ulcers may form, or allergies may aggravate and maintain the maladjusted nerve processes. Usually these chronic diarrheal illnesses occur periodically. They are reactions to experiences and changes in one's living conditions. Diarrhea is not the only symptom. As a result of the inflammation and overstimulation of the intestine, mucus and blood are also passed and there is pain. Everyone knows about the cramp-like pains which occur with temporary diarrhea. It is intestinal colic which causes the pain, and the same occurs in chronic diarrhea complaints. These pains cannot be cured with aspirin. There is a very good remedy for them, which reduces the intestinal nerve activity. This is atropine, made from deadly nightshade (belladonna). Diet forms an important part of the treatment. In the chapter on Man and his Food on page 109 you can find in the section on "People with Weak Stomachs" just how you can help yourself in illness of this kind.

Mental-Nervous Causes

When these illnesses are seen, and during their relapses, the doctor notices over and over again certain emotional situations. One is the appearance of an insurmountable inner or external obstacle against the fulfilment of an obligation. This may be of a physical nature (for example, with a woman who feels it her duty to present her husband with a child), or it may be a moral or even monetary obligation. The second emotional situation is when one is frustrated in one's ambition to achieve something which demands concentration and determination. One's failure affects one's bowels. Generally adult patients with colitis also show fear. They have not progressed beyond a certain stage in their childhood development. This is made clear by the following example, which really happened and was carefully investigated.

A young woman with colitis who had recovered after three months' medical treatment had been married for six months. One Sunday morning she had a sudden serious relapse and diarrhea started again. The psychotherapist was able to elucidate the reason the next morning. The woman's husband had asked her, half jokingly and half in earnest, about the money he had lent her for her trousseau and when he was going to get it back? The young woman was inwardly worried about this and could not really believe it was a joke. At the same time she had not got the money to be able to fling it angrily on the table in front of him. Her diarrhea started again. She reverted to the emotional mechanism of her youth. When in the course of treatment this connection became clear, the diarrhea stopped—without diet or repayment of the money.

Of course it is not always possible to remove the wrongly guided mental-nervous excitement as easily as that. At times it requires great perseverance, which the patients are only rarely able to muster. They do not like to be helped. "Help" can constitute a moral obligation, which aggravates the illness. But perhaps it is better, before starting any treatment, of whatever kind, to find out about the actual nature of the complaint, as we have shown here. It becomes increasingly obvious that the modern doctor is no longer a mysterious "medicine man," and, indeed, does not want to be regarded as such. Treatment is a joint affair between doctor and patient. That is why people are greatly interested in modern medical science, and for that reason this book had to be written. There are no mysterious or infallible remedies which can perform miracles. Illness demands an understanding of one's own ailments and co-operation with the doctor who is exerting himself on one's behalf.

THE COMPLAINT OF "ALWAYS FEELING TIRED"

While we know that tiredness can be a symptom by which many illnesses are recognized (T.B., for example), in the great majority of cases tiredness and lack of concentration occur as an independent psychosomatic illness. "I fall asleep at work." "In the afternoon I can no longer concentrate." "In my shorthand course in the evenings I just cannot take in anything more." We are accustomed to such complaints every day from our acquaintances. There is also generally low blood-pressure, slight giddiness, somewhat irregular heart action, and "nervousness."

Mental-Nervous Causes

For the sufferer to understand this illness and to be able to help himself, he should recall how, as a child, he could go on reading forbidden crime novels in secret with a flashlight under the bedclothes for hours on end without getting tired. Yet at school, after reading two lines of a school book, he would be overcome by a violent attack of yawning. Pleasure in his work can make a research worker quite oblivious of his tiredness and need for sleep, if he is working on an exciting problem, while on another day he cannot fill up a tax form because of a feeling of "run-downness." People who have to address envelopes all day and every day have to overcome an inner resistance against it. They have to make a game out of it, otherwise they could not keep it up for long. This may be a triviality. It may even be the pleasure derived from the speed of one's writing. But there is a limit to the possibilities of enlivening "soul-destroying" work and there are many occupations in which this disadvantage cannot be overcome. This is a defect of our civilization, which for the present can scarcely be avoided.

Manual work is almost always better for one's health as the work of the muscles themselves counteracts the "tiredness."

Tiredness and Blood-Sugar

It becomes clear and obvious that the "tiredness" is dependent on the interest which one derives from work and on the zeal with which one carries out activities. These sensations stimulate the sympathetic nervous system, and the blood-sugar, so extremely important to the efficiency of the brain cells, is kept high. No cell becomes so easily weak as the nerve cells of the brain when insufficient glucose is brought by the blood. While the remaining parts of the body valiantly go on working, the nerve cells of the brain faint. The body behaves as though it were time for the peace of one's nightly sleep. The brain cells half faint, and bang!—one's head is on the table. All this happens because the activity is not "exciting" or is being undertaken reluctantly; because the sympathetic nervous system is not sufficiently stimulated and therefore too little adrenaline is injected into the blood, while the hormone, insulin, which causes the blood-sugar to fall, is increased. This results in the hormonal opposite of diabetes, the illness of tiredness. This can become so deep-seated and such a habit that even relaxing in the evenings and occupying oneself with interesting things fail to counteract it.

Prevention

However, this does not happen to everyone with a boring and soul-destroying daily job. You can stick to that sort of thing for eight hours if you devote the rest of the day to more active pursuits—physical training, for example. The adrenals then have to secrete quantities of adrenaline, whether they like it or not. Muscular work compels a sensible balance in the vegetative nervous system. This occurs also in an exciting game, such as chess. Exertion banishes tiredness, but it must be exertion which is undertaken with real interest and pleasure.

Almost any hobby is all right. Even secretly playing with the children's toys when they are in bed may give one pleasure. There were many things which we longed to do in our childhood and yet never did. You are never too old or grown-up to make up for this omission. Just have a try. You can do the silliest things quite sensibly. It is not "childish." It is a tonic to counteract lack of concentration and getting tired easily and against getting old! Believe me for the sake of your own efficiency. All these stupid little things can be covered by the rather high-falutin term "creative." Indeed, in no other psychosomatic illness can you do so much for yourself as in the illness of tiredness, and you may take my word we nearly all suffer from this up to a point.

Alcohol is quite the worst thing. A small drink or two may help to put a person right, and then may be taken in the evenings, but only as a means to an end. If coffee interferes with sleep, its use should be restricted in the evening. I dare not mention cigarettes. Whoever could manage that? But start to cut down by five and then three. When you have come down from twenty to ten, you will notice that there was a bit of chronic nicotine poisoning which was responsible for part of the tiredness.

NEUROTIC TIREDNESS

Unfortunately there are people who feel an insurmountable aversion when they have to perform even light duties. They really have to force themselves the whole time. Reproaches and abuse are of no avail; indeed, they have the opposite effect. Perhaps they are people who have chosen quite the wrong occupation or were obliged to do so. Whatever they have to do, even something dictated by their own reason and conscience and concerning their own immediate interests, the result is always the same; their eyes automatically close. These people are often highly intelligent, but they never really get anywhere, much to their own surprise. Neurotics are, however, not educable. Otherwise they would not be ill. Only great changes in their personality can restore the proper working of the vegetative nervous system and organs. Of course, the younger the person, the easier this is. The ability to learn helps him to acquire new modes of behavior. Help by others is possible by means of psychotherapy. Sometimes a surprising change comes in a short time and sometimes it takes a long period of work. Often a recommended change of occupation does the trick.

11. What Psychotherapy Acualtly Is

THE MAGIC OF MEDICINE

In the broad sense this is half the battle in any form of medical treatment. It goes without saying that confidence and faith in the doctor's knowledge and ability are essential for any cure. It has been proved by experiments that the doctor's faith in the effectiveness of his own drugs and treatment is also an indispensable factor. Present-day pharmaceutical research is hard put to eliminate this personal element.

Although various doctors may possess the same knowledge and ability for treating an ailment, the doctor who uses "psychotherapy" often has greater success. It is the effect of psychological factors which invests the naturally optimistic, confidence-inspiring doctor, who is himself never ill, with the superior powers of a healer. It is this which makes the doctor's name a genuine and in some cases indispensable part of the cure and the free choice of a doctor on the part of patients one of our inalienable civic rights. But it is also this which has been responsible for the amazing success of charlatans and other murky aspects of medical science, in which the other essential part—the proven medical techniques—has been neglected. The effect of patent and quack medicines is rooted in this "magic of medicine," partly because traditional medical science in the past 100 years—in the "scientific age" —was at pains to deny their existence. Thus patients could not be made to see that modern drugs were or could be much greater "wonder medicines" when not deprived of their magic.

Nowadays this magic is no longer based on "faith" alone, but on the knowledge of the amazing effectiveness of modern drugs.

AND WHAT IS PSYCHOTHERAPY?

But of course this "magic of medicine," the existence of which cannot be denied and which is often unjustly termed "suggestion" (implying that one is not ill, but hysterical), is not what is actually meant by psychotherapy. Psychotherapy is the scientific probing into the mental causes of illness and possibilities of treatment, such as we have already encountered in previous chapters in a number of illnesses. It is the step from tentative groping to the application of sure knowledge. One no longer depends on the chance of a favorable effect of the doctor's personality, but sets about understanding the laws of this natural phenomenon and putting them into practice. For this influence of personality is a natural phenomenon, a part of our human nature, and is not something mysterious with which only some people are endowed. It is quite simple and straightforward. The human language, which enables us to understand our own personality, is used with great effect as a method of treatment.

FALSE MOVES

Day in and day out, our minds and bodies are affected by language, the sense of words, and by the feeling and expression of intonation and accompanying gestures. It is therefore easy to realize its potential qualities as a powerful instrument in medical treatment. This scientific method has evolved since the end of the last century. It is based on the fact that there are processes and memories in the human mind of which we are not consciously aware. No one knows everything about himself and few care to probe into the deeper recesses of the soul, where unwelcome desires and experiences lie dormant. No one likes to have to answer for all his actions. Sometimes mailing a letter is "forgotten," or a slip of the tongue makes one rather ridiculous, or an object is mislaid and one cannot "remember where one put it." In short, one's mind does not always function as it should. Something from one's subconscious upsets it and one becomes surprised and angry with oneself. It is noticeable how unreasonably angry one becomes when reproached by anyone for such a "ridiculous" false move.

With their customary scepticism some research workers set about elucidating these strange failures, and the amazing result of their investigations was that there is always a definite purpose underlying these false moves. Two opposing impulses cross in the human mind. For instance, a young man put an important letter in his coat pocket, hung his coat in the wardrobe, and then looked for the "mislaid" letter for four weeks. It contained personal papers which were necessary for his wedding. In this example the marriage soon went on the rocks. But in this case it was quite certain that the conflicting intentions were unconscious. The young man had not knowingly rejected the idea of marrying the girl for any reason. He was really convinced that this marriage was the right one for him.

CONSCIOUS AND SUBCONSCIOUS

These simple examples open up a whole new vista of the human personality, something like that described in the section on "The Brain and Its Peculiarities" on page 91. Not only do irrational and false moves become understandable, but also senseless dreams begin to make some sort of recognizable sense. Above all, however, mentally sound people learn to understand the delusions of insanity and the incomprehensible actions of people suffering from mental disorders.

In neuroses the emotions are kept below the surface as a kind of mental defense mechanism called repression. They cannot be completely controlled and invariably have to find an outlet. The patients appear "affected" because their emotions are never quite suited to the occasion. Just as normal people occasionally inadvertently say "good-bye" instead of "hello," so hysterical people have a strange compulsion to laugh when others would weep, and vice versa. Any healthy person is liable in a minor degree to an emotional distortion such as this. There are times when we cannot "let off steam" in the office or at home because of having to control our tongue in front of a superior (who is the source of our annoyance), or because of having to give in to the wife for the sake of peace. Then a trifling incident may later cause us to give vent to our feelings, and fly off the handle like someone gone berserk, simply because, for example, a stranger happens to tread on our foot in the train—a thing to which we would have reacted with "Careful!" had we been in a mentally balanced state. We have transferred our emotions from the actual person who has upset us to another, "innocent" object. This is another kind of mental defense mechanism called displacement. It is neurotic behavior in an otherwise mentally sound person. It is not a very satisfactory thing to do, however, for although one's annoyance is temporarily dissipated and one "cools down," part of the anger remains unassuaged and waits for further explosions; furthermore, it becomes divorced from the original cause—the superior in the office or one's wife. One has buried one's head in the sand and repressed the real source of irritation. Actually one becomes unaware of it. It becomes an impulse, driven back into the subconscious, which upsets our mental efficiency. This is rationalization, or intellectualization, of a problem and it is immaterial whether "noble" feelings like politeness or consideration at home, or cowardice and fear of one's superior in the office, are responsible. It is in any case the "inner cage-bars" that have compelled us to adopt the line of least resistance.

CONTENT OF THE SUBCONSCIOUS

So you should not be surprised to find that your repressions may include the most impossible and repulsive things—things which one has deliberately thrust far away so that they remain undisturbed in the depths of one's soul.

There remains as a reversed image of what is customary; the negation of "that which one would like to be." A longing for tenderness and devotion may also be buried there—something which one has put aside because of having to go through life the hard way and without scruples. In everyone there are such "undigested remains," which date back to early youth. Therefore we should not be horrified if sexual urges and desires, sometimes in a fantastic form, are predominant in our subsconscious. These urges can easily upset our conscious planning of life. We must necessarily control them if we are to keep our emotions stabilized. However, we are particularly badly prepared for this task because the facts of sex are always hidden during childhood. We do not gradually grow up to meet these difficulties, but are brutally precipitated into a world of complicated rules and emotions. Our own incipient sexual stirrings in childhood may be rebuked, our questions either not answered or even punished. We take far more trouble teaching our children to swim than preparing them for the sex matters that will dominate their adult life. These conditions are admittedly better now than fifty years ago.

AGGRESSION

In our upbringing, the ability to assert oneself and to do the things one wants, suffers the same fate as sex. As an adult it is not practicable to be as docile and obedient as many parents still imagine the ideal well-behaved child should be. Luckily most children are able to compensate for this and thus escape this danger. They maintain their ability to get their own way, to do things on their own initiative and to be aggressive or destructive in play. But this is a perversion of aggression. The word means: to set about something. However, the object of aggression is not destruction just for its own sake. That is only the most primitive outward expression of aggression. Children who come up against an unsympathetic adult world and who are not allowed to say or do things of their own accord, may give vent to their aggression in the destruction of toys and other things, and in the torture of animals. If they are also so unfortunate as to love the parents who so restrict them, their life is virtually ruined. Not being allowed to do anything becomes an uncanny inner compulsion—a matter of conscience, which they are unable to overcome. They do not know why they invariably fail whenever they are required to take aggressive action. They are weighed down by a morbid conscience, of which they are unaware—"inner cage-bars," which render them unfit for life.

"UNDIGESTED REMAINS" IN THE MIND

At first glance it would therefore seem that one's fate was sealed. You cannot wipe out the past and pretend that it has never happened. You may therefore say that it is surely better to let well enough alone and leave things undisturbed in one's subconscious. What can anyone do with these crazy desires and emotions deep down inside oneself, even if one understands something about them? Should you go and shoot your father simply because you once wished your father dead during your childhood? It seems preferable to be ill than a murderer. How can one expect a young woman to grasp that every time she embraces her husband part of her soul is embracing her father; that her own husband represents a substitute for this unfulfilled and unfulfillable desire. What should she do about this criminal wish even if she understands it? The answer is simple and quite obvious. She can overcome it once she realizes that she is no longer a child, in whom that wish was born. She can overcome what seemed to her at the time just as incomprehensible as it was pressing. She can overcome her "conscience," which punishes her for this "forbidden" desire by making her frigid in her husband's arms. She can be happy only when she has "digested" the "undigested remains" in her subconscious. These are always due to mistakes in upbringing, which come about as a result of ignorance or the effect of our parents' own neurotic behavior. Man was not born to suffer, but can be harmed in the process of mental and emotional development.

Thus it is the task of psychotherapy to unearth these "undigested remains"—the hopeless confusion of repressed desires—and to help people to assimilate and overcome them. Unfortunately this takes time and is a tedious process and patients strongly resist it. They have, as it were, got used to the disturbing elements in their subconscious, even though these have been wrongly and incompletely repressed. If they have now to probe deliberately into this carefully subjugated territory, the fear that they may be overwhelmed by their hidden urges invariably holds them back.

MAKING THE SUBCONSCIOUS CONSCIOUS

But the will to recognize one's subconscious desires is not sufficient in itself. It cannot be done unaided as there is a strange world deep down in the depths—a world of thought associations, which the untutored cannot understand. It is the primitive world of superstition and magic, where it is logical to believe that, by eating the heart of one's slain foe, one acquires his courage. These are the crude beginnings of human thought which still exist in everyone's subconscious. The trained psychotherapist knows this "language of the subconscious" and deduces the connections of the repressed "remains" from the symptoms in the adult. He knows how to analyze the strange sign language of the subconscious.

DREAMS

Dreams are regarded by some psychotherapists as the most tangible expression of the subconscious. However, recent research indicates that dreaming is not necessarily restricted to humans but occurs in many species of animals, including cats and dogs, whose subconscious minds have thus far defied psychoanalysis. It has been suggested by some behavioral psychologists that dreams represent an effort of the subconscious mind to sort through recent events and experiences and attempt to fit them into a mosaic of memories from previous experiences. In prehistoric times, the subconscious activity of analyzing new experiences and storing them for future use may have been vital for human survival in a hostile environment. Modern man's survival, on the other hand, frequently depends upon understanding of words, numbers, and symbols rather than hunting food and hiding from hostile elements with the result that the mental images of the modern sleeping mind may be more complex and the individual's repressed fears and desires more difficult to interpret. One type of psychotherapy seeks to understand the troubled mind by studying one's dreams and nightmares.

Repressed desires can penetrate the open spaces of the soul in sleep and manifest themselves in hallucinatory wish-gratifications of the strangest kind. As a simple example, a hungry sleeper dreams that he is eating a chop. However, simple cases are rare and the desires underlying the gratifications dreamed are usually incomprehensible. It is an art to find one's way through this confusion. But psychotherapeutic treatment, with its analysis of dreams, awakens the train of associations into the lost depths of one's subconscious past that are causing harm. When expressly asked by the doctor to tell everything one can remember about a dream, a spate of ideas and memories follows and these explain the dream. This spate of memories bridges the gulf between the patient's early past and the subconscious wishes of his adult life. It is then possible for the patient to cope better with his repressed desires than he could in his immature early childhood. He tries, with the doctor's help, new and more adult ways of behavior in life. He tries to come to a new understanding with the world, which he had failed to do when he first encountered the world through his parents.

BASIC RULES

The most difficult rule to follow in psychotherapy is to divulge everything, no matter how senseless, irrelevant, embarrassing or indecent. This is the sort of "letting oneself go" that we all scrupulously avoid because of the fear lurking behind it. When danger from outside threatens, the body prepares for immediate action with emotions of terror. We human beings adopt exactly the same behavior to counter dangerous inner urges and instincts that threaten to invade our conscious life. This is terror—the fear of the unknown. The fear has a paralyzing effect. Our conscious personality impedes the freedom of our actions and defends itself with a fear reaction against being overrun by conscious urges.

THE PSYCHOTHERAPEUTIC SESSION

Dream interpretation and "free associations" are a part of a system of psychotherapy developed around the beginning of this century by Dr. Sigmund Freud, a psychoanalyst who practiced this method of treatment in Vienna. In psychoanalysis the patient lies (or sits) relaxed in a quiet room—preferably in such a way that he cannot see the doctor, who sits behind him. The patient talks. The doctor is almost entirely silent. He only prompts and gives the necessary explanations when the spate of "free associations," stimulated by a dream or a mistake, slows down. He confines himself to an occasional "Perhaps this may be the connection?" His surmises are followed by a question mark in the hope that sudden and swift recognition will dawn on the patient. The doctor's art is to see the connection and await the right moment for making his suggestions. It is, of course, useless for him simply to give the patient his own explanation of a symptom of illness or a character trait. The patient must always come to realize these things himself, and this is possible only when he has become strong enough to face up to the truth about himself. If instructed too early by the superior knowledge of the doctor, the patient's knowledge obstructs the emotional understanding of himself that is so necessary.

DEMOLISHING THE "INNER CAGE-BARS"

These psychotherapeutic sessions are not without fear, pain and tears. Repressed emotions, revived in recollection, are admitted to consciousness and are, so to speak, unloaded. This is, however, only one aspect and not the whole purpose of the work, which is the release of all the mental energy tied up in unnecessary internal struggles and constant tensions—in other words the demolition of the "inner cage-bars" which have cropped up so often in this book. The personality is liberated from its fetters so that it can deal in an adult fashion with the urges which surge up from the subconscious depths. In other words, the personality is untrammelled and free to follow its own pattern of life without crippling inhibitions. People then behave decently, not because they are afraid of their conscience, but because they agree with their conscience. The incomprehensible, morbid and unconscious part of the conscience known in psychotherapy as the super-ego—the "inner cage-bars"—has vanished. It no longer causes illness because it no longer diverts mental energy or allows constant tension to creep into the nervous system and influence the person's behavior.

PSYCHOANALYSIS

Formal, or Freudian, psychoanalysis still has a place in psychotherapy. But other methods have evolved in recent years, some based on Freud's original techniques and others representing approaches to treatment developed by psychotherapists who oppose the Freudian viewpoint toward mental ills. One system, founded by Alfred Adler, proposes that personality problems are related to self-preservation rather than sexual matters. The problem becomes manifest through an effort of the patient to overcompensate for an inferiority feeling, in the view of Adler, who coined the term "inferiority complex." Another psychotherapy pioneer, Carl Jung, who added the terms "introvert" and "extrovert" to the language of psychology, developed a concept that mental illness frequently could be traced to conflicts of religious beliefs and what he called the "racial unconscious," or experiences associated with one's heritage. Jung's technique involves word-association tests and "slips of the tongue" in revealing the inner conflicts of a patient. Karen Horney and Eric Fromm developed treatment methods based on cultural conflicts or the demands of society as opposed to the demands of nature.

Since World War II, Group Therapy has become a popular approach to the treatment of mental illness. Group therapy differs from the traditional method in which the patient discusses his problems in privacy with a psychotherapist by encouraging a group of patients with emotional or neurotic disorders to "talk out" their problems with each other while the therapist functions as a moderator. While the therapist directs the group, patients with similar problems frankly analyze and interpret the neuroses of other members of the group and each is helped while helping others. In addition to solving personal emotional problems, the patient learns to relate and participate with individuals from other walks of life so that he can function more effectively in society.

Psychodrama is a type of group therapy in which mentally disturbed patients "act out" their problems on a stage. Some of the patients may serve as spectators while others play the roles of actors or actresses. According to therapists who use psychodrama, both actors and spectators gain insight into their emotional ills through this technique. And in some cases, an individual patient may prefer to use the stage to reveal his personal conflicts as in a nightclub or vaudeville setting.

Play therapy has been used successfully in treating children with emotional disorders. The child is placed in a room, alone or with other children, with access to various dolls, doll houses, and other toys. Through the child's imaginative play, in which he may assign the roles of mother, father, siblings, and himself to the dolls, he reveals the sources of his fears, desires, or frustrations.

Occupational therapy is a more structured and adult version of play therapy in which the patient is given supplies for painting, carving, or drawing whatever may help to express a clue to his neurosis. Other handicraft types of work also are available, usually, such as weaving or woodworking. As in group therapy, the patient mingles with other disturbed persons and develops empathy for others in discovering that he is not the only individual with a troubled mind. Still another benefit of occupational therapy is that the patient gains confidence in himself through achieving certain goals, such as completing a bookbinding or woodworking project.

Reality therapy is based on the concept that personality development in childhood is normally modified by demands of parents and other adults so that the individual becomes "unreal" by the time he reaches his own adulthood. The therapy is directed toward helping the patient to find his "real self" and to escape from the pseudomorphic personality that he has acquired in order to earn the love of his parents.

Encounter groups, primal therapy, assertive therapy, graphotherapy, shock therapy, and hypnosis are among other approaches developed and practiced, sometimes in combination with other methods, by various therapists. Insulin shock therapy, for example, may be used with music therapy as an adjunct. Or insulin shock may be used in combination with electric shock therapy. The choice of methods, as in the treatment of organic illness, usually is selected according to the type of mental disorder, the general condition of the patient, and the experience of the therapist in treating similar cases.

LARGE TOWNS AND UPBRINGING

Earlier generations were more fortunate. Their children had more freedom. They could go out in the open air and observe nature. Sexual processes in the animal kingdom were always available for study; when they tried to relate these to human processes the observation of animals enlightened them. There were always numerous children, and parents only occasionally intervened or reprimanded them. They grew up freely. Today we and our children live under more congested conditions than former generations, and for that reason we must know more because we have far more opportunity of doing harm through our ignorance. It would not be a bad thing to incorporate study of the development of a child's mind, as revealed by recent research, as a final-year subject at school. By this a great deal of harm might be avoided for the next generation.

MENTAL HYGIENE

In the past half-century, knowledge has been acquired in all branches of medicine that has been made possible only by studies of the interaction of the mind and body. As a result of co-operation between psychiatrist and physician, a whole series of illnesses of unknown causation could be understood and effectively treated for the first time.

These sections on "Psychosomatic Medicine" (page 232) and "Illnesses Which Originate in the Mind" (page 249) deal with this revolutionary and epoch-making knowledge in so far as deemed necessary for the purpose of this book. These illnesses are a particularly rewarding part of our work, as I discovered in my years of experience of enlightening laymen in regard to matters of health. In many cases understanding helps patients along the way to recovery. Once you have grasped the obvious fact that body and mind are one and belong to each other and that illnesses of the "nerves" have nothing to do with a weak will, you do not try idiotically to overcome your "weakness," which would only make you more ill. Of course this cannot be done in a day. It takes time. But knowing about these things is just as important as the basic knowledge of infectious diseases and their prevention, which we all possess —i.e. that we must keep ourselves and our food and dwellings clean. This is physical hygiene. What has been written here about illnesses of mental-nervous functions is the foundation of mental hygiene, which can save us from equally serious and protracted complaints. It is something that few know and that everyone should know.

Physical hygiene is a matter of protecting oneself and others against infectious diseases. Mental hygiene is a matter of protecting oneself against ailments such as high blood-pressure, stomach ulcers, over-functioning of the thyroid, asthma, heart disease, colitis, rheumatism and numerous other complaints— and how to protect children from errors and defects of upbringing, which make them liable to mental and psychosomatic illnesses.

12. On Begetting Children

It is easy to become a father, but to behave as one is very difficult" is an old saying and one which on the whole is still true. Motherhood is quite another proposition. We know that it is the more laborious part of parenthood. It involves every part of a woman, and that is saying a great deal. It is either the beginning of a new phase for the body or denial of its fulfilment. Only too often do we forget the significance of this denial on the part of the woman. Her physical and mental sex processes reach completion only with the birth of the child and in breast-feeding it. In spite of all talk of equality, there is a difference, and the mother is the more important partner. The least that a person deserves is a thorough understanding of the physical and mental processes of sex life. Enlightenment on matters of sex is necessary for healthy family life. It does away with the old male prejudices about woman's position and relegates man to his rightful position. So we are going to try to give a complete picture of the normal process of sex.

How It Happens

First of all there must be two people; one with healthy and mature testicles and the other with ovaries in the same state. In the testicles there are mature seed cells ready to be released. In the ovaries there are egg cells which are capable of being fertilized. One of these becomes detached and lies in the Fallopian tube ready to meet the sperm.

Secondly there are sex hormones in both partners' blood. In a woman their composition fluctuates rhythmically with the menstrual cycle, while in a man they are more even. Without these hormones there can be no "love," no sex interest.

Thirdly there is a feeling of longing and loneliness in both sexes and an urge to come together. This comes directly from an instinct and can take on a thousand different guises. In women it takes the form of an instinctive desire to be attractive in gesture, demeanor and voice and a longing to be touched. Men are bent more on impressing themselves upon women and possessing them, by force if necessary. Underlying all this there is a feeling of longing, being lonely, and painful incompleteness. We can leave the poets to describe all the forms which these various emotions take—it is their stock-in-trade.

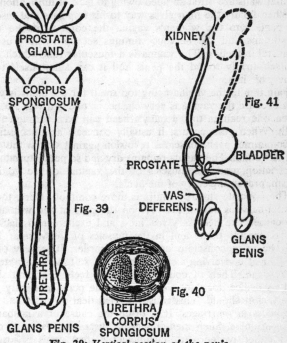

Fig. 39: *Vertical section of the penis.*
Fig. 40: *Transverse section of the penis.*
Fig. 41: *Male genito-urinary organs.*

The nervous tension of these emotions paves the way for the act of sex. The distribution of blood is directed to the sexual organs. This is obvious in the male. The blood-vessels

which supply his genital organs become so dilated that there
is an increased blood supply to the penis so that it can become
erect. The penis is distended with blood. The penis consists of
tissue, known as erectile tissue, in the hollow spaces of which
extra blood is contained. A similar thing happens in the female. Her erectile tissue is situated in the labia, on each side
of the vaginal orifice, and in the clitoris.

Another indispensable effect of this sexual excitement is
the secretion by the female of mucus which lubricates the
vaginal orifice. In cases of rape, when disgust and horror prevent any sexual excitement on the part of the woman, the
vaginal walls are often abraded owing to lack of lubrication.

When finally the man gives way to his impulses and inserts
his penis into the woman's vagina the contact of the two
sex organs and the nervous stimulus set up by it cause a
pleasurable feeling. The vagina is a muscular tube which can
fit itself firmly round the penis and it can adapt itself to a
variety of sizes.

Pain due to the vagina being too small for the penis is very
rare because the vagina is very elastic, as one can well believe
when one realizes that a baby's head can pass through it at
birth. When pain occurs, it usually conceals an unconscious
or sometimes even conscious revulsion against sex on the part
of the woman. The vagina remains dry and so pain is produced
by friction, and the muscles of the vaginal orifice go into
spasm, preventing entry of the penis.

The opposite state of affairs is more common. Here, too, a
mental-nervous sexual disorder on the part of the woman is
the cause. The necessary readiness and excitement is lacking
in her erectile tissue and in the muscles of the vagina. This
may be an unconscious emotional disorder. It is very often
the fear of conceiving a child. The body, so to speak, pretends
to be dead. Then of course the vagina feels wide and slack
and its orifice does not close around the penis as tightly and
firmly as it should. This causes a great deal of upset and unhappiness in marriages. It is often the cause of a husband's
unfaithfulness. Such mental-nervous discrepancies may occur
with either partner. An insufficiently erect penis is just as
much a hindrance as an insufficiently taut vagina, and this,
too, scarcely ever has physical causes. It is almost always the
outcome of a mental disorder, even if only a temporary one.
A pessimistic, timid mood prevents the necessary firmness in
the male.

This question is so important that one should immediately

consider taking steps to overcome the difficulty. Let me repeat once more that anatomical differences in the size of the male and female sex organs almost never upset marital happiness (the normal vagina is 3–4 in. long and the normal penis about 6 in. long and 1–1½ in. across when erect). When unconscious emotional disorders are responsible for the organs being badly prepared for the sexual act, one can improve the local conditions without resorting to psychotherapy. The muscles of the vaginal orifice are voluntary ones and therefore amenable to will-power. For this reason they can be trained, like any other muscles. They can be strengthened, and this helps a great deal—perhaps many a marriage may be saved in this way. Things such as this about which one does not speak can have dire effects, sometimes more so than open quarrels waged with curses and tears. So take courage and discuss these matters if they are not satisfactory. There is nothing sinful or vicious about this.* On the contrary—by sensible preventive measures one can avert the tragedy of a disappointed marriage partner becoming addicted to vice, be it alcoholism or sexual immorality. It is better that we should revise our conceptions of cannubial "pleasure" rather than give rise to unhappiness because of false modesty.

THE SEXUAL ACT

The preparatory swellings and muscle tensions in the genital organs of both sexes are necessary to produce sufficient stimulation conducive to the completion of the act of sex. One should not regard the whole business in a disinterested way or as though it were a disagreeable duty that has to be performed. This applies to both partners. To do so is equally detrimental to the health of both sexes and does one's marriage partner the worst possible service. It is more harmful to one's marriage than the occasional complete refusal to have sexual intercourse. (The latter is not grounds for divorce, as some people erroneously believe, but applies only when the refusal is consistent.) In fact, it is sometimes better to avoid intercourse if you are not in the mood for it. On the contrary —abstaining can occasionally increase your own excitability so you can subsequently give your partner more complete satisfaction again.

Unfortunately we are accustomed to glossing over these matters with false modesty and do not devote our conscious attention to them. Many women still have the feeling that they must submit to the "beast" in man, as "duty" demands it. They have the utterly false feeling of complete passiveness, which, looked at crudely, means simply regarding themselves as no more than a means for man's self-gratification. It amounts almost to being bought in exchange for the housekeeping money. One must revise this state of affairs, for without real union in marriage there can be no marital faithfulness and the way to "sin" is paved. All sexual intercourse with a partner who does not inwardly enjoy it or, because of a mental-nervous disorder, cannot enjoy it, leaves an empty feeling. On looking at the matter more closely, it is a feeling of having been cheated.

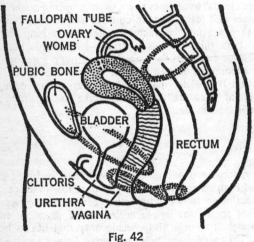

FALLOPIAN TUBE
OVARY
WOMB
PUBIC BONE
BLADDER
RECTUM
CLITORIS
URETHRA
VAGINA

Fig. 42

Sagittal section of the female pelvis (dotted rings show important muscles).

It is a blow to masculine pride if one's wife remains cold, even if the husband feels that he has had his "pleasure." An undigested mental remnant remains, which disturbs him and makes every other woman appear to him as a temptation, and there is a secret longing to try and see whether things would not succeed better with them. There can never be real satisfaction when only one of the partners achieves this. A wife can hold her man only if she herself is satisfied and not by merely submitting to him—and certainly not with reproach and tears.

However, let us return to the normal procedure. The nervous stimulation brought about by the friction of the genital organs in sexual intercourse causes a violent surge of emotion. This delicious tension increases until it reaches a peak, where in ideal cases the hitherto voluntary controlled movements of the pelvis in both partners become automatic; muscles and erectile tissue of the sex organs themselves stretch to bursting-point, and finally, with rhythmical muscular contraction, the man's semen is released. The ultimate crescendo of feeling that marks the release or ejaculation also is known as orgasm. A similar response, without ejaculation, occurs in the woman.

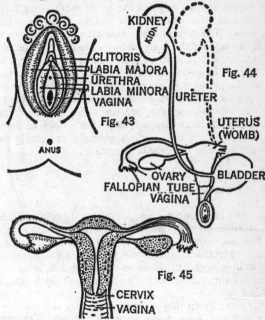

Fig. 43: *Diagram of the vulva.*
Fig. 44: *Female genito-urinary organs.*
Fig. 45: *Diagram of the womb, Fallopian tubes, ovaries, and vagina.*

The sperm cells travel rapidly, for their size, and about one percent of the hundreds of millions of sperm ejaculated by the male during coitus can be found within the womb only three minutes after the sex act. The mobility of the sperm is aided by chemical changes in the cervical mucus following ovulation. The female orgasm during coitus is quite complex and, according to recent research, may involve both the vagina and the clitoris, which is situated just above the vagina. The clitoris is a small collection of erectile tissue situated at the front of the junction of the inner lips of the vulva. It contains numerous sensory nerves and is the masturbation organ of small girls. The organ corresponds to the male penis and may increase in size during the initial phase of sexual excitement. However, it does not become erect like a penis; in fact, it withdraws as sexual excitement continues while the walls of the vagina become swollen with blood, reducing the opening of the vagina so that it grips the penis more firmly. During actual orgasm, the walls of the vagina undergo waves of contractions. The womb also undergoes contractions as do muscles throughout the body of the woman. Once the peak of sexual excitement is reached, the contractions occur, like the male orgasm, in an involuntary manner. After the orgasm is reached, the changes in anatomy and physiology revert back to the pre-excitement stage, unless sexual excitement continues, in which case the orgasm cycle can be repeated. Psychological factors also are important. Fear of having a child, for example, is a serious obstacle to female orgasm and one which can scarcely be overcome.

WHAT IS NORMAL?

Excessive intercourse does not cause detectable ill-health. With sensible people things are adjusted automatically. If there has been excess, excitement wanes, and that is that. This can vary very much at different times. With a young couple madly in love intercourse can be extremely frequent.

Statistics show that, on the average, men up to the age of thirty-five years have sexual intercourse about three or four times a week. From then to the age of fifty the average number of orgasms goes down to twice a week. This includes married and unmarried men, homosexuals, and those who predominantly practise masturbation. Taking the married ones only, the figures show that, at the age of twenty, intercourse takes place five times a week, and from then to fifty-five the figures gradually but steadily drop to twice a week. An average of seven times a week is found in not quite 10 per cent of all men, including adolescents (at least according to statistics compiled in the U.S.A.). After fifty years of age this applies to only two per cent, and so a lot of the boasts heard in taverns and clubs should be taken with a pinch of salt.

Probably the figures would be higher if one's sexual efficiency were not hampered by mental inhibitions. Voluntary abstinence may not be counted as a mental inhibition of this kind. The sections found on page 93 and also on page 228 deal with the influence of abstinence on one's mental efficiency.

These figures give one information about normal masculine sexuality. There are not many statistics for women, but it is likely that they are similar to men in this respect. There is, however, one main difference. Their sexual needs vary periodically in intensity. In the physiological sense one must accept as normal an increased desire in the first days after menstruation when the discomfort of premenstrual tension is ended. However, this is not the same in all women. The time of greatest sexual need can occur at any phase of the sexual cycle, including the days of the monthly period itself. However, sexual needs can vary in any woman.

INCREASED SEXUAL NEED

With some women the need for increased sex may not be genuine but rather an expression of a lack of satisfaction with the acts of sex she has experienced. In the great majority of healthy women and men sexual craving takes on an unpleasantly urgent character after any involuntary abstinence of more than fourteen days. But here too the law of "usually" must be applied. By and large one can depend upon it that the body itself will restrict the frequency of sexual intercourse. Incidentally, the body is much more efficient in this respect than one imagines, as every married person probably knows from his honeymoon. There are no fixed rules. Great frequency (e.g. over twenty times a week) makes one suspect that satisfaction derived from the act is incomplete. A remnant of excitement remains to provoke fresh stimuli. That is pronounced in all forms of sexual behavior which makes one partner insatiable because there is no real satisfaction.

POSITIONS FOR SEXUAL INTERCOURSE

This is a matter of personal taste and therefore it is idle to discuss what is "normal" or "abnormal." Judging by the anatomy of the genital organs, the "normal" thing would be for the penis to be inserted from behind. At any rate the vaginal orifice can be most easily reached from behind, and both sex partners then have the greatest freedom of movement. The natural curve of the vagina in this position adapts itself to the curve of the penis most completely and so this position is perhaps more conducive to conception than any other.

In primitive man the customary position seems to have been one in which the woman squatted over the man lying on his back. At any rate the oldest picture depicting the human sexual act shows the couple in this position. Also in pictures derived from the oldest human civilizations (Central America, India, China, and Mesopotamia) and from classical times, this position is the one most frequently depicted. It would appear to be particularly favorable for producing female orgasm. Here she plays the "active part"—a role which some men in our Western civilization still resent. Nevertheless, it is from this position that the woman is better able to guide the complicated process in such a way as to meet a need for compatibility in sexual intercourse. And for psychological as well as medical reasons, the position in which the man lies on his back frequently is recommended for intercourse when the woman is relatively frigid. But, unfortunately, sexual practices can be influenced and modified by cultural backgrounds of husband and wife. In such cases it is wrong to endanger one's marriage because of masculine resentment with the sexual position. Marriage partners must occasionally have an earnest heart-to-heart talk about such things as in this way they can avoid much distress.

The usual position adopted in our present Western civilization is not the natural one, but an artificial one, which has become a habit. Erotically speaking, it has the advantage of a more tender and intimate contact of both bodies and corresponds to a traditional concept of masculine superiority in that the man lies on the woman. Many non-Western peoples find this way of performing the sexual act distasteful. It is a good thing, if one uses this seemingly most convenient position, to raise the woman's pelvis by the use of a pillow.

Laymen are inclined to grossly overrate the importance of knowledge concerning different positions. This is not important. All that matters is the fundamental capacity for love of both partners and their simultaneous and complete satisfaction. It is only during pregnancy that the usual position should obviously be modified, because of pressure on the woman's abdomen.

There are great differences between the various social classes with regard to being dressed or undressed during intercourse and as to whether it takes place with the light on or in the dark. In general men find nakedness an added attraction, and the same applies to lighting. With men vision plays an erotic part which should not be underrated. Women who are not inhibited sexually feel an "instinctive" need to exhibit themselves to their beloved. Statistics show that the upper social classes of the population have greater freedom in these things. According to one statistical study, 90 percent of people in academic professions have intercourse naked, while only 50 per cent of the working classes do so. These differences apply to an even greater extent to the positions used for intercourse. Seventy-five per cent of poorer people stick rigidly to the conventional position, while among educated people nearly 50 per cent "experiment." There are good reasons for this, since "frigidity" among educated women is regarded more as a disorder to be overcome than in other circles, where it is inclined to be accepted and no attempt made to deal with it.

It must be mentioned that touching the genital organs with the hands or mouth before intercourse is no longer regarded as a perversion since large-scale investigation shows that the former is done by 80 per cent of all married and unmarried persons, while the latter is customary in almost half of all marriages between educated people and in one-quarter of marriages between uneducated ones. It could, however, cause disaster in marriage if one of the partners were disgusted because the other expressed such a desire. It is difficult to say whether or not such habits are desirable.

In order to avoid misunderstandings between marriage partners, they should know about the average duration of the sexual act. In about three-quarters of men orgasm takes place within two minutes of insertion of the penis. In a considerable proportion the time is less than a minute, and this in many cases is unsatisfactory from the woman's point of view, above all if she is at all frigid. For this reason a number of men learn to delay their own orgasm. But it is questionable whether this voluntary control of a natural function, in itself automatic, is good when ejaculation avoidance is carried to extremes. One relatively harmless side effect is that the sperm may be forced into the man's urinary bladder. Ironically, some men who suffer from psychogenic aspermia can maintain an erection indefinitely without ejaculation, but they experience no sexual satisfaction.

Another thing should be made clear at this juncture. The sexual urge of a normal woman is not extinguished with the change of life. With the menopause all is not over, as many people wrongly believe (see page 230). So one need not be self-conscious or regard oneself as unnatural if, despite "advancing years," one still feels sexual desire. This is what happens in all healthy people. Love does not stop.

Some readers may be surprised that we have dealt in such detail with these intimate matters. They may perhaps feel that in a book on health we should have confined ourselves to a few remarks about physical harm incurred through sexual intercourse and its morbid perversions. We have been detailed because we realize—and stressed it at the beginning of this chapter—that a complete knowledge of everything pertaining to sex life is an indispensable foundation for mental stability.

It is not only disorders of a purely mental nature that can originate from ignorance of these matters. Mental-nervous disorders of this kind often form the starting-point of psychosomatic ailments—the most widespread group of illnesses known to human beings. With our ancestors things were different. Their methods of upbringing, as has already been stressed over and over again, were quite different from our present-day measures. The large family of children living outdoor lives were able, despite their upbringing, to develop into healthy people. Their knowledge was derived directly from nature and from older playmates. Their sexuality was only rarely inhibited. Nowadays, in large cities, with fewer children in the family and under constant supervision, things are quite different. Many children become victims of their upbringing. One simple difference is that formerly a child (on account of its greater freedom) was only caught in the act of doing something wrong every tenth or hundredth time, whereas the present-day town child is probably caught almost every fifth time it does something it shouldn't.

This change in our conditions of living compels us to devote ourselves more intensively to sexual matters and to questions of upbringing from the medical point of view. This does not mean that medical science is immoral or that people are more immoral. They simply live differently and old customs and habits no longer apply.

CONCEPTION

The actual biological and instinctive purpose of the sexual act is conception, and there is no escaping this fact. Everything in the bodies and souls of two healthy people strives for this in their union. This can be recognized in the woman's emotions by her need to receive and to give herself completely to the male. In man it manifests itself in the need to give everything, to be generous, and in longing for the

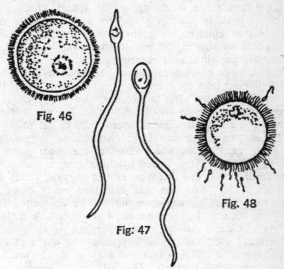

Fig. 46   Fig. 48

Fig: 47

Fig. 46: *The female egg.*   **Fig. 47:** *Sperm.*

Fig. 48: *Penetration of female egg by sperm.*

woman's tender surrender.

In the sexual act the seed cells (sperm) released by the man reach the womb almost directly during intercourse. Although some experts claim they are helped along by activity of the female organs, the semen ejected by the male contains hundreds of millions of living sperm which are highly motile and reach the womb in a few minutes by their own power. They wriggle forward quickly, propelled by their tails, and can travel 70 times their own length in one minute.

The chemical secretions of the vagina are highly unfavorable for the seed cells (except during phases of the monthly period). After one hour in the vagina they have usually lost their ability to move. Outside the body they can live for days if kept cold; at a temperature of 98.6 degrees they can last for fifteen to eighteen hours. In the neck of the womb they live for two days, in the womb itself twenty-four hours, and in the Fallopian tubes for about two days.

There is some doubt about the role of the female orgasm in insuring fertilization of the egg by the sperm. The vagina is the worst possible "storage place" for sperm. Despite this the majority of children are probably produced without female orgasm. By shutting off her emotions, the woman does not safeguard herself against conceiving a child.

If a female egg which is capable of being fertilized is ready in the Fallopian tube or womb, or if it is released from the ovary within two days after intercourse, then the sperm cells can penetrate it and bring about fertilization. For this it seems necessary for a large number of sperm cells to get near the egg. An enzyme is released from disintegrated or possibly from living sperm cells, which dissolves the outer covering of the egg. This enzyme, called hyaluronidase, is indispensable to fertilization. The discovery of this enzyme, which occurred about 30 years ago, has explained many cases of childlessness which previously could not be accounted for. Taking into account the varying content of a counter-substance (anti-hyaluronidase) in the female organs, it is possible to understand such mysterious happenings as the fact that both partners of a childless marriage may be able to produce children with other partners. The balance of enzyme and counter-enzyme was unfavorable in them, but not with other partners when they marry again.

Other causes of childlessness are due to obstructions in the spermatic duct of the man or of the Fallopian tubes of the woman. A frequent cause of this is gonorrhea, although many other kinds of bacterial infection, including tuberculosis, can result in Fallopian tube obstruction. Gonorrhea is not always diagnosed at an early stage in women, allowing tubal inflammation to remain undetected. (See p. 163.)

If a sperm cell succeeds in penetrating a female egg which is fertile, it then amalgamates (its head is virtually only a cell nucleus) with the nucleus of the egg cell to form the new creature. This decisive stage—the actual fertilization—takes place from some hours up to two days after copulation. The child's sex is always determined by the sperm. There are "female-producing" and "male-producing" seed cells in the sperm of every man, which invariably contains both kinds of cells.

The view held by laymen that boys are produced out of one of the two testicles and girls out of the other is wrong. It is also erroneous to believe that the two ovaries of the woman have a similar significance. All egg cells, regardless of their origin, can be fertilized to produce either male or female embryos.

It is not possible to determine beforehand the sex of the child. The most one can say is (and here again one is obliged to fall back on the law of "usually") that some statistical studies show that children conceived in the first half of the monthly period are girls and in the second half boys. Studies also show more boys are conceived but more male embryos also fail to survive. It may well be that the mucous membrane of the womb in the last days of the fertile days (normally the fifteenth to eighteenth day) is better prepared for the lodgement of the embryo.

Another strange observation has been made about predetermining the child's sex. In times of war and in illicit sexual relations very many more boys are born than girls. The only common factor in both circumstances is the fact that sexual intercourse is much less frequent, but has a more intensive character. The man on leave and the lover are, generally speaking, more passionate than the everyday husband. Perhaps by artificially creating such conditions the sex of the child may be influenced. In any case there can be no harm in voluntary abstinence from time to time in order to give one's connubial love a new impetus.

There may occasionally be medical reasons for determining the sex of the child prior to delivery. For this purpose, some drops of amniotic fluid are aspirated from the womb with a needle and syringe. The fluid contains cells detached from the mucous membranes of the child. Examination of these under the microscope allows one to determine the sex. There can be very few occasions when this is necessary and there might be grave psychological consequences resulting from disappointment if the practice were used inadvisedly. The process of birth might well be more difficult if the mother consciously resented the child not being of the desired sex. But the new-born child can engender love that smothers any disappointment originally felt because the other sex was desired.

Women who know and observe their bodily feelings particularly well maintain that they already know when they have conceived, hours or the day after copulation. This interesting contention has not yet been checked scientifically. But it is certain that the hormonal processes in the pituitary, the ovaries and the mucous membrane of the womb change in a very short time. About two weeks after the first missed period, pregnancy usually can be diagnosed by blood and urine tests.

It is quite probable that this change manifests itself much sooner in the woman's mental-nervous state. It is the beginning of the normal change in character in the healthy woman during the time of pregnancy, the beginning of a time of inner peace and serenity, of heightened joy and a feeling of comfort in one's own body, but also a time of increased susceptibility to illnesses of all kinds. The purely "female-maternal" side of the woman is predominant. Progesterone, the hormone of the second half of the monthly cycle, also dominates pregnancy.

BIRTH CONTROL

The sex urge consists not only of a longing to be sexually excited but in many adult men and women a frequently repressed desire to procreate. The true function of the natural sex urge is to continue the lineage of the species, whether in humans or other animals. And Nature's method of insuring continuation of the human species is through the temptation of sexual excitement. But man has since very ancient times devised techniques of birth control that would permit enjoyment of sexual excitement while limiting somewhat the risk of unintentional procreation. Some of the earliest known drawings by cavemen show males wearing penile sheaths.

Penile sheaths, or condoms, are still used by a large proportion of modern men even though recent studies published by the Planned Parenthood Federation of America show that the rate of failure for this birth control device is about 10 per cent per year. Still less effective is the diaphragm; some 17 percent of women using that method become pregnant within a year. Even the oral contraceptives, which are highly promoted as the most fool-proof method of birth control, have a failure rate of four percent in the first year. The IUD, or intrauterine contraceptive device, results in five percent unwanted pregnancies per year, according to the study.

Overall, the survey of the use of birth control among many thousands of married women in America in the 1970s revealed that approximately one-third of all couples who employed the use of contraceptives in order to enjoy sexual activity without the risk of parenthood did conceive a child within five years. On the other hand, the rate of unwanted pregnancies was only about half the number of the previous decade, before general public education about birth control was started. Also, despite the rate of failures, and the risks of side effects from oral contraceptive use by some women, most doctors agree that the hazards of unwanted pregnancies both to individual mothers and to the community in general require a better understanding of the conflict between the urge to enjoy sexual activity and the strong natural drive to procreate.

It is noteworthy that recent surveys of Roman Catholics show they are now as successful in preventing unwanted pregnancies as people of other faiths. And the rate of failure of the rhythm method of birth control is only 20 percent, which is nearly as effective as use of a diaphragm. And either technique is twice as effective as douching.

Beyond moral reasons against birth control, there are practical considerations to be faced. The increase in hygienic conditions of living has resulted in (1) a great reduction in infant mortality and (2) has considerably prolonged people's youth and also the time of their procreative ability. The change of life in women now starts on an average a good ten years later than it used to. (3) Wars and epidemics no longer take their toll of life as much as formerly. (4) Thanks to improved medical care, stillbirths and miscarriages are rarer. (5) Owing to our changed conditions of living, children nowadays are a source of great expense, whereas in former times they grew up virtually free of cost in the country and provided valuable additional labor. So they used to be a real blessing, while they now constitute a burden, however delighted one is to have them. (6) Despite all efforts the sex urge has refused to be controlled. Limiting one's family by complete abstinence over many years is a demand which no married couple can fulfil. (7) The largest number of children known to have been born to a single couple is sixty-nine! (This includes twins, triplets, and quadruplets.) Modern living conditions would soon equal or even beat this unique record if we did not practice birth control. (8) All told we should multiply at least six times as quickly as our great-grandparents if we did not use birth control.

It is sufficient to bear these facts in mind in order to appreciate the necessity for birth control. There is no need to conjure up fantastic visions of over-population and mutual cannibalism! One need not start working out figures or studying economics. It is simply impossible to do without birth control.

FERTILE AND NON-FERTILE DAYS

Since the idea of voluntarily restricting sex life on the part of any appreciably large proportion of people is purely theoretical and possible only in one's imagination, the fact is that the vast majority use contraceptives when they have sexual intercourse. This is in a way a perversion of the sex urge, but it is inevitable that people will do so, and it is an important task of this book to rob this practice, forced upon us by necessity, of any harmful aspects, detrimental to health.

Having read the contents of this book so far, we already know that, according to the law of "usually," there are regularly recurring periods of greater and lesser fertility in a woman's monthly sexual cycle (see also page 226). The desire for a child can be fulfilled by having sexual intercourse on definite days, and the size and spacing of the family can be planned by avoiding sexual intercourse on these days.

In a normal woman the most fertile days are always from the thirteenth to the sixteenth day of every twenty-eight day cycle. The days are always counted from the first day of the monthly period. There is also a good likelihood of conception from the ninth to the twelfth and from the seventeenth to the eighteenth day. So the time when conception is most likely extends from the ninth to the eighteenth day of the twenty-eight-day cycle.

In women whose cycles last a longer or shorter time all dates change by exactly the amount the cycle is prolonged or shortened. This of course applies only when periods are regularly shortened or prolonged over many months. To make things plain, the fertile and most fertile days indicated in the following chart are for cycles of twenty-four to thirty-two days.

Cycle length in days	Fertile time	Most fertile time
24	6th-14th day	9th-12th day
25	7th-15th "	10th-13th "
26	7th-16th "	11th-14th "
27	8th-17th "	12th-15th "
28	9th-18th "	13th-16th "
29	9th-19th "	14th-17th "
30	10th-20th "	15th-18th "
31	11th-21st "	16th-19th "
32	12th-22nd "	17th-20th "

The time when conception is most likely is usually the time of "follicle rupture"—the moment when a mature egg leaves the ovary and is ready for fertilization. To be quite certain of being helped by the chart, you must first keep a written record of the length of your own cycles for a period of some months. (To rely on memory is inadequate.) If the time varies between twenty-eight and twenty-nine days (one day later than previously), then the fertile days will run from the ninth to the nineteenth day, and the days when conception is most likely from the thirteenth to the seventeenth. If the cycle is more irregular, this simple chart will not be able to help you.

Cycles of longer than thirty-three to thirty-five days often have no "follicle rupture" and therefore represent a non-fertile period. Women with occasional shortened cycles probably tend to release eggs from their ovaries under the influence of particularly satisfying sexual intercourse or other mental or nervous excitement.

One can greatly simplify the fixing of these dates by keeping a regular check on one's temperature for several months. The temperature should be taken every morning with a clinical thermometer under the tongue and recorded. The dates of the monthly periods should also be noted. Then (apart from any feverish illness) one will always find a rise in temperature of about half a degree roughly in the middle of the cycle. The temperature goes up about half a degree with the "follicle rupture," and stays high until the next period starts. If you ascertain in this way, for example, that the fifteenth day is the one on which the egg is released, you can deduce the most fertile and relatively fertile days by reckoning two days before and two days after the date of egg release.

This regular variation between fertile and non-fertile days is more reliable when sex life in marriage is regular and even, i.e. when long periods of absence enforced by the husband's or wife's profession do not result in periods of intensive love-making alternating with periods of abstinence. When sex life is regular, the dates are more likely to be reliable. Any form of excitement such as holiday journeys with a change of climate, being greatly in love, wedding nights and the like, upset the regular hormonal processes. The same applies to feverish illnesses and to all external influences which, as we learn from experience, may bring about a change in the dates of one's monthly periods. Every woman knows best herself which influences affect her. The more stable a woman's emotional life, the more can she depend on fixed fertile and less-fertile days with clockwork precision. Erratic people's hormones also behave erratically. For this reason every woman is advised to check her period dates and body temperature for months before relying on her fertile and less-fertile days. But here it must be emphasized again that biological laws are not 100 per cent reliable. None the less, by understanding one's own body and by careful observation one may sense a deviation in time if one has learned to interpret the corresponding symptoms. This is all learned during the period of observation, when the period dates and body temperature are checked.

Undoubtedly this method of limiting one's family by paying attention to the natural change of a woman's fertility—"the rhythm method"—is regarded by many as a sensible one. But for others, the release of the natural sexual urge may be hampered. Spontaneity which comes naturally must be restrained at times to conform with a calendar. These periods of restraint can, in turn, lead to a buildup of tensions which may strain the marital relationship. And the urge does not necessarily diminish as the partners mature. The nearer a woman is to the change of life the more difficult for her is the inner renunciation. The "urge to conceive" is not always lessened by the presence of children already in the family. On the contrary— in many cases this helps to arouse it.

This method of observing the woman's likely days of conception, devised by Professors Knaus and Ogino, is the kind of birth control traditionally accepted by the Roman Catholic Church. Those who follow the practice should be aware of the personal demands required to make it effective and accept the fact that the rhythm method, even when followed as conscientiously as possible, may not prove reliable.

OTHER METHODS OF CONTRACEPTION

Probably the most primitive method is the one of withdrawing the penis shortly before the male orgasm and release of sperm. If practised constantly this can cause mental-nervous disorders even in the most robust person. It is the worst and most dangerous interruption of the urge, and perverts most strongly the emotional purpose of the sexual act. From the medical point of view I cannot warn you too strongly against it. The woman in particular suffers as a result. The man generally has a sort of orgasm, even though incomplete, but the woman usually remains entirely unsatisfied. Just at the moment when one's emotions cry out for the most tender union, the act is interrupted and perverted from its essential purpose. This practice, which is regularly carried out by many couples in ignorance of other methods, has caused untold suffering and broken up countless marriages.

An almost equally ineffective method is the vaginal douche directly after intercourse. It is not very reliable as a birth control measure for the reason that sperm can travel to the uterus from the vagina at a remarkably rapid pace. Even if douching is carried out immediately after ejaculation by the male partner, it is possible that water flushed through the vagina, with or without the addition of a mild disinfectant, will arrive too late to prevent fertilization if the woman has just ovulated. Douching also demands a promptness on the woman's part which is not compatible with the peaceful bliss she might otherwise enjoy after sexual intercourse. It is, of course, out of the question for strict Roman Catholics, as are other "artificial" birth-control methods. They include the condom, or sheath for the penis, made of thin rubber or animal membrane, and the cervical cap and cervical diaphragm for women. These devices serve as mechanical barriers against the tide of sperm that would otherwise be free to travel from the penis of the male to the woman's Fallopian tubes. Spermatocidal foams, creams, or jellies sometimes are used instead of or in addition to the mechanical devices. Injected into the vagina before intercourse, the substances kill the sperm. Spermatocides and mechanical barriers are more effective than douches or withdrawing the penis as birth-control methods. Still more effective, however, are the oral contraceptive pills and the intrauterine contraceptive devices, or IUD's. The oral contraceptives, now used by millions of women, contain estrogens or progestogens, alone or in combination. They mimic a woman's natural hormones to suppress ovulation. IUD's are plastic or metal coils implanted in the womb to prevent implantation by a fertilized egg.

ABORTION

Since the 1973 U.S. Supreme Court decision, women in the United States are permitted to have an abortion during the first six months of a pregnancy. And the deliberate interruption of a pregnancy by surgical removal of an embryo or early-stage fetus from the womb is no longer considered a criminal act. Historically, laws against surgical abortion, as contrasted with natural or spontaneous abortion in which an unborn child is lost through miscarriage, were passed in the 19th century when abortion procedures were much more dangerous than they are today.

A primary concern of the past was that many doctors were reluctant to violate the law by performing an unauthorized abortion and women wishing to terminate a pregnancy usually had to resort to the services of persons who were willing to perform abortions even though they were not trained in medical skills. There were great physical dangers in illegal abortions, including the possibility of an infection of the pelvic organs, septicemia, and death from excessive loss of blood. Usually there was little regard for the necessary cleanliness (sterility) observed in proper operations, and unskilled hands using unsuitable instruments can easily cause serious damage to the reproductive system, leading to hemorrhage. Improved techniques developed in recent years, however, are relatively safe, efficient, and quick. One device now in rather common use is called a vacuum aspirator. It can remove the embryonic material from the inside of the womb by suction in less than 10 minutes.

Not all abortions were illegal in the past. An abortion previously could be authorized if doctors decided that the health of the pregnant woman was so poor that the birth of a child would endanger her life. The more recent legal attitude is that abortions during the last trimester, or last three-month period of pregnancy, must be restricted to cases in which the health of the mother would be seriously threatened if the pregnancy were allowed to continue. But during the first two trimesters, the decision of whether or not to abort a pregnancy can be made between the woman and her doctor without violation of the law.

Despite the more liberal legal attitude toward abortions, there are a few laws of nature that still prevail and which need to be considered by the woman contemplating an abortion. One is that a surgical abortion can be performed much more easily during the first few weeks of pregnancy. In the early stage, within perhaps 21 days after a missed period, a doctor can insert a tiny plastic cannula into the uterus and remove the embryonic material with a minimum of pain and complications. This procedure may be similar to dilatation and curettage (D & C) in which the lining of the uterus is scraped free of an implanted embryo or the embryonic material removed with a vacuum aspirator, or both. This relatively simple procedure can be performed in a doctor's office or clinic. But as the pregnancy is allowed to continue, the abortion technique becomes increasingly difficult and risky. After about seven weeks, a larger cannula usually is required, the cervix must be dilated, and there is a greater chance of bleeding and infection, even when the abortion is performed under surgically sterile conditions.

After 12 weeks, when the pregnancy has entered the second trimester, the unborn child is no longer an embryo but has developed to the stage of a fetus. During the second trimester, an abortion is even more complicated and risky for the mother, even though the procedure is handled in a hospital rather than in a doctor's office. A common technique for fetal abortion involves the injection of a saline, or salt, solution into the uterus; the effect of the salt solution is to produce labor and expulsion of the fetus. An alternative second trimester procedure is abortion by hysterectomy, in which the uterus with fetal contents is removed by surgery. A hysterectomy, obviously, also ends forever the risk of pregnancy in the woman but it also is a more expensive procedure and carries with it a greater hazard of infection, bleeding, or other complications.

Healthy women can endure a great deal and most can get over an abortion without physical ill effects. But some women seem unable to get over an abortion without suffering mental harm. Many psychosomatic illnesses have been attributed to the effects of abortion and numerically they exceed the physical ill-effects. Remorse may be particularly severe in a religious person because of a loss of pregnancy by one's own volition. On the other hand, abortion frequently offers a woman a reasonable means of terminating an unwanted pregnancy. Before legalization of abortions in America, pregnant women usually were forced to accept such alternatives as marriage to the father of the child, or another husband willing to accept responsibility for the offspring, enrollment in a home for unwed mothers, a back-alley illegal abortion shop, or, in some cases, suicide. Even after bearing an unwanted child, the mother frequently risked abandoning or battering the child, alcoholism, and other forms of anti-social reactions. And women of lower-income status traditionally experienced greater difficulties in resolving the conflicts of an unwanted pregnancy than did women of adequate financial security. Thus, although there may still be some controversy about the propriety of liberalized abortion laws, the pregnant woman today undoubtedly has more, and perhaps better, choices of action than were available in the past.

SEXUAL DYSFUNCTIONS

The human sex urge is a much more complicated business than one is inclined to think. In previous paragraphs we have learned about the great significance of its relation to the urge to procreate, but this by no means exhausts all its aspects. Sexual desire is not produced solely by contact of the genital organs. We all know the power of the kiss to produce sexual desire. But there are races among whom kissing is not only never practised but is regarded as indecent—a sexual perversion. Nor does kissing amount to the whole of love-play. Sexual desire may also be heightened by the slight pain of a gentle bite. Probably every normal man feels a need to press a woman painfully against him, and the woman equally has a craving for the gentle use of force. Especially in men, pleasure is derived from looking at pretty girls, as can be seen from the illustrated magazines exhibited on every news stand. In the same way the desire to excite and entice her man by exhibiting herself more or less undressed is one of the normal urges of a woman. Fashion bears this out. All these things add up to the more or less developed composite features of our "normal" sex urges.

However, if people come to a standstill in their sexual and mental development, then such individual component parts of the urge may take on an obsessional independent character. Some people can feel sexual desire only if they are beaten, hurt, or otherwise humbled, and this is known as masochism.

The opposite, a feeling of sexual desire aroused only by actively inflicting pain on one's partner (or also when one utters degrading words of abuse—the infliction of mental pain), is called sadism. This can even develop into lustful murder.

When sexual gratification is complete just from looking at an undressed female, the male is described as a visophile.

The opposite behavior in men who have a compulsion suddenly to expose their sex organs in public, usually to little girls, is known as exhibitionism.

People who feel sexually excited only when they handle a piece of clothing or an intimate article of use belonging to the opposite sex (women's shoes or underthings are often among these) are called fetishists.

Maturbation is not a sexual dysfunction in the strict sense as one can hardly call the behavior of 90 per cent of all men dysfunctional. It is apparently a normal stage in our sexual development under present-day conditions of life. It may best be defined as an expedient for satisfying a sex urge, which for social reasons cannot be done otherwise. The practice may continue in marriage, with the wife participating, in sex play. Married men and women who feel no desire when they have sexual intercourse, but who have an orgasm when they masturbate, are not entirely unknown. Homosexuality—love between two men (or two women, when it is called Lesbianism)—is not uncommon. It is, as it were, an over-extension of the male spirit of camaraderie, common in bars and clubs, to the province of sex. The feeling of friendship and understanding experienced by normal men among themselves becomes, in the homosexual, invested with physical sexuality. A similar difference exists in ordinary relations between men and women—the difference between the pleasurable company of a congenial member of the opposite sex and being madly in love with one physically.

So homosexuality in some degree is also a component part of the normal sex urge, but the majority of people do not recognize it as such because it is diverted from the purely sexual to higher aims among men (or women) in a way corresponding to their individual natures.

Homosexuality between men but not between women is regarded as a criminal offense in some states. But homosexuality among men is quite common. According to some statistics about 40 per cent of all men have had single or repeated homosexual experiences. Among unmarried ones this figure even reaches 50 per cent round the age of thirty. Men with an academic education are less addicted than other classes, but there is no explanation for this as yet. By far the majority of homosexual men and women maintain normal (heterosexual) relations as well. Only 6 per cent of men are exclusively homosexual.

Beastiality

This means sexual relations with animals and naturally occurs predominantly among the country population. In adolescents this, like masturbation, is a substitute for normal intercourse. Only in rare cases does bestiality take on an independent character, to the exclusion of normal sexuality, thereby becoming dysfunctional.

All sexual dysfunctions are in the last analysis mental disorders, even if those concerned (as is usually the case) do not feel themselves to be deranged. Above all, genuine homosexuals cannot be made to feel that there is anything wrong with them. Their sexual feelings and behavior have become such second nature to them, as indeed ours have to us, that only in rare cases is it possible to change their sexual attitude by psychotherapy. They lack any awareness of being abnormal.

PERSONAL HYGIENE OF THE SEX ORGANS

Nature could not cover the sex organs with thick skin because they are intended to feel sensations. For this reason they should not be touched with unwashed hands or otherwise exposed to disease organisms. The female sex organs are especially vulnerable to infectious diseases that may be transmitted from the environment or spread from other parts of the body. Sex organs should be cleaned regularly with lukewarm water; too much soap should be avoided because it can be harmful to those tissues. The vagina normally keeps itself clean by the activity of helpful bacteria.

Any discharge that goes on for any time demands medical

attention. It should be cleared up. It is not a normal condition and must be dealt with. Some discharges are from mucus of the cervix or from normal shedding of cells of the vagina and need no particular treatment. Itching and odor are rarely associated with such discharges and there are no pus cells involved. Inflammatory discharges, however, nearly always require examination and treatment by a doctor.

A common cause of such discharges is an infectious organism called candida. Such infections have become increasingly common in women using oral contraceptives and are difficult to control without interrupting use of the pill.

A more serious discharge, of course, may indicate the presence of an abnormal growth. For this reason, personal hygiene should include regular pelvic examinations by the doctor. A Pap test of cells normally shed by the cervix can detect the beginning stages of cancer as much as 10 years before the more serious symptoms appear. A pelvic examination also may reveal the presence of a gonorrheal infection. Although that venereal disease in men is easily detected by a milky discharge from the penis, there are obvious symptoms in most women. A swab of the cervical or urethral area usually is required to collect exudate that can be examined in a laboratory to determine if a woman has gonorrhea.

During the monthly period women must of course pay special attention to cleanliness. It is not sufficient merely to use sanitary napkins. A deodorant soap or a baby powder can increase one's sense of personal security.

All these sections have great significance from the point of view of health. Knowledge of these matters not only averts unhappy marriages, but it is also an essential part of mental hygiene. One still cannot estimate the extent to which impairment of the sex urge is responsible for the most common illnesses—psychosomatic disorders. This applies not only to women, but also to men, who consider themselves to be so much more "robust." We must not forget that of the twenty to twenty-five children which a healthy married couple could produce without birth control, only two or three are in actual fact born.

THE PELVIC EXAMINATION

Beginning about the age of puberty, and certainly no later than the time when a young woman nears the end of her second decade of life, she should begin regular visits to her doctor for examination of her pelvic organs. Regular gynecological examinations should occur about once a year for a younger woman, and examinations twice a year are recommended for women after they reach the age of forty. Because the reproductive organs, located in the pelvis, generally are concealed by nature to protect them better from the environment, the development of abnormal tissues can occur without the knowledge of the woman. And although it is possible for a woman to conduct her own examination in a superficial manner, the doctor is much better equipped to diagnose abnormalities with the aid of laboratory facilities.

The pelvic examination should be scheduled for a day immediately after a menstrual period ends. Among other advantages of visiting the doctor at that time is that any unusual symptoms of menstruation are more like to be fresh in the mind. And the doctor may want to ask questions about the flow and symptoms, such as pain or discomfort that may have been associated with it. Some doctors may ask about the number of tampons or sanitary napkins used during menstruation.

Although the woman wants to be clean when she reports for a medical examination, she should not douche before visiting the doctor. In fact, some doctors prefer that the woman not douche for several days before a pelvic examination. The reason for this admonition is that douching simply washes away specimens that the doctor may need for determining the presence of certain infections or the early stages of a cancerous growth. However, it is helpful for purposes of the examination if the woman has been able to empty the lower bowel, which also is checked during the examination. The patient will be asked to empty her bladder at the start of the examination; a full bladder can make it difficult for a doctor to examine carefully other organs in the pelvic area.

In addition to examining the pelvic region, the doctor will want to examine the breasts while the patient is in various positions as well as checking blood pressure, lymph nodes, and other aspects of female anatomy and physiology. A study of organs outside the pelvic area frequently reveals clues to problems that are related to reproductive physiology —such as abnormal effects produced by the use of oral contraceptive pills. If the woman has cysts of the breasts or if the female members of her family have been treated for breast cancer, the doctor may want to obtain X-ray pictures of the woman's breasts.

Questions may be asked about types of contraceptives used and patterns of sexual behavior. The patient should not be embarrassed by such questions because the information, which will be held confidential, also can reveal otherwise hidden clues that will help the doctor make a proper diagnosis. Even if the woman has intercourse with more than one man, that information may be an important piece of the jigsaw puzzle from which the doctor forms a complete picture of a woman's gynecological health.

In the actual pelvic examination, the doctor will inspect the genital area outside the vaginal orifice for lesions related to viral infections or abcesses of the small glands of the vulva which help to lubricate the vaginal orifice during intercourse.

In the area of the vagina and cervix, using an instrument called a speculum to hold the vaginal walls apart, the doctor will look for any abnormal tissues in the lining of those organs, such as cysts or tumors. If the woman suspects she may be pregnant, the doctor should be advised. Otherwise, the doctor will make a similar examination of the lining of the uterus. This is done by pressing down on the abdomen with one hand while inserting the fingers of the other hand to feel the lining of the womb. Later, he will inspect the rectum, of the lower bowel, for abnormal growths.

A sample of cells normally shed by the cervix will be taken for a Pap test, to determine the possible presence of cancer. The doctor also may take with a cotton swab a smear of secretions from several areas, particularly the urethra, the vagina, and the cervix, to be examined in a laboratory for possible evidence of a gonorrheal infection. Doctors formerly took specimens only from the vagina for gonorrhea tests but more recent evidence indicates that a woman may be infected with the venereal disease yet have no gonorrhea organism in her vagina. So, a more thorough examination requires obtaining specimens from several different genital areas.

Gonorrhea may be present in women without presenting symptoms although the disease is easily detected in men. But another kind of venereal disease, trichomoniasis, thrives in the opposite way—the infectious organism can produce complaints in women but no symptoms in men. It is marked by a discharge and irritation in the vagina, but it can be controlled by antibiotics. However, as in the case of gonorrhea, both the male and female sex partners must be treated to prevent reinfection.

Another disease that may be revealed by a pelvic examination is moniliasis, which is produced by a yeastlike fungus called Candida albicans. The organism produces, among other symptoms, a thick white discharge in the vagina; it is related to the throat inflammation known as oral thrush. Because moniliasis is affected by hormonal changes in the woman, it is most common in pregnant women and those who use hormonal oral contraceptive pills.

The regular pelvic examination is an important preventive health measure, of course. But it also provides an opportunity for the woman to discuss gynecological problems with her doctor and to seek advice regarding medications to relieve the discomforts of menstrual periods or the advisability of using one of the newer contraceptive techniques.

NORMAL PREGNANCY

SYMPTOMS OF PREGNANCY

Pregnancy begins with fertilization—the moment when the head of a sperm cell amalgamates with the cell nucleus of the egg cell. An embryo comes into being, which grows on the mucous membrane of the womb, through which it absorbs directly foodstuffs necessary for growth.

This minute collection of cells, which can be seen only through a microscope, already secretes substances which effect changes in the body of the mother. The mother's pituitary secretes different hormones and the monthly periods cease. The mature mucous membrane of the womb is now urgently needed—at last it fulfils its real purpose and is no longer passed out with each monthly period. It does occasionally happen that the first period after pregnancy starts is not completely suppressed, especially when conception takes place in the few days before a period. It may then be that the embryo is still in the Fallopian tube. Very rarely the periods go on for some months, although they are scanty. This does not harm the child, but in this way a pregnancy may only be discovered in the course of medical examination.

Normally, however, the cessation of monthly periods is regarded as a symptom of pregnancy. This symptom may be unreliable in women who tend to have longer menstrual cycles (over 30–35 days), and who anyway occasionally miss a period. Periods may also cease when there is distress or want (captivity, flight, great uncertainty), when mental stimuli cause the pituitary to inhibit the release of mature eggs.

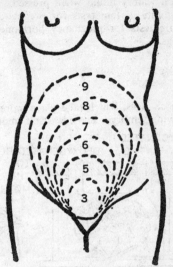

Fig. 49 .

Diagram showing the heights of the fundus of the womb during the various months of pregnancy.

Further symptoms of pregnancy are: nausea or sickness (very common, but less so in women who are quite healthy sexually and hormonally). The appetite is not affected. Sometimes giddiness occurs (this was probably more common in former times, at least judging by novels, according to which husbands first became aware of the sweet secret by the sudden fainting fits of their wives). There may be a sudden craving for unusual food. But urges to eat unusual foods should not be allowed to interfere with sound nutrition. In most cases, a more effective substitute can be recommended by the doctor. If, for example, one has a desire to eat chalk, it would be better to ask the doctor to prescribe calcium tablets. Change of mood may occur; in some women this produces moodiness and irritability—in healthy ones there is withdrawal of interest from outside things and an increased sense of contentment with themselves. There is darkening of the skin over the genitals and of the nipples and appearance or darkening of a streak running vertically from the navel to the genitals.

The breasts enlarge and from the second or third month onwards exude a watery liquid when pressed.

The only absolute certain tests for pregnancy in the first three months are tests for pregnancy hormones carried out on mice or frogs.

THE EMBRYO

During these changes, which take place more or less regularly, the growing embryo embeds itself more and more

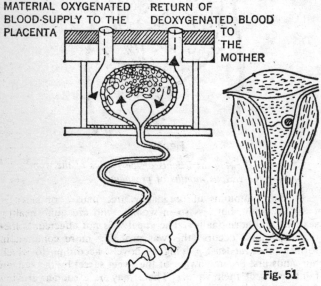

MATERIAL OXYGENATED BLOOD-SUPPLY TO THE PLACENTA

RETURN OF DEOXYGENATED BLOOD TO THE MOTHER

Fig. 51

Fig. 50

Fig. 50: *Diagram of the foetal circulation.*
Fig. 51: *The fertilized egg has embedded itself in the lining of the womb.*

firmly into the mucous membrane of the womb. Influenced by hormones, this womb mucous membrane becomes increasingly thicker and more richly supplied with blood. Eventually it forms, together with part of the embryo, the placenta—an organ provided with blood-vessels and blood exchange surfaces, which supply nourishment and oxygen to the embryo as well as removing its metabolic waste. This organ of exchange remains connected with the developing embryo by means of the umbilical cord. (The embryo is called by its Greek name up to the third month of pregnancy.) The blood in the vessels of the umbilical cord is pumped by the embryo's own heart, which has already started its life-long beating during the first month. The mother's blood does not come into direct contact with the body of the unborn child. Between the two sets of blood-vessels there is a dividing wall, which among other things prevents any bacteria present in the mother's blood from infecting the embryo (but not viruses) (see page 187).

THE FETUS

The embyro quickly develops into a fetus, the Latin word for offspring. By the end of the first month this is not yet quite half an inch long. The brain, eyes and hands begin to take shape and the heart starts to beat.

At the end of the second month the embryo measures one inch and already can move (though this is scarcely perceptible) its body and shoulders.

By the end of the third month its size is already four inches and it is called a fetus. This is a critical time. When miscarriages occur they usually do so at this stage of pregnancy. The child's movements can still not be felt for certain and the doctor's stethoscope cannot yet detect the heart-beats from outside. The precursors of the sex organs have developed and can now be recognized as male or female. The eyes already move behind the lids, which, however, are still closed.

By the end of the fourth month the length is six inches and its movements can be felt. An impression of what these are like can be gained by putting the hands on the cheek and rubbing the tongue along it inside. In its movements the fetus reflects the mother's emotions so far as these can be conveyed by hormones in her blood. For example, it becomes lively when more adrenaline is secreted, as during fright or sudden excitement. The fetus does not feel the fright as such, but only the restlessness and increased tension conveyed to its nervous system and muscles by adrenaline. If it is firmly wedged by taut abdominal muscles, it cannot move at the time and becomes lively only once the mother's tension dies down. The fetus prefers to carry out its gymnastics in the evenings, when the mother lies down to rest and the abdominal muscles are relaxed. The stimulus to movement may be derived from the change of position, for it is now lying in a different way. The mother's abdomen gradually begins to become prominent. This is a happy time for the mother.

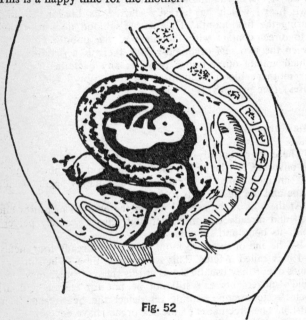

Fig. 52

Vertical section of the pelvis showing the young fetus in the womb.

At the end of the fifth month the child measures ten inches and its heart-beats can be heard from outside. The heart beats about twice as quickly as that of the mother.

At the end of the sixth month its size is twelve inches and the child's movements can be started by noises from outside. The child hears. In view of the fact that new-born children have a highly developed reaction to moods and emotions, which they can sense from the speaker's tone of voice, we could say that there already exists at this stage mental contact with the outside world.

Under favorable conditions a fetus measuring thirteen inches can already live if born prematurely in the seventh month. Miscarriages of this size have to be registered as births, even if the child is stillborn.

At the end of the seventh month, 14 in.
At the end of the eighth month, 16 in.
At the end of the ninth month, 18 in.
At the end of the tenth month, 20 in.

DURATION OF PREGNANCY, DATE OF BIRTH

The months of pregnancy are "lunar" months of twenty-eight days each from the last monthly period. Altogether there are 280 days. The calendar can be used as follows: subtract three months from the date of the beginning of the last period and add seven to ten days. You then know when to expect the birth, though this is only approximate. (For example: last monthly period April 2nd; 3 months back = January 2nd + 7–10 days = 9th–12th January.) For the child the date of birth is not so critical as is generally imagined. It is true that this is the time when it first sees light. But it could have seen light some months before. It is true that birth is the moment at which the supply of the body switches over from the placenta to the baby's lungs and stomach. But it has had the ability to do this for about two months. The body of the child tends to adapt before it actually has to perform new functions, although each child develops at its own rate. In general, the mental and physical achievements of the child can be counted from the time of conception rather than from the date of birth. As the premature infant grows, he gradually catches up to the achievement levels of a normal child. By the age of two years, a premature infant should compare quite favorably in development with a full-term child.

LEADING A SENSIBLE LIFE DURING PREGNANCY

Pregnancy is a normal and healthy condition. The birth of a child should leave a woman as physically fit and efficient as she was before. Pregnancy is the final outcome of physical sexual maturity. Nowadays pregnancy and labor no longer constitute any appreciable risk to women. Nowhere has medical science succeeded more completely in safeguarding a natural physical function from dangers. Fatal puerperal fever, which years ago caused half the deaths in childbirth has virtually been abolished.

We have, however, one legacy from the past: fear of the pain of childbirth and fear of its dangers. Both are fundamentally superfluous. Giving birth to a child is the less painful the better a woman is prepared for it, and above all, the less she fears this pain. "Suffering" in childbirth is nothing to boast about. It should be the ambition of every woman not to have suffered.

In order to achieve this, we must discuss pregnancy and birth a great deal more frankly than was formerly regarded as decorous. Above all, one must realize that pregnancy and birth are the most important part of the sexual urge. It involves mental-nervous processes which start with sexual intercourse.

Mental-nervous disorders of sex life occasion disorders in pregnancy and birth. No feeling in a pregnant woman is more unnatural, more "ill," than shame and fear because of her condition. This works against the normal, hormonally conditioned contentment with oneself—the whole physical preparation for pregnancy. These are "inner cage-bars" which make one ill. The feeling that one is making a sacrifice for others by giving birth to a child is also something unnatural and harmful.

For many women an important objective is to have a child for her own sake, for her own fulfilment and happiness. She feels this desire as a healthy and instinctive goal of her relationship with her marital partner, to be a mother. For this she is vastly superior to man because she is able to bear a living creature, which goes on growing and which makes her the most indispensable part of mankind and the human family.

So take courage and look at the world in its proper perspective. You will save yourselves and your children a great deal of sorrow and pain. Take pregnancy for what it is: the natural fulfilment of the female act of sex and her most complete and supreme achievement, of which she may justly be proud. In the depths of the mind where the instincts originate, everything is simple and natural in all women, even when the "inner cage-bars" clamp down on perception and they cannot feel these things. It is easier for women to have a simple understanding of their nature than for men. Women are more closely linked to the true nature of sex instincts by their body's monthly preparation for pregnancy than is the case with the more even, less well-defined sexual drive of men.

And here we have the foundation of all mental hygiene during pregnancy—the growing awareness by the woman of her importance. This is absolutely necessary for painless childbirth. Do not act contrary to nature, but with it.

DIET DURING PREGNANCY

There is little more to be said about diet during pregnancy than was already stated in the chapter on diet (see page 217). There is no need to go to any great trouble with a "pregnancy diet," provided one eats sensibly. There is an increased demand for calcium—which we tend to get too little of anyway—and vitamin D, which at other times is not so vital to adults. Extra supplements of both should be taken—a few drops of halibut-liver oil daily and calcium tablets crushed and dissolved in milk. (But the ideal way is to make one's own vitamin D by sunbathing.)

Moreover, pregnancy is a time when one can and should rely on one's instinctive tastes. A desire for sour things is best satisfied by vegetable and fruit juices, less well by vinegar, pickled herrings or pickled cucumber. The quantity of liquid drunk should be greater than usual. After all, one has to excrete the waste matter of two people through one's kidneys and this is more important than "eating for two." The additional calories required are negligible—at most 5–10 per cent more than usual, which is so little that one would hardly notice it. The extra protein needed for the growing fetus is also slight—less than one ounce per day, the amount of protein in a half can of tuna—or about 10 percent more than normal consumption. In fact, a pregnant woman need eat only a little more than usual if she lives sensibly and takes the necessary basic minerals and vitamins regularly in her diet. If, however, this is not the case and she tries to eat much more than usual, she will become fat and unshapely and will make unnecessary difficulties for herself when the child is born. Unless the doctor expressly orders it, the quantity of protein in one's daily food should not be reduced. As much as four ounces of actual protein a day is recommended (about 12 to 16 ounces of meat, cheese, or eggs must be eaten to obtain four ounces of actual protein). Liver should be included occasionally.

There are divergent views with regard to the amount of liquid to be drunk during pregnancy. At one time it was believed that the quantity of liquid in the womb (in which the fetus floats and which protects it from bumps) was increased in a harmful way by drinking a lot during pregnancy. But there is no experimental proof to support this claim. However, it is unanimously agreed that drinks taken should include fruit and vegetable juices. It is not so much a question of the quantity of liquid as of the mineral content of the drinks. Above all, do not eat any unnecessary fat. Fat does not make one strong, but fat.

EXERCISE AND OTHER BODY AIDS

Man has adopted the erect position. His scaffolding of bones and the arrangements of his internal organs are, however, still constructed for the four-legged animal from which he evolved. This is particularly apparent in pregnancy; women who have to sit or stand a lot at this time suffer from swollen feet. This is simply due to the fact that the weight of the child and womb presses on the veins in the lower part of the pelvis all day. The blood-flow from the legs back to the heart is obstructed and the feet swell. This sort of thing does not happen in the four-legged animal as the womb and fetus do not press on the back of the abdominal wall. When an expectant mother makes a practice of walking for one to two hours every day, much of this is cancelled out. The blood-flow through the legs functions better, the more the leg muscles contract. Of course, suitable footwear, with heels neither too high nor too low, is essential. In addition the pressure exerted by the womb is varied rhythmically as a result of the up-and-down motion of walking. So the movements of walking are an excellent form of exercise. Ordinary housework, too, with its constantly changing movements, is preferable to any sitting or standing form of occupation. Naturally there should be a pause for rest at times—but always lying down! Sitting is useless during pregnancy. Work that has to be done on the floor should be done on the knees and hands. Do not kneel bent backwards. The four-legged position is the basic exercise of pregnancy gymnastics.

What has been said about the upright position of human beings causing pressure by the womb on the pelvic veins, applies also to the strain on the abdominal wall muscles. Here again sitting or standing all day is bad. This has nothing to do with the strength of the abdominal muscles, which can be trained by sport or exercises, but one cannot check the harm due to stretching, which comes about when the muscles are resting. Here, too, the deterioration in blood-flow as a result of immobility plays a part. Stretching of the abdominal wall is not insignificant in pregnancy. In the later months its area is almost doubled.

All told, the special effects of the upright posture and our civilized mode of life demand that the body be given support during pregnancy. This is even more so if one has to go on working after the fifth month in a sitting or standing occupation. Usually a simple pregnancy belt, which supports the abdomen by raising it, is sufficient. Since some women wear a girdle or corset anyway, one can select a suitable supporting garment. Pregnancy corsets can nowadays be made just as fashionable and as elegant as ordinary belts. Nylon is not only used by the fashion industry. You can be particular when choosing medical requisites also.

It is false pride to think that your body is trained in such a way that it does not need assistance of this kind. It is all very well if you can walk about the whole day long in the open air. But if you have to sit or stand, then help is needed, and the abdomen must be trained. But how?

(1) *Basic exercise* (Fig. 53): Go down on all fours every evening.

The important time for pregnancy exercises is from the fourth month onwards, except for the last four weeks before the birth, when one must use moderation. Mild crawling exercises are, however, part of a natural rest for the intestines. In the middle months of pregnancy the crawling exercises can be varied using one's imagination. The exercises must be done regularly—every day. For childbirth nothing is more important than the muscles of the pelvic floor and the abdomen.

The *crawling exercises* consist of:

   (a) Walking on hands and knees—left leg and right arm together, etc.

   (b) Just the same, but using right leg and right arm together.

   (c) Walking on hands with legs stretched.

   (d) On knees and hands, with elbows bent outwards ("crocodile walk").

   (e) On knees and elbows.

   (f) Dragging stretched legs after one, forwards and backwards.

(2) Stomach-swing. On all fours draw the abdomen in and release it, in turn. You can become very skillful at this. Some

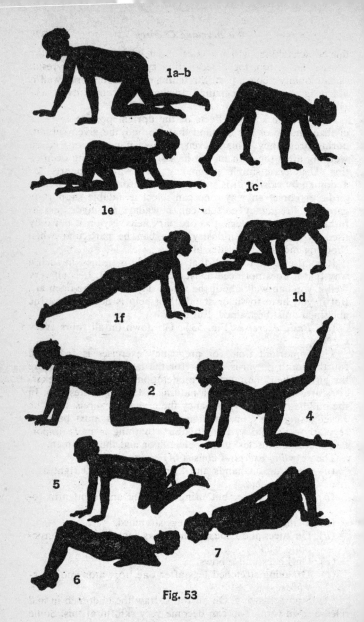

Fig. 53

women can move their abdomen to and fro sideways, thanks to the strength of its muscles.

(3) Knee-stretching. On all fours separate the legs as widely as possible and draw them smoothly together again. A light or spongy bed mat and a smooth floor are required for this.

(4) Leg-throwing. Kneeling on all fours, one leg is kicked up backwards and kept for a moment as high as possible. Then the same is done with the other leg and repeated for each in turn.

(5) Crawling and gripping with one's feet. When crawling, a large ball or cushion is gripped between both feet. This exercise can be done only on a soft carpet, and it is excellent training for the pelvic floor. It is easier, though less effective, to grip a firm cushion between the knees while crawling.

(6) Raising the pelvis. On one's back with the soles of the feet firmly planted on the ground, the body is raised so that only the head, shoulders and feet are touching the floor.

(7) Pressing together and stretching the knees against the resistance of the hands (only if exercises 3 and 5 cannot be done).

(8) Breathing exercises, kneeling and standing. When breathing in, spread out the arms sideways, and when breathing out bring them together again in front of you.

Well, this is quite a full program, but it should not be overdone, at any rate not at first. We are not trying to break any sporting records, but are simply concerned with exercise—that is to say, a program of exercises designed to strengthen muscles which are otherwise not used much. In this sense walking does not constitute exercise. It is physical activity without gymnastic value. The daily program should take up five minutes at the beginning, later fifteen to twenty minutes at the most. More than this can be harmful and it is up to you not to overdo things.

It is a myth, and one which is widely believed, that abdominal muscles hardened by sport complicate birth. The answer to this is: any natural process can be painful if muscles are used wrongly. Athletic training does not protect one from fear of childbirth, and it is this fear which causes the pain. It causes muscles to become taut, when they should actually be loose. It hampers the expansion of the "birth channel" and has nothing to do with strength of the muscles.

SEXUAL INTERCOURSE DURING PREGNANCY?

One question remains to be answered, as it is of interest to many people. May one have sexual intercourse during pregnancy or should one abstain?

Scientific data on this question are few, but two things are known: most mammals do not do so, with the exception of monkeys, who have intercourse up to a period which corresponds to the seventh month of human pregnancy. The vast majority of human beings do have sexual intercourse.

We are dealing with a question as to whether a common habit has harmful consequences or not. In some, sexual interest declines somewhat during this time, with others this is not so. In women, even, it is not unknown for them to experience an increased sexual need during pregnancy. The mental relaxation produced by intercourse and the feeling of a closer tie with the man on account of the coming child are responsible for the removal of inhibitions. An increased capacity for love results, although the purely biological urge has become weaker.

Sexual intercourse in marriage has lost its primary character of mating and fertilization and has become a symbol of tender devotion. It assures the pregnant woman of her husband's love, and that is something extremely important at that time, when a woman unconsciously fears that she may lose her husband, because she may no longer interest him sexually. This is not because of the coarsening of her figure, as some people believe. A man's tendency to turn away from his wife is much more deep-seated. Man's natural function in reproduction is fulfilled once he makes a woman pregnant. One can get on better once one realizes this. The man can more easily sort out his muddled feelings and emotions with regard to his pregnant wife. Tenderness increases and sexual interest declines and the attraction of other women becomes greater. This is nothing unnatural, monstrous or base, but just a simple fact based on instinct. Heaven forbid that one should do all the things one secretly longs to do! However, the better one understands these things, the easier it is to remain happy. Any real pangs of jealousy experienced by women become blunted in pregnancy. Her own feeling of fulfilment, which has something victorious about it, outweighs all fear of competition.

The husband should be encouraged to have a share in the

positive experiences of pregnancy—in the growth and movements of the child. Men sometimes take great interest in this (and are secretly proud). It helps them to become good fathers. Becoming a good father is difficult if nine months of a complaining wife make you labor under a sense of guilt. Help your husband to become a father. He cannot feel the growth of the child himself. He is a useless creature in this respect. Let him try to take part. It is as important to help your husband to become a father as it is to do pregnancy exercises and to eat the right food. The task arises again with each new child. Our children need fathers, and fathers are trained during pregnancy.

This is more important than the question about sexual intercourse during pregnancy. From the medical point of view there is no objection. The rule is, of course, that no pressure should be put on the woman's abdomen in the last months of pregnancy. The position in which the man lies behind the woman is recommended by some obstetricians; the woman also may lie on top of the man or in some other comfortable position. In the last weeks of pregnancy, any additional pressure on the mother's abdomen tends to compress the aorta and inferior vena cava, two major blood vessels in the abdominal cavity. This in turn can cause faintness in the mother and restrict the oxygen carried to the fetus through the blood. In the last fourteen days intercourse must really be forbidden, because the date of the birth cannot be calculated with complete accuracy. For this reason the risk of spreading infection immediately before the birth is very great.

A common fallacy, derived from old superstition but still believed by some, must be exploded. Sexual intercourse during pregnancy is not necessary for the development of the child. The male sperm contains nothing needed by the growing child.

THE BIRTH

First and foremost the act of childbirth is hard bodily work. The expression "birth-pangs" is unfortunate as it conveys an impression of passive endurance—suffering the process of birth. In reality childbirth is work on the part of the body—active work—as the far more appropriate term "labor" suggests. The body itself creates the "pains"—the muscular efforts by which the child is thrust out of the womb.

The idea that childbirth need cause suffering seems to be

based on the biblical injunction, "In sorrow shall you bring forth children." This belief may account for the suffering experienced by women of Western culture in contrast to the easy, spontaneous way of delivery that is the rule among primitive races. For this reason we shall try to abolish the expression "pain" in connection with the natural process of birth. This may sound revolutionary, but we cannot otherwise free ourselves from the suggestion of fear contained in this and other sayings. We will, therefore, deliberately avoid the expression "pain" in this connection and use instead the word "contraction" (which, by the way, is an accurate description of the work done by the womb). Also, because of tranquilizers, analgesics and anesthetics administered to the mother during delivery in a hospital, it is unlikely that she will feel any unbearable pain.

WHEN THE TIME HAS COME

The first symptom of approaching birth manifests itself four weeks before. About this time the womb becomes lower in the body by about the breadth of a hand. The mother's breathing becomes freer and easier. Her body curves more sharply in the lower part. If you press carefully the upper abdomen with the flat of your hand, you can feel that the upper limit of the womb is lower than before and is now approximately the breadth of a hand above the navel. Then birth will occur in another four weeks.

The first direct symptoms of approaching birth manifest themselves in restlessness and a feeling of pressure in the groins and small of the back—similar to what most women feel when their monthly period starts. This is due to the growing tension of the womb muscles and womb ligaments. Gradually this becomes rhythmical—waxing and waning in intensity—and painful. The first labor contractions have started.

Then it is an idea to have a bath—or at least to wash carefully from the navel down. It is time to prepare calmly for what is to come. On an average the first baby takes about twenty hours; subsequent babies take about twelve hours. If a woman is to be confined in hospital, she has plenty of time. If she is having her baby at home, she can let the doctor know that she has begun her labor.

The womb has a long job to do. By repeatedly contracting itself, it stretches its exit—the neck of the womb and its orifice. As it contracts, the pressure inside it becomes higher and higher. The child and its protective coverings are squeezed together. The liquid in which the child is encased pushes itself forwards with its coverings and paves the way for the expansion of the womb canal. It looks like a great bubble of water and is sometimes called the "bag of waters." Things are of course becoming somewhat more unpleasant. Some blood-stained mucus is expelled ("the show"). The contractions come every two to five minutes and last about half to one minute.

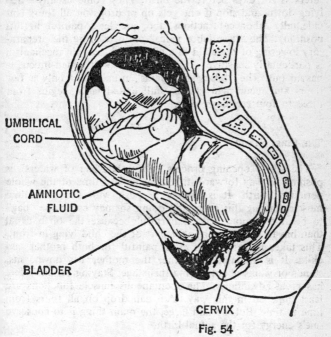

UMBILICAL
CORD

AMNIOTIC
FLUID

BLADDER

CERVIX

Fig. 54

The child in the womb just before birth.

The intervals between the muscular contractions of the womb are necessary for the child to recover. If anything, it is worse off than the mother. With every contraction it is put under violent pressure and its blood and oxygen supplies are reduced, because the blood-vessels in the womb wall are squeezed shut. We adults would refer to the feeling as one of suffocation. Being born is not an enjoyable process—even though the head is protected from direct pressure There are some doctors who trace the origin of fear to the experience gone through in these early hours before the first breath.

If the intervals between single contractions last longer (up to ten minutes) and the contractions become shorter—something is wrong, and medical attention is required.

This should not be confused with "false labor pains." These are mild contractions, which may happen at not quite regular intervals for days before the birth. They come usually when lying down, and stop if one gets up or drops on all fours (incidentally labor contractions, too, are least painful in this position). The "false labor pains" are caused by the preparatory lowering of the child in a woman whose pain mechanism is particularly sensitive. At times even blood-stained mucus is passed out. The "false labor pains" usually last only a few hours and recur many times until actual labor begins from three to fourteen days later.

THE FIRST STAGE

The whole opening process, when the "bag of waters" is pushing its way forward, takes the longest time of the whole period of birth. It is useless to push with the abdominal muscles during this time, and doing so may cause the "bag" to burst too soon. This is harmful because the birth canal then has to be dilated by that part of the child lying in front. This takes longer and is more painful for both mother and child. It is immaterial whether the mother lies down, sits, stands or walks about during this stage. Staying on one's feet has great advantages. The spontaneous muscle functions are least impeded in this way. You can drop on all fours from time to time. But, by and large, the main thing is to conserve one's energy for the actual birth.

THE SECOND STAGE

When the mouth of the womb is sufficiently dilated, the "bag of waters" bursts. A fairly large quantity of watery liquid suddenly gushes out. This marks the beginning of the second stage of the birth process—the period of expulsion, when the child forces its own way outwards. Normally the driving wedge is the head. That is a very annoying condition for the poor infant thus thrust into life. Later one is reluctant to rush at things head first. During the period of expulsion the little skull is driven, with each contraction, deeper into the "birth canal." One must try to visualize this. Perhaps by thinking of it one can lessen one's own fear of the pain of the process and thus cause the muscles of the pelvic floor to reduce their resistance. This must happen. After all, two people have to go through the process of birth together. It is by no means certain which of them suffers most. Incidentally, the mother's pains are less if she does not resist the natural process of things.

To ease the movement of the child through the vaginal orifice, the doctor attending the birth may make a small incision to widen the opening. The incision, called an episiotomy, also helps prevent accidental tearing of the tissues around the opening during passage of the baby's body.

The contractions affect all the body muscles—above all, of course, the abdominal muscles. They instinctively squeeze as well. Now one needs strong abdominal muscles—an athletic past pays good dividends. Now there can be no more holding back. Nothing matters any more. If you must scream, then do so between the contractions. Pushing is indispensable for completion of the birth process.

The "period of expulsion" must be supervised by a trained helper—nurse or doctor—and what they say, goes.

With each contraction the child's head penetrates further and further out through the vaginal orifice. The child opens the door to the world itself with the back of its head. At the last decisive moment you stop pressing and the womb muscles take over the work again. Otherwise birth occurs too quickly and something splits. The doctor supports the perineal muscles lightly with the hand and with one final contraction of the womb the head emerges—face downwards. The eyelids are swabbed with sterile cloth. Rapidly, the body slips out and the child is received by the doctor.

THE THIRD STAGE

After about three to five minutes the circulation through the navel cord stops. The navel cord must be cut. The child's own breathing through the lungs starts with its first cry.

But this is not the end of the birth process. During the next half to one hour the afterbirth comes out. This is the placenta, the tissue through which oxygen and foodstuffs are exchanged between mother and child. This piece of flesh (about as large as a soup plate) is, of course, attached to the navel cord.

HELPING ONESELF IN URGENT CASES

It can sometimes happen that in exceptional circumstances the doctor or nurse cannot arrive in time. For this reason the rudiments of midwifery should be known to everyone. This is part of one's general education. There is less to it than one thinks.

The first rule is cleanliness and still more cleanliness.

Large quantities of warm water are required—and clean sheets. Tap water and clean sheets fresh from the cupboard are almost free from bacteria. Note that freshly shed blood is quite clean. Only when it has been exposed to the open air for a long time do bacteria develop in it. Hands which were clean and become covered with fresh blood are still sterile.

The bed must be placed so that it is accessible from both sides. If available, a waterproof covering should be placed under the clean sheets. The skin and hairs surrounding the vagina are washed carefully, but thoroughly, with warm soapy water and a clean cloth.

The person delivering the child must keep his or her hands scrupulously clean. The finger-nails should be cut quite short and the hands and forearms should be thoroughly washed— each side for five minutes—in very hot, soapy water, using soap and a brush—above all, wash in between the fingers. Even if no more dirt can be seen, go on washing. The helper of course has the sleeves rolled right up. An apron (or a sheet) should be put on and tightly tied round so that it cannot fall off. After washing the hands, do not touch your clothes any more. The washed hands are not dried on a towel but held up and shaken until they are dry.

This thorough handwashing is not required until some little time after the waters have burst. This is all watched from outside. You must not put your hands in to feel how far advanced things are or to pull.

Previously we indicated exactly when the mother has to push. Before the time for this comes she is encouraged not to use her muscles actively. Do not press with the hands. The most important thing is to talk to her encouragingly—"Open up quite wide, let it come—give way—it will hurt less," is the tenor of the helper's words. It is very important to control your facial expression. Do not show fright if a lot of blood is shed or let the woman see if you are embarrassed. Nothing could render the confined woman's work more difficult. Above all, do not prattle about "being brave" and "everyone has been through it." It is of no concern to the woman in labor what other women do or have done. She is there with her own experience—only the immediate present is important for her—nothing else matters.

When the "waters" have burst, the woman should lie on her back with her knees bent and grasp her thighs from outside with her hands. Then she should push with all her might. When the head becomes plainly visible, so that it will shortly emerge, you must apply the brakes and tell the woman to stop pushing. Let things come slowly. If you can, support the perineum—this is the area between the vaginal orifice and anus—during the last pains with a clean hand laid flat. Slight counter-pressure on this helps the head forward. However, thousands of women give birth without this being done.

CUTTING THE CORD

This is the most important part of the layman's knowledge of midwifery. About five minutes after the child has been born, the cord is tied in two places, about three inches from the child's abdomen, and cut between these two places with scissors or a knife, which have been boiled. By boiling we mean that the instruments must have lain in bubbling, boiling water for ten minutes. Before the boiling they can be knotted in a handkerchief or table napkin. Then they can be taken out clean more easily after being boiled and when the water has been poured away. For bandaging the part attached to the baby, small pieces of sterile wrapped bandages are best. Of course little strips of linen can also be used if they have been boiled. Nothing must be handled except by the person delivering the child, who has made his or her hands sterile by washing. One more thing—rust is not dangerous provided that the instrument has been sufficiently boiled after being rubbed previously.

TREATMENT OF THE NEW-BORN BABE

First of all the child's mouth is cleaned gently with a sterile finger, round which is wrapped a boiled piece of linen or a sterile muslin swab. Then it is lifted by its legs with one hand and, if the first cry does not come automatically, given a mild slap on its bottom. If it has already cried, well and good. There are, however, other ways of seeing that it is breathing properly. If its breathing does not get going properly, first put a cold, wet cloth on its forehead, then on its chest, and rub it. Clean the mouth once again and, putting the child on its back, apply artificial respiration with both hands on the sides of the chest. A child breathes very much more quickly than a grown-up.

The eyelids are carefully wiped with wool and sterile water and the child is bathed. The water should not feel hot to the elbow. Then bandage the navel and put the child in its cot. Of course the bandage on the navel must be sterile. If nothing else is available, pieces of cloth can be dried in the oven, after having been boiled—take care that they do not char. Of course they should not be put on the dirty floor of the oven, but left in the pan in which they were boiled.

THE AFTERBIRTH (Placenta)

Nothing happens to the mother for a little while after the birth. She rests until the womb recovers its strength and ejects the afterbirth. When the afterbirth has come out, it should not be thrown away, but left until the doctor comes, so that it can be seen whether it is complete.

Then let the mother and child sleep, after the mother has been carefully washed. But take care that nothing touches the vaginal orifice during washing. Infection must be prevented.

THE FIRST DAYS

For twelve to twenty-four hours absolute quiet is essential in every case. The infant is hungry, but is well enough provided for. The mother thinks of her figure and follows the instructions of the doctor. The general trend of treatment is to start active movement as soon as possible and to get up as soon as possible—but only in accordance with the instructions. Foot movements and careful raising of the pelvis are the very first exercises. They help to keep the blood circulating and prevent inflammation of the veins and thromboses. The young mother usually knows by instinct how much she can manage.

After twelve to fourteen hours the child is put to the mother's breast for the first time. If the breast is too distended, the child cannot get anything out and the breast must be milked a bit by hand. Actually it almost always works—only one woman in fifty cannot feed her baby at all. The size of the breasts has nothing to do with their functional ability—especially not the size of the breasts before pregnancy. What makes them large then is only fat and not milk-gland tissue.

The vaginal discharge (lochia) is no cause for alarm. It is secreted by the place where the placenta was torn off from the womb. It soon loses its early blood-staining and is supposed to have a peculiar, stale smell. If this discharge smells foul, then the doctor must be consulted. It lasts for two weeks or longer. The mother's temperature immediately after birth is usually somewhat raised (by about one degree). This persists for some days and is due to the absorption of the blood and tissue remains from the interior of the womb. Temperatures of over 100 degrees Fahrenheit must be due to abnormal causes and should be investigated.

All organic changes quickly revert to normal when the mother feeds the child herself. Breast-feeding can help the mother regain her figure by regulating the calories needed for the baby and her own ideal weight.

BREAST-FEEDING

The milk of every species of animal has a different composition and is the best imaginable food for the babies of that particular animal. Mother's milk has a different composition from cow's milk. In addition it has other advantages. It is always provided in a sterile form and at the right temperature straight from its source. It need not be boiled in order to insure sterility. Cow's milk contains fairly large quantities of bacteria, which can cause illness unless it is pasteurized before delivery.

Breast-feeding is the safest way of feeding an infant, because the danger of intestinal disorders caused by bacteria is virtually non-existent. Breast-feeding is the most convenient way of feeding an infant, because it takes the least time for the mother and is less trouble and worry. Breast-feeding is not exhausting. It is a secretion process out of a gland tissue there for that purpose. Breast-feeding does not sap the strength of the mother's body. The milk is produced from the ordinary constituents of the mother's diet. To cover this she should eat about 25 per cent more than usual. For this reason the mother's diet does not cause any difficulty if she eats sensibly. She is best guided by the directions given in the chapter on nutrition. Extra calcium and vitamin D, as during pregnancy, are needed. The quantity eaten is governed only by appetite. If, however, the diet is not a balanced one, she will get fat, because the body, with its increased appetite, searches indiscriminately for the substances necessary for the milk and its own requirements. The rest turns into fat.

Breast-feeding is the best cosmetic method for quickly restoring an attractive figure. It is the last part of the physical sexual process. It gives pleasure and a special kind of proud satisfaction. It is not a "sacrifice" made for the child, but woman's natural function. Breast-feeding does not spoil the breasts if they are treated properly before and during the puerperium. Women whose breasts were small before pregnancy find that breast-feeding generally gives them greater firmness. Gland tissue is firmer than fat. Of course it is important to give the heavy breasts proper support during pregnancy and breast-feeding.

Mother's milk is not some special "juice" to be invested with superstitious ideas and theories. It is a suitably composed watery solution of a number of chemical substances, which serves as an ideal food for the infant. The child does not take in any character qualities with it. These come to the child in quite a different way. Many substances taken by the mother, including nicotine in tobacco, caffeine in coffee, tea, and cola drinks, and drugs in medicines, are secreted into the milk and should be used cautiously during breast-feeding.

Milk is nearly 90 per cent water. For this reason one is terribly thirsty while breast-feeding. Plenty of liquid must be drunk—preferably fruit and vegetable juices, but also cow's milk. The milk's composition is not affected by food taken by the mother. It is the natural purpose of mother's milk to make the infant independent of the chance fluctuations of food eaten.

Duration of Breast-feeding and Feeding Difficulties

The child is breast-fed up to the fifth month, if possible. You can change over gradually to cup-and-spoon feeding. This is done in addition to breast-feeding, which simplifies the problem of weaning. Babies lose interest in the breast in time—sometimes from one day to another. You must then allow them a much more varied diet than one is inclined to imagine children should eat. It need not all be sweet. But most foods that appear on the parents' table, with the exception of highly spiced foods, can be offered to a six-month-old child in a chopped-up form. The child will tend to choose foods that are good for it and to reject what is not good for it. This has been proved by large-scale observations in which 36,000 meals freely chosen by a large group of children of this age were examined. Now of course you cannot, as was done in the experiment, offer your child fifteen different sorts of food every day and leave it to choose. But you can, without loss of time, simply offer the child everything from your table. That takes one minute daily and one avoids all feeding difficulties.

Breast-feeding difficulties are almost always the result of insufficient knowledge. The nurse or doctor must show one how to suckle the infant at first. It is fed according to an approximate timetable—every four hours with a nightly interval of eight hours—as, for example—6, 10, 2, 6 and 10 o'clock. You must stick to a timetable. By doing so you accustom the infant to time-conditioned feeding reflexes. It is, of course, not sensible to wake a child simply because it is its exact feeding time. Usually it is punctual after a few days. But if it wakes up ten minutes late, you should wait for it. Another time it may be hungry a quarter of an hour earlier. It would, of course, be equally idiotic to let it scream for fifteen minutes with the clock in one's hand. The child's feeding timetable must not become a matter of rigid principle. Only with the early morning feeding must one take care that this does not slip back into the night, otherwise there is the devil to pay. The infant sleeps most of the day, anyway, but the mother's sleep is all too short. At each feeding the child may feed from each breast or, sometimes, only one breast is drained. This takes fifteen to twenty minutes, with intervals to get its breath. Falling asleep with the nipple in its mouth, because the child is too lazy to drink, is overcome by holding its nose. If the child falls away, it is put back to the breast again. The child is held as comfortably as possible. Suckling is strenuous. After each feeding the breast is milked with the hand until nothing more comes. It must be pumped quite empty, in order to be properly full again in eight hours. The breast is easier to suckle at the beginning of a feeding and less so afterwards, and no one will exert himself if it is possible to avoid doing so. Certainly no infant will do so! In such things they are even lazier than adults. Infants are also human beings. Not every scream indicates hunger. In the summer it is just as likely to mean thirst. Boiled water, given in a spoon, works wonders. An infant may well get too hot in its many layers of clothing. This is just as likely to make him uncomfortable as being cold. Furthermore, he has no other means of expressing himself except by screaming. You must be sympathetic. After all, the little chap has to lie wrapped up for hours and cannot move. You try it. How soon do you feel a crease or even a knot pressing? What should the child do? It can only scream. Take it up. If something feels uncomfortable (or too tight), re-wrap it. A damp diaper which stays warm is generally not unpleasant, but if there is a stool in the diaper, most infants get annoyed. Such screaming is not due to hunger. A person with a sensitive ear can differentiate between the hunger scream and the discomfort scream.

If an infant screams immediately after feeding, that scarcely ever means that it is hungry. The act of sucking and grasping the nipple with its mouth gives it pleasure. It is almost the infant's only pleasure, and if this is denied it, it curses—but not for long. When it is over-fed it cannot scream because the distended stomach presses on the diaphragm and prevents deep breaths. While awake an infant needs something small to stimulate and train his eye movements, because, for him, practising and being active have already begun. This object could be just a simple piece of wood, or a celluloid doll or rattle. It must be within range of the infant's eyes and it should not be the same one every day. Bright colors such as colored curtains have a soothing effect as they satisfy the infant's visual needs. He curses if his face is turned away from the light. So all screaming is not hunger, but can be complaint. This is no reason to give it more food.

The new-born babe's weight goes down in the first five days of life by as much as one pound. This is normal and it is not a sign of insufficient feeding. Only after ten or fourteen days does it regain its weight at birth. Any delay in this increase in weight must be reported to the doctor. Do not give it extra feedings without the doctor's advice.

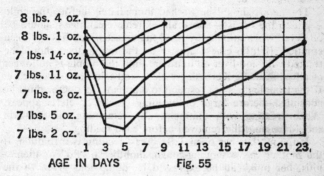

Weight curves of four healthy new-born babies.

A screaming infant can almost always be calmed by feeding, above all when it is fed with the breast or bottle. This is not proof that it was hungry before, but only that it enjoyed being nursed!

Being fat is not synonymous with being healthy. Artificially fed children can easily be made fatter and rounder than breast-fed infants. But that indicates wrong feeding and is certainly no reason for pride.

CARE OF THE BREAST

There is actually no need for special care of the breasts. They should be washed every day with soap and water and well rubbed. By brushing the nipples during pregnancy their skin is hardened so as to be able to cope with the business of suckling.

A suitable "bra" is of great importance. It must meet three

demands. Firstly it must carry the breast and relieve it of its own weight. The breast must not be lifted or otherwise pulled out of its natural shape. Secondly, the "bra" must be able to be opened in front, so that the child can be given the breast without difficulty. Thirdly, it must be washable (and washed often!). Little patches of clean cotton should be placed between the "bra" and nipples. These protect the nipples and absorb any milk which dribbles out, thereby preventing the clothes from becoming soiled.

The hands should be washed immediately before the child is put to the breast—above all, extreme cleanliness should be observed when milking by hand the breast which has not been emptied. If little cracks appear on the nipple they should be treated with cod-liver oil ointment until the nipple is no longer at all painful. Be increasingly clean and take the utmost care. If the trouble does not respond to ointment the doctor must be consulted, before large or bleeding cracks or clefts appear. When treating with ointment, any remaining on the skin should be carefully removed before each feeding.

If the mother has open T.B., breast-feeding is forbidden. If the mother has whooping-cough, diphtheria, "flu" or meningitis, her milk can be expressed by pump and given to the child.

If the mother has typhoid, scarlet fever, measles or chickenpox, she may go on feeding the child. The danger of infection is less than that of suddenly changing over to artificial feeding, since by the time the mother's illness has been diagnosed, it is a pretty safe bet that the child is also infected. The doctor decides in individual cases. Resumption of the monthly periods or mild infectious fevers do not necessitate stopping breast-feeding.

If a new pregnancy starts during lactation the child should be weaned.

If the infant gets a cold, it finds difficulty in sucking. During this time the breasts should be emptied by pump so that the supply does not diminish and the milk is given with a spoon.

One obstacle to breast-feeding is maternal aversion to feeding her child in this manner. If the mother's state of mind is such that she is reluctant to use this method, no special effort should be made to convince her that breast-feeding should be tried; aversion alone can prevent success. Medical reasons for not breast-feeding include: tuberculosis, diabetes, heart disease, mastitis, or badly cracked nipples. Avoiding breast-feeding sometimes helps more to develop the maternal instinct (which is so indispensable for the child's development) than vain attempts at breast-feeding in spite of the woman's inner resistance. In such cases the doctor must supervise the child's feeding. He must prescribe not only the composition of the food, but also the quantity permitted. Extreme cleanliness is one's duty when artificially feeding infants. It means a lot of work to bring up a child on a bottle as safely as is possible when it is breast-fed. It can be done almost as well if one carefully observes all the rules. In order to give one an insight into the difficulties, here are the differences between cow's milk and mother's milk:

	Cow's milk	Mother's milk
Protein	3.7 per cent	1.9 per cent
Fat	3.5 " "	3.5 " "
Sugar	4.5 " "	6.6 " "
Minerals	0.7 " "	0.2 " "
Calories per ounce	25 " "	25 " "

So it is clear that cow's milk is made for quite a different young living creature than mother's milk, and, judging by the higher quantity of protein, one which grows more quickly—i.e. the calf, as opposed to the human infant. Judging by the different distribution of the kinds of protein, cow's milk is also made for a different kind of stomach from that of the human infant. The quantity of minerals in human milk is not only less, but also differently distributed. Both kinds of milk contain antibodies—only in cow's milk they are for calves' illnesses and in mother's milk for children's illnesses.

In order to make cow's milk a more or less suitable infants' food, one must add an equal amount of water, and add to each pint 1½ ounces of sugar (preferably glucose) and ¾ ounce of fresh cream. Even then one is giving cow's milk protein, which does not always agree with sensitive infants' stomachs unless it has first been dried (dried milk) and then re-dissolved. It is better to get one's doctor to prescribe a reliable dried preparation of a recognized infants' food and to use fresh milk only in accordance with his instructions.

The science of artificial feeding has shown great advances recently. Fifty years ago the death-rate among artificially fed babies was 20 per cent. With efficient medical supervision and intelligence and care on the part of the mother, this is now no longer the case.

Here is a chart to show what the baby gets through:

Age	Calories	Quantity of milk in ounces per day
2nd week	350	16
4th ”	445	20
12th ”	580	27
20th ”	700	33

CARE OF THE INFANT

This is a science which children can learn by example and at school. Playing with dolls would be much more amusing if parents would only show children how to put on a diaper and rompers, and explain why all that is necessary. What is still better is being allowed to watch and lend a hand with baby brother or sister.

You must get someone experienced to show you just how it is done. For this reason only a few tips will be given here—ones which are often not remembered and which simplify life.

Firstly a young infant needs parental love if it is to thrive. In other words, it is not insensitive. It is true that it does not react to words or gestures, but it does so very much to tone of voice and to tenderness of touch when handled, and to all the many unconscious emotional expressions which we adults also use to communicate with one another.

Secondly the rule is cleanliness of parent and child. Mere good intentions are not enough. Hands must be washed every time before putting on diapers, breast-feeding and washing the infant.

An infant is bathed every day. The temperature of the water should be 90 degrees Fahrenheit. Special care is given to the washing of its buttocks, sex organs, and groin, and a mild soap and wash cloth should be used. All soap must be carefully removed from the skin with a second clean wash cloth. Children with a particularly sensitive skin can be rinsed in a second basin. When drying, do not rub, but dab. Rubbing harms the still sensitive infant's skin. Every trace of moisture must be removed from any creases in the skin. (Its own little towels should be very absorbent.)

The sex organs are cleaned with cotton wool moistened with olive oil. In girls the vulval lips are separated and the front part wiped clean. In boys the foreskin is carefully drawn back and the part underneath carefully cleaned.

After the bath do not sprinkle powder on the child's skin.

Powder your own hands and then rub them on the baby's body. Powder made from potato or rice starch is not suitable as it gets lumpy when damp and then irritates. Talcum is the correct foundation for children's powder.

The infant is never bathed just after a meal and never immediately before going out or being put out in the open air. When the diaper is soiled by feces, the worst is removed with a corner of the dirty diaper and the infant is washed with a wash cloth specially reserved for the purpose. Soap should only be used if one cannot possibly manage otherwise. Always wipe from front to back, especially in girls. With children who have sensitive skins, water should be avoided entirely and cleaning should be done with cotton wool soaked in olive oil. If a rash appears on the skin, at once apply a mild ointment, which should always be kept handy—something like a simple zinc ointment. This prevents the rash from spreading. Cleaning the child's head is a separate matter. Washing the scalp should not present any problem. The wash cloth must not be rubbed over the child's eyes, which are wiped from inside outwards with cotton wool soaked in water. If necessary the nostrils and ears are cleaned out using cotton wool dipped in oil, which has not been rolled into too much of a point. Before cleaning an infant's ears for the first time, try it on your own to see how sensitive they are!

Finally a few remarks about putting on diapers. The most important thing to remember is that an infant needs exercise in order to develop well. After all, it has been busy kicking inside its mother's body for four or five months. One should not drastically interrupt muscle exercises which were begun before birth, now that life is starting. Therefore restrict the infant as little as possible. Every child should at least have a holiday from its diaper once or twice every day and should be able to kick freely to its heart's content for some time. From the start one should lay it on its stomach in order to develop the throat and neck muscles.

For a diaper it is best to use square cloths, which are folded as shown on page 350. By doing this you get more layers from the same piece of material, and can, in addition —unlike the customary way of putting on diapers—strengthen the front in boys and correspondingly the back in girls. Besides, the child's freedom of movement is less impeded. Rubber pants should not be used as they retain perspiration.

It is usually possible for the infant to be kept dry only just before or after feedings. If the infant has passed a stool in its diaper and screams because of this, it must be changed right away. The child should very soon be given greater freedom. Instead of tightly rolling it in a diaper, one can easily make a waterproof "diaper carrier."

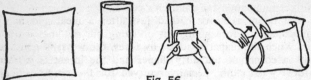

Fig. 56

It is best to use cellulose for the inner layer, though expensive. It is very much more pleasant as it is less liable to chafe than diapers, which always contain traces of detergents. On top of this comes rompers. In winter the whole thing can be put in a flannel bag.

The infant's cot or basket should have a firm mattress. Between this and the sheet put a rubber sheet. A pillow is bad. It is best for the infant to lie quite flat. There is always a danger of suffocating with feather pillows. On the other hand it is a good thing to pad the head-piece of the cot by fixing a hard cushion to it. This prevents the infant from banging its head when it kicks.

As soon as the mother is up again, the infant should have its own room, or at any rate should be away from the mother's bed at night. This is a great help in training it to keep quiet at night. Children and even infants react to emotional excitement, which they can tell from sounds and the tones of voices.

An infant needs fresh air. From the fourth week onwards it can be put out of doors, even in the winter (unless it is very cold) provided it is well covered and protected from the wind. It should be out for half an hour to start with and then remain up to two hours. Until you are experienced, you should at first frequently check the warmth of its face and hands.

In the summer sunbathing without clothes is advantageous, as sun rays cause vitamin D to form in the skin. This vitamin protects them from rickets and should be taken additionally in the winter to be on the safe side. (But give only small quantities. Too much can be harmful.) And take care with the sun. An infant's skin is sensitive. Let it sunbathe only for a very short time at first; and the face must never be directly exposed to the sun, otherwise the infant screams. If possible, the child should be put out of doors, protected from the wind, every day in the summer. A balcony is sufficient—but take care that the child does not get over-heated.

TRAINING IN CLEANLINESS

It is not advisable to start this in earnest before the ninth month. Of course one offers the toilet before this, once the child can sit up and once one has noticed the times when it usually empties its bowels. The child should not be put on the toilet until it is able to sit on it unaided. Training it to be clean by force before nine months old, and especially punishing it, leads to lifelong mental injury and is tantamount to wanton physical mutilation. The only permissible training measures are unobtrusive rewards, and making it obvious that the child has done what was expected. It is wrong to punish the child, if it lapses during the early months. An angry or a sad face is one of the worst punishments. One must take care that the child experiences no disadvantages or unpleasantries while it is learning to be clean, such as having its buttocks cleaned too roughly. A little care and thought is of great value.

Everything can be achieved very easily once you really understand that controlling the functions of the organs of evacuation has to be learned, just like walking. No one would dream of forcing a child to walk by punishing and beating it. The child is trying out its own body, and its efficiency in passing excreta. We adults are accustomed to regarding excreta, etc., with exaggerated disgust. But try to imagine how we could cope with this sense of disgust if we were not able to control these functions. It would be ghastly. But this is just what happens to a child if its parents try to enforce cleanliness too soon. Once the child learns by punishments or scolding that it can play up its parents by wetting its bed, the situation is very serious. It may be the start of a bitter struggle—the outcome of which is generally years of bed-wetting. This tragedy is disturbingly common. Widespread investigations suggest that one in every three or five children is so affected. This is due to the absolutely stupid but widely held view that reproaches and spankings can influence such unconscious processes as the nervous stimuli of bed-wetting. It shows complete lack of knowledge and understanding of one's own child. It is the parents who have failed in getting the child clean, and not the child. If the child is seen before the age of six, a single psychotherapeutic interview is usually sufficient to find out the real cause and remove the disorder —provided that the parents have the sense and insight to change their harmful attitude.

SEXUALITY IN CHILDREN

In children playing with sex organs has nowhere near the same significance as in adults. Harm can be caused by adopting a wrong attitude of shame. First of all the facts:

Every normal boy has the ability to erect his penis from the day of birth onwards. Observation has shown that the excitement leading up to this occurs when an emergency situation calls for extra effort—e.g. when the child experiences difficulty while feeding at its mother's breast or from the bottle. Corresponding excitement with little girls cannot be so well observed, but it is probably just as common. People who see anything indecent or punishable in this must have excessively dirty minds. But there is also no cause for embarrassed giggling. Both these things can make the child unnaturally sex-conscious.

Reliable observations on several hundred children (boys) have shown that one-third of all children in the first year of their life are capable of producing a "lustful" orgasm, comparable to that of grown-ups. The percentage rises to 80 per cent at about the age of ten. About 70 per cent of all boys have already masturbated before puberty. In girls the figures are believed to be somewhat lower. Masturbation does not cause physical harm or injury in adults or children. However, serious harm is caused by adults drawing children's attention to sex at an early age (0-5 years) by punishment or other behavior (surprise, embarrassed astonishment, pretending not to notice). By so doing they make an artificial distinction between sex and other everyday things, and, as a result, playing with the sex organs acquires a sexual character. Parents who use their imagination and can put themselves in their children's position and leave them to themselves without resorting to punishment or indicating amusement, act for the best. Then the children usually lose interest in the game, which never meant much to them anyway. They have to investigate all parts of their body, and they do so quite impartially. But if the grown-up's attitude makes them aware that the game has a special significance, they occupy themselves more intensively with it, and finally discover methods which lead to real orgastic pleasure and which, as one can understand, they therefore persist in doing.

It should go without saying that adults should not stimulate children's sex organs. This can happen quite unintentionally by rocking a child on one's knee, etc. If one notices the corresponding excitement, it is best to stop without comment and without showing any emotion. The danger for the child of such stimuli, which may pass unnoticed by the adult, is infinitely greater than when the child itself plays with its sex organs. It is an obvious, sexual activity with a partner and it is not for nothing that such rocking games are very popular with children.

But by and large it can be said that children who are not disturbed when playing with their own private parts remain what they are—pure and innocent—while others, who encounter a conspicuous attitude on the part of their parents or grandparents, are spoiled by it. From a medical point of view this would not be a bad thing except they retain lifelong mental ill-effects and inhibitions, which only too easily result in psychosomatic illnesses, and these affect the body—quite apart from the capacity for love later on when the child is grown up.

One thing one must impress upon oneself. Excitement occurring in small children, similar or comparable to the sexual excitement of adults, is not a sign of illness or sexual precocity, but a normal form of self-expression which is noticed only if children are closely observed. It is immaterial whether these games or "bad habits" are defined as sexuality. One must just realize the scientific facts given here and abide by them, in order not to cause any harm. It is one of the most important things in the upbringing of children, and unfortunately a lot of mischievous nonsense is printed about it.

Some of you may wonder why so much space has been given to these matters. But if one wants to help one's readers to avoid suffering and illness, there is nothing for it but to treat in great detail questions about which such erroneous views are held.

THE CHILD

Children who are healthily fed and are not suffering from any other defects have fundamentally greater powers of resistance to illness than grown-ups. They are only at a disadvantage in one respect: their body has not yet learned to deal with the various infectious diseases. Incidentally this is true of other things. A child's abilities are greater at birth than those of adults. All they lack is knowledge. This applies as much to their astonishing quickness in grasping things, as to their ability to resist illness. If properly fed, their bodies are incredibly vigilant. They deal promptly and vigorously with all threats from bacteria and all their defensive measures are brought into action. This is why children often run a temperature for the slightest reasons. Fundamentally this is a good thing since this reaction prevents worse things happening.

THE SUSCEPTIBLE CHILD

For this reason all mothers should remember that a temperature in a child is not a bad sign. On the contrary, it shows the child's body's readiness to fight.

If you look at the matter in this way, you will see that a child's health is threatened by two things. The first are the infectious children's illnesses, known to us all (measles, scarlet fever, diphtheria, etc.), against which the child's body has not yet learned to defend itself. (See chapter on Infectious Diseases, page 132.)

The second are the various forms of allergy and sensitivity. These include nettle-rash, repeated nose and throat catarrh, bronchial catarrh, asthma, and feeding disorders. Some children are always falling ill, because their defense mechanism does not work efficiently. The defenses are set in motion too easily and for that reason quickly become exhausted. The most important part of the treatment of a child susceptible to illness is a sensible adjustment of the child's diet, which should in general be light. (Generally speaking grown-ups imagine that children need double the amount of food that is really necessary.) On the whole fresh milk is harmful. The diet of a child like this should be supervised by a doctor, preferably a pediatrician, since "over-sensitivity reactions" (pages 266 and 268)—so called food allergies—very often occur. The skin symptoms can be caused by different kinds of animal protein—eggs or milk or cheese or fish. It might just as well be oatmeal or flour, potatoes or tomatoes.

Once it has been discovered which food causes these reactions, one must exclude it and, in accordance with the instructions in the chapter on nutrition in this book, choose as nourishing a diet as possible. You should try and get away as far as possible from "children's food" and introduce as much grown-up food as you can. All "food tonics," which are expensive, are useless, since they constantly draw the child's attention to his "special condition" and thereby aggravate it. The idea that he is sickly and not able to do things like other children takes root in the child's mind and can have a harmful influence on him in later life. The only thing that is allowed and really does any good are vitamin preparations, which should of course be given to the child not as medicine, but as a delicacy. Children usually love them.

It is fundamentally wrong to adopt the attitude that "my child has low resistance. I must be particularly careful with him." It is useless to consult a different doctor each time the child has something wrong with him. You should consult a pediatrician and really follow his advice. A doctor is not a "miracle man," who can tell at a glance the right thing to do in a particular case. He must try out various treatments from case to case until he finds the right one, and he can only do this if the child continues to come to him. He cannot tell immediately whether a particular child is allergic to eggs, fresh milk or white bread. These have to be tried out, and it takes time and requires understanding on the part of the parents.

It may be that forbidding fresh milk and going over to dried milk may solve the problem at the first attempt. But it may also be that one has to go on experimenting with different kinds of food, trying each in turn. But above all else stick to it and do not go to another doctor after a couple of weeks, only for him to have to start the laborious business of experimenting all over again. The doctor is bound by the law of "usually." He invariably starts by suggesting the cause that most frequently occurs. People who break off treatment never get anywhere by constantly changing their doctor.

These many and varied symptoms constitute the greater part of children's non-infectious illnesses. They are all that we associate with sickly, susceptible children. These children run a temperature easily without infection and it is not always possible to find out the actual cause of the trouble. In such cases it is a good thing to introduce a "fruit and vegetable juice day." The squeezed juices should be well sweetened.

The Normally Developing Child

Growing is the child's main business—growing physically and mentally. This growth follows a definite set of laws. Every newly acquired ability and power must constantly be tried out, grasped and assimilated; in other words, a child must be allowed to play untrammeled in order that his body and

DEVELOPMENT OF

Age, Length, Weight	Sleep in hours	Calories, Amount of Food, Kind of Food
4 weeks. 21-22 in. 7-8 lb.	18-20.	400-500 cal. 5 feedings.
16 weeks. 24-25 in. 11-12 lb.	15-18, generally from 6 p.m. to 5 a.m. The rest in three daily naps.	600-650 cal. 5 feedings.

THE CHILD

Excretions	Activity and Interests	Social Behavior
During 24 hrs., 1-3 or even 4 stools on waking. Some children scream if they lie wet. The kind of screaming can be distinguished from hungry crying.	Looks at lights and windows. Likes to turn its head to one side. Gets annoyed if its head is turned away from the light. Bright colors calm it. Sunlight falling directly on its head causes great discomfort. Light and bright colors (red and orange) are of great value.	Looks into one's face if one comes close enough. When it cries in the evenings the child calms down if it is picked up and laid on a table where it can kick and listen to voices and watch lights (1-2 hrs.). This craving for light and colors is greatest between six and eight weeks. It is certainly as important as the craving for food.
1-2 stools, sometimes a day is missed (no laxatives needed). Often children tend to go at a certain time, and by observation one can sometimes catch them at the right moment. But this usually does not last longer than a week.	Head movements, kicking, turning on one side, reaching for objects, catching hold of its own hands, sucking its thumb or finger. All these are popular forms of exercise. A toy hanging on a string is the height of bliss. Voice exercises are tried (single vowels). Light disturbs the child's sleep in the evenings.	It wants to be taken notice of, especially in the afternoons and evenings. It likes to be talked to, so much so that it may cry if left. In its "playtime" it lets itself be taken out of its crib or basket and deposited on a couch. It likes to sit very much. The father or brothers and sisters are more suitable for satisfying the child's social instincts than the

DEVELOPMENT OF

Age, Length, Weight	Sleep in hours	Calories, Amount of Food, Kind of Food
28 weeks. 28-29 in. 15-16 lb.	14-17, generally from 6 p.m. to 6 a.m.; usually waits half-hour before crying for its food in the morning. Two to three short naps in the course of the day—preferably out of doors.	700-750 calories (3-4 meals). Pulped fruit and vegetables and meat fed with spoon. Drinks out of a cup. Bring in meals ready as children are very impatient.
9 months. 30-31 in. 20-21 lb.	12-14, generally from 6 or 7 p.m. to 5-7 a.m. In the mornings and afternoons, naps; for preference in a closed room. It usually plays contentedly before the	750-800 calories (3-4 meals). It likes to eat everything that is offered if the quantities are not too large. It is best fed with a spoon and given drinks out of a

THE CHILD—*cont.*

Excretions	Activity and Interests	Social Behavior
		mother, who is always associated with its feeding.
One a day (in the diaper), usually in the mornings. Only some girls submit to the toilet. Most children resist. There are great differences between boys and girls with regard to urination. Girls last out up to 2 hrs. and often go on the toilet then. The amount of urine and wetting is great.	Prefers to lie on its back again. It kicks and catches hold of its own feet and puts them in its mouth. It observes with interest the movements of its own hand. It takes off its shoes and stockings. It does not put its hands in its mouth so often. It prefers playing with string, paper, soft rubber toys and rattles which it bites. It has a large vocabulary of different sounds which it produces contentedly for itself. It does not need company so much.	It likes to be shown things by grownups and can cope with several people at the same time. It likes to be handed things and likes hearing rhythmic words. It is beginning to be shy with strangers, especially in new surroundings. Four weeks later the child can easily be over-excited. Laughter which is closely followed by crying can serve as a warning. Exercise is much appreciated.
1-2 stools a day. Some children go on the toilet regularly, if one catches them at the right time. Girls are often dry the whole day if, for example, they are	The child now has many sounds at its disposal —"Papa," "Mama," and other two-syllabled words. It often laughs at its own noises, particularly high notes. It ex-	Now it is better for only one person to attend the child, although it is good to let it participate in the family life from the playpen. It is still shy of strangers and

Age, Length, Weight	Sleep in hours	Calories, Amount of Food, Kind of Food
	first morning meal for 1-1½ hrs.	cup. It manages with the fingers if anything falls off. (Don't punish it for doing this, but let it do it—vital exercise in independence.) It can eat virtually everything (offer!) if it is chopped finely enough.
1 year. 31-32 in. 21-22 lb.	12-14. Night sleep is 11-12 hrs., generally only one daily nap before lunch. Impatient after waking up. Give it a cracker to quiet it. Breakfast ½-1 hr. later.	850 calories (three main meals). Preferably fruit juice in the afternoon. After waking up from every sleep a piece of toast or cracker is very popular. The children are very eager to feed themselves, for which patience and a cover of oilcloth are necessary. (Table manners are learned at the earliest three years later, and then by watching others.)

THE CHILD—*cont.*

Excretions	Activity and Interests	Social Behavior
put on the toilet directly after their afternoon sleep, or at definite intervals.	amines closely individual toys. It plays with its cup as though it were drinking. It chews objects. It is very mobile. It crawls, pushes and fetches things. The child must no longer be left unattended on a bed or table as it can easily fall down. It is not afraid of water. In warm districts the children learn to swim easily.	strange voices. It delights in trying to stand. All kinds of activity are not only useful, but also very pleasant.
Successes on the toilet are now rarer than before. The children resist being made clean and are usually "dry" in the day and occasionally at night as well, if put on the toilet directly after they wake up in the night and in the morning.	They try to stand, and like leaving the playpen. They enjoy putting hats, baskets or cups on their heads. They often throw things out of range and are then annoyed. Especially popular: putting smaller objects (buttons, etc.) into boxes or cups.	It needs company very much. It takes a particular interest in moving objects, i.e. cars, people. Its own toys no longer satisfy it completely. It loves to be chased when crawling and hides behind chairs. It hands things to grown-ups, but expects them back at once and gets annoyed if the things which it has thrown down are not brought back again. It gets very

DEVELOPMENT OF

Age, Length, Weight	Sleep in hours	Calories, Amount of Food, Kind of Food
15 months. 32-33 in. 22-23 lb.	As 1 year. Some children wake at night and are quieted down most quickly if they are allowed to look out of the window, or if something is put in their hand, or if they are given something to nibble like a cracker. The daily nap is now generally an ordinary midday sleep.	900 calories. Children are eager to eat by themselves with their fingers. Some children show considerable skill with the spoon, even if they hold it wrong way around. The appetite is largest at midday and in the evenings and is on the whole good.

THE CHILD—*cont.*

Excretions	Activity and Interests	Social Behavior
		angry if anything is taken away from it. Reacts to "No" (but not regularly). Shyness with strangers may disappear.
1–2 stools a day. Sometimes a day is missed. Resistance to the toilet grows gradually less. If put on the toilet at favorable times, it works, but at times it still fails. The same applies to lying dry. Some children wet their clothing directly after they have been taken off the toilet. It is nonsense to make them sit for hours or even to punish them. The only success is for the child to run about in wet clothing without saying anything. Some children now are continent up to 3 hrs.	The child amuses itself quite happily and contentedly in the mornings, but as the day goes on it loves more and more stimulus and variety. Favorite toys: balls, spoons, cups, boxes, and games where the pieces are made to fit into each other. It chases balls which it has thrown away.	Generally shyness with strangers has by now vanished. The child is bent on investigating its immediate surroundings. It takes pleasure in noises, also sudden barking of dogs, roaring of airplanes, thunder, etc. The child copies grownups' gestures—coughing and blowing one's nose. It demands everything it sees. Of special interest: wastepaper basket. It takes everything out and generally leaves it lying about. It likes looking at picturebooks. Undesirable actions are interrupted by picking up the child and putting it elsewhere.

DEVELOPMENT OF

Age, Length, Weight	Sleep in hours	Calories, Amount of Food, Kind of Food
1½ years. 33–34 in. 23–24 lb.	As 1 year. After an exciting day occasional waking up in the night. Calm it by talking to it, giving it a drink or putting it on the toilet. Putting it to bed is made easier if the child is allowed to take a toy (such as a teddy bear or its own shoe) into bed with it. Midday sleep as for 15 months.	950 calories. The appetite is poorer than three months ago. Changing preference for individual kinds of food. Most children can eat with a spoon by themselves and can drink unaided out of a cup. Bits of meat, pear and similar firm foods are put straight into the mouth with the fingers. The handle of the spoon is held horizontally in the whole fist and is put into the mouth with the elbow held horizontally (it can't yet be done differently). The child is easily distracted when eating.
2 years. 34–35 in. 25–26 lb.	Night sleep approximately 10–11 hrs. It does not us-	1,000 calories. The appetite is good to middling. The

THE CHILD—*cont.*

Excretions	Activity and Interests	Social Behavior
A difficult time, as the times when the child's bowels move change greatly. Children who "go" directly after meals are more easily accustomed to the toilet. In the course of the coming three months there are many "setbacks," often combined with diarrhea. Some children are only successful on the toilet when they are quite naked. Dryness is generally not yet achieved, although most children like going on the toilet if they are not put on it too often. Much depends on catching the children directly they wake up. There is not much point in waking them at night since they usually do not last out anyway.	It is very active and constantly changes its own toys. There is much climbing and pushing about of chairs. Curtains must be very firm. Old papers which can be torn up are a good safety-valve. Some children refuse to stay in their playpen. A garden is ideal and sand one of the best toys. In the course of the next 3 months their activity diminishes and the child takes more interest in people again. Falling and bumping itself become more frequent.	It likes to help with the cleaning and washing up and sometimes fetches Daddy's slippers. It likes to take things back. It does not play with grown-ups the whole time, but usually only in the evenings before going to bed. In the course of the coming three months it develops a sense of property, i.e. what belongs to the other members of the family and what is its own. It likes to be in the kitchen and participates in all the chores. The child reacts more strongly to grown-ups and demands more of them. It is influenced by praise and correction. It takes advantage of the discovery that grown-ups will come if called by their names.
This is the time when the children feel proud if they	The children are quieter when playing and stick to it	Adapts itself better in the home than before and realizes

Age, Length, Weight	Sleep in hours	Calories, Amount of Food, Kind of Food
	ually go to sleep before 8 or 9 in the evening. If it sleeps at midday the night sleep is shorter. For the sake of convenience it is therefore not good to let the child sleep too long in the middle of the day. Night sleep is "sensitive." The child likes to dawdle when going to bed. It is not good to keep the child out late at night. Sleeping has been difficult for about 3 months. It is very good to stick to a certain routine when putting the child to bed.	main meal is at midday. Not too much at breakfast. The children are definitely "choosy" and like firm food in large pieces, such as whole potatoes, etc. It is wrong to force certain kinds of foods on them at this stage. Some children eat quite alone and are better left alone in their own room or at their own table where they are not observed.
2½ years. 35–36 in. 27–28 lb.	Peace at night depends on how long the child sleeps in	1,050 calories. Appetite changes rapidly. On the whole

THE CHILD—*cont.*

Excretions	Activity and Interests	Social Behavior
succeed in getting to the toilet in time and with success. Many want to be left alone while performing. Sometimes success is achieved if the children are allowed to run about near the toilet with their clothing down at the appropriate time. Usually call to stool is announced. In most cases the children are dry in the daytime, but there are always lapses. On an average girls are dry at night considerably sooner than boys. In some cases it helps to get the children up at night, but not usually. If a child has lasted out and refuses to have a diaper, one must take a risk for once, otherwise one can cause opposition.	more than before. Mobile toys, such as bikes and cars, or mechanical kitchen utensils are of special importance to the children. Bricks and other things which fit into each other are also important. Miniature books, little bottles, etc., are collected. Outside, sand still thrills them and they can now use the spade more effectively. Splashing about with water adds to the attraction. Running, climbing, and pulling carts.	what belongs to others and what it may not touch. All the same, it likes to possess things and takes charge of everything and claims it. Outside the house it is the other way round and the child is generally shy and gives in. Now it is very shy of grown-ups again. It likes to help in the house. But if left alone it can make a great deal of untidiness. It likes to run on steps or low garden walls if held by the hand. It seeks the company of others, above all of older children, and plays with them. There is less friction if either only the father or the mother devotes his or herself to the child. When both are there, difficulties crop up.
Number of stools varies greatly—one to two a day. More	Speech has quite taken possession of the child—and it	The pedantic sense of order and tidiness can be very

Age, Length, Weight	Sleep in hours	Calories, Amount of Food, Kind of Food
	the middle of the day. The time it falls asleep varies between 6 o'clock and 10 o'clock, but it is not good to put the child to bed after 8 p.m. There is generally a going-to-sleep ritual, which should be observed if one wants to save time. The midday sleep is often a problem.	a definite meal, either at midday or in the evening, is especially good. The child still has definite preferences for certain dishes, which rapidly change. It often asks for tidbits between meals, which one may give it, if one takes into account that the child's appetite will of course be smaller at mealtimes. If necessary fruit or fruit juice with crackers should be offered the child at definite "between meals." It is better not to let it see sweets. Don't worry if the appetite is poor for a few days. This will right itself.

THE CHILD—*cont.*

Excretions	Activity and Interests	Social Behavior
and more frequently the child misses one or two days (for heaven's sake, no purges!). It only rarely has an "accident" in its clothing now. Children prefer to go alone and climb onto the grown-ups' lavatory seat. They like to be alone while performing. The child is usually dry in the daytime by now. Most children go alone, above all if suitably dressed, so that they can manage themselves, with the help of a stool placed near the toilet, etc. Many girls can last up to 5 hrs., but sometimes they still come too late. They are very fastidious even if only a little drop goes over the edge. At times there are difficulties when using a strange toilet. The child likes to watch others when	goes by leaps and bounds. It talks incessantly. Even when it is alone it tells stories. Individual toys cannot hold its interest for long and are left lying about, while a new one is taken up. Playing with toys does not last long. If the child makes too much noise running about, it is a good thing to put it out to "let off steam." It is useless to try to make it tidy up first. The playing requisites for out-of-doors are similar to what they were six month ago.	trying for the rest of the family. All furniture, etc., must remain in the same place and position. It is not good to shift the furniture in the house at this stage. The child sees to it that everyone puts away and hangs up his or her things properly. With itself, on the other hand, it is still extremely lenient in this respect. That is a passing phase. Life in the family is made simpler if one gives in to the child's demands with humor. And it is in any case quite a good thing for grown-ups to learn to put their jackets on a coat-hanger properly. The children like to run little errands. Usually they plainly prefer one parent, but their preference may change according to the need of the moment. Great need

Age, Length, Weight	Sleep in hours	Calories, Amount of Food, Kind of Food
3 years. 37–38 in. 30–31 lb.	While the child's daily habits show greater maturity, it remains for the most part where it was at 2½ years with regard to sleeping. The "going to sleep" ritual again loses its significance. Many children now stay quietly at home by	1,100 calories. The appetite becomes more settled. Breakfast achieves a greater significance. The appetite at midday is correspondingly less and is good again in the evening. Children like to drink milk again (4 small cups of

THE CHILD—*cont.*

Excretions	Activity and Interests	Social Behavior
in the toilet. Wetting during the midday sleep is now more frequent. A few children last the whole night. Some wake up and call. By taking the child out at 10 p.m. there is a fifty-fifty chance that it will be dry in the morning. If children protest, one should, however, refrain from doing this. Diapers and rubber sheets are still the best way of guaranteeing the child's physical and mental comfort at night and of reducing the amount of washing.		for society. Shyness with strangers has generally been overcome. It is better to let the child play with one other child, and an older one for preference. It is sometimes a good thing to hide the child's favorite toys if another child comes to play. This makes it easier for the children to adapt themselves to the company.
By now the stools are generally regulated. Most children go to the toilet by themselves and only ask for help when they are finished. The bowels move once or twice a day. An occasional day is missed. Most children are now dry	Three-year-olds are very self-sufficient. To please the grown-ups they clear away after playing. Their imagination is more lively. Colored boxes of blocks are an important part of their training. Climbing and swinging can occu-	Very helpful in the house. When playing with other children all is well usually only for 20 or 30 minutes. Then they start to quarrel if not under supervision. Even if supervised, playing with children of the same age is scarcely suc-

Age, Length, Weight	Sleep in hours	Calories, Amount of Food, Kind of Food
	themselves, if their parents tell them that they are going out (if necessary the day before). If that is not successful, another attempt must be made later on. Waking up is difficult. The children are often tired and grumpy in the mornings.	milk supply about 400 calories and therefore considerably reduce the quantity of solid food that can be expected to be eaten at meals). The child's tastes do not change as they did. Meat, fruit and milk are often preferred. The child likes something to chew. Some children can already hold their spoons correctly. Children eat best if left alone.
4 years. 40–41 in. 34–35 lb.	Going to bed is relatively easy and many children of 4½ go of their own accord. A definite time for going to bed should be introduced, if necessary with an alarm clock set at the right time.	1,300 calories. Appetite at the beginning of the year mediocre. At 4½ it is usually good to very good at times. Individual meals are equally important. Favorite dishes are requested repeatedly.

Excretions	Activity and Interests	Social Behavior
in the daytime and at night without having to be taken out. Occasionally there is a lapse in the daytime and some children lapse once or twice in the week at night or for a whole week consecutively.	py them for hours. The child takes an interest in its "baby period" and realizes that it has already grown. When it is 3½, it often invents an imaginary playmate, for whom it keeps a place at table, etc. Many children like to play at being animals. The children are now more attentive when listening to stories.	cessful, 5–6-year-olds are the best playmates. One can recognize two types: those who play alone and at home and who do not like sharing; and the opposite type. Generally speaking the mother is preferred. The child likes to refer to her and itself as "we." A new phase of self-consciousness has begun. The child likes to make simple decisions between two alternatives, i.e. "Will you come in at the front or round the back way?" is a valuable trick for luring the child inside.
Children are normally clean and dry at this age. Only a few children bed-wet and a very few need to be taken out between 10 and 12 p.m. It is difficult for them to go to sleep again after-	The child prefers to play with children and not alone. It arranges its toys in gigantic piles. When drawing and scribbling, the child uses up a lot of paper and drawing materials. It is proud to show oth-	The 4-year-old is a positively sociable creature. It can be surrounded by playmates all day long, and may not be so keen to help in the house. It makes comparisons between home and conditions else-

DEVELOPMENT OF

Age, Length, Weight	Sleep in hours	Calories, Amount of Food, Kind of Food
	Usually the light has to be left on for ¼ hr. while the child looks at a picture-book in bed, etc. It is an advantage to change over to a bigger bed. Only a few children sleep in the middle of the day at this age. They amuse themselves in bed or in their room at this time. The whole period of sleep seldom exceeds 12 hrs.	This rights itself when the child is 4½. For most children it is a good thing to be allowed to sit at the family table. They cannot, however, converse as they are too taken up with the business of eating.

mind can develop normally. Playing is just as important for children as a job is for adults. The child begins life happily with the right ideas. Growing, learning, eating and sleeping are all a pleasure. We all know that with the passage of years

THE CHILD—*cont.*

Excretions	Activity and Interests	Social Behavior
wards. If bed-wetting persists, a psychotherapist with experience of children should be consulted when the child is 4½ years. This difficulty can usually be overcome very easily.	ers its efforts—drawings as well as buildings made of blocks, etc. Sometimes the child clears up alone, but it is better if the grown-ups tidy away the child's toys when it is not there. The child does not like to limit itself to one room, but one can come to an agreement with it with regard to definite times for being alone. The 4-year-old is glad to be granted new privileges and keeps to the rules. If kept under too much there is a danger that it may kick over the traces altogether. Four-year-olds then like to run away from home.	where, whereby home always comes off best, and it likes to boast about it. It likes to emulate its parents' methods of upbringing when with its playmates and is inclined to boss others when playing. Nevertheless, all is usually well. The children play at being a doctor and housewife. Two children play better than three together. If possible, supervision is a good thing. Family excursions on Sunday are now the great thing. It is usually best with father only. Imaginary playmates, etc., lose their significance. The child's play is more closely related to reality.

a lot of that pleasure will wear off, but we must do all we can to postpone this as long as possible.

This can best be done by parents not bothering about "how fat?"; "how big?"; "how often and how much food should a child eat?"; "how often and how much sleep does it need?"; "how forward?"; or "how backward?" at every stage of the child's development. In this way they get fixed ideas as to what a child "must" do or be like and this can easily be detrimental to its normal, healthy physical and mental development.

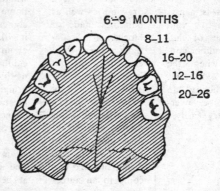

Diagram of the milk teeth showing when they are cut.

All these questions are so vital for the child's health that one ought actually to devote a whole book to them. However, here we must confine ourselves to compiling the necessary knowledge in a chart (page 356ff), bearing in mind especially the law of "usually." Every child is different; it is an individual with its own personality. One can best tell whether it is thriving by seeing whether it is healthy and lively and not by constantly fetching the scales and tape-measure.

UPBRINGING AND HEALTH

In the congested conditions of present-day life in the towns, our children have been brought up in a way which is sometimes harmful. We still behave as our own parents and their ancestors were taught to behave. But the world is no longer what it was when such methods were correct and sound. We can no longer simply pick up our children from the garden or field after the day's work and give them a spanking as a precautionary measure and a necessary part of their training, if I may express myself in such exaggerated terms. We live at far too close quarters with them for us to be able to afford not to understand the world they live in. For that reason children are in the awkward predicament of always living with "almighty gods" (for that is what grown-ups appear to them), whose actions they generally cannot understand. The more these "gods" love and cherish and sacrifice themselves for the children, the worse the mental strain may become for the latter.

So there is nothing for it but for us to try and put ourselves more and more in their position and to learn more about their world, which we have lost. Decades of intensive research have in the meantime taught us the essential things about this world. We need only to put this knowledge into practice. Anyone with children should set about this. The chart can help even though it is necessarily imperfect, as can well be understood. Mere knowledge alone is not sufficient. Many things connected with our views and actions in regard to children occur automatically, without our thinking about them—tone of voice, facial expression, and similar things which are difficult to control, and we can overcome these only by showing special tolerance and indulgence to our children when we cannot understand their actions. This can be easy for us if we remember that many peculiarities are not permanent "bad" qualities, but rather passing phases in the child's mental development. Something which annoys or shames us in a child of two has gone of its own accord six months later. The less we punish the child and forbid it to do anything, the more certain we may be that it will stop doing it. We must never forget that we are very much on top of our children these days and drastic interference leads only to trouble and unhappiness for us, unlike our ancestors, who were free to run wild out of doors in childhood and forget their problems amid the beauties of nature.

As we now know only too well how much our physical health in later life depends on the mental health of our childhood years, we ought really to add a whole supplement on the upbringing of children to this book on health. This, however, is impracticable, and so we can go closely only into one single aspect of the problem which is a source of consternation to many and which only emphasizes the necessity for a change in our methods of bringing up small children.

BED-WETTING

According to the few available statistics (owing to the embarrassing nature of the subject it is difficult to get hold of them, since parents generally hide the matter) this occurs in about a third of all children living in towns. It can be said that bed-wetting is a neurotic illness if a child is not absolutely dry at night by the age of four. Before this it should not be regarded in that light unless there are other indications to that effect. Physical causes for it are extremely rare and can easily be recognized by a doctor. In cases of mental defect due to injury to the brain, or in diabetes in children, bed-wetting can occur. But all other surmises with regard to organic reasons have not been confirmed.

It is as well for a parent to know about the functions of the bladder and kidneys in the body and how their voluntary and involuntary control affects the child's mind and nerves. It is essentially a question of growth rather than of training. To spank a year-old child for "messing" in the night is acting just as illogically as trying to train it to eat hard crusts of bread by spanking it. You must wait until it has teeth and they grow in their own time. What really happens? The infant, as everyone knows, empties its bladder, like its bowels, when it has to. The bladder remains comfortable until it is filled by urine from the kidneys. When the bladder wall is stretched a nerve impulse automatically opens the muscle at the bladder exit. The infant's body only slowly learns the difference between night and day. It sleeps in the daytime just as it does at night. Later, in grownups, the kidney "goes slow" at night. Hormones and nerves reduce the excretion of water. The kidney concentrates salts and waste matter, which have to be got rid of, more strongly at night so that there is room enough in the bladder for the nightly quantity of urine. Sleep does not have to be interrupted in order to pass water at the same intervals as in the daytime. This nightly work of concentration and conserving water on the part of the kidney could not be performed by any of us at birth. We had to learn to do it unconsciously. It started when we realized our ability to stop this automatic opening of the bladder when full. We learned to check the muscle. This is just as simple or just as difficult as learning to ride a bicycle or any difficult exercise in balance. No one can take a bicycle and say, "Now I want to be able to ride a bicycle." Far from it. One must practice hard. Mere will-power alone is not enough. The difficult muscles have to learn to function automatically, so that one can keep one's balance on the wobbly vehicle without thinking. Of course this is easiest when one enjoys learning to do it.

This applies more than ever to the small child, who can have no understanding of social necessities. But the child is proud of its achievement. It gets a kick out of conquering another automatic muscle, and it is this satisfaction which enables the child to include the "full bladder" among other stimuli which may disturb its sleep and cause it to wake, i.e. hunger, noises, etc. Actually it is not the ignoring of the full bladder but decreased secretion by the kidney which takes place at night and which enables children and grown-ups to last out the night. If anyone reads an exciting book in bed, he generally has to get out of bed once more before going to sleep. Excitement in the evening fills the bladder in children also. Excitement of the sympathetic system increases the kidney's excretion of water.

If a child is forced to learn a thing at a time when it is not sufficiently advanced physically to do so, it detracts from the pleasure which the child ordinarily feels and things go wrong. And there is also another important factor. One does it to please the parent, who is quite justifiably fed up with still having to wash diapers. And the parent makes it quite plain that it is far more pleasant when the diaper is dry. In this way the parent and the parent's love become involved in bed-wetting and this can cause the whole process of development to break down. So let us assume that a child has grasped that its parent is pleased when the diaper is dry. It cannot, however, keep the diaper dry since it has not yet learned to control its bladder, and so it fails. The parent's patience is exhausted and he or she becomes angry, slapping the child as if it could understand about naughtiness. Or the parent makes a sad face, which is probably worse. Or the parent scolds the child, which is just as bad. The child learns that it can punish its parent, who gets angry and sad when the diaper is wet. It also learns the opposite, i.e. getting dry, with slaps. It has learned to do this to please Mother or Father rather because it could do so by itself and be proud of mastering it. The slightest emotional fluctuation on the part of the parent manifests itself in the child's diaper. It becomes the barometer of the parent's emotional life. We cannot get away from the impression that the child wets its bed out of naughtiness and we begin to spank it and to adopt other methods of punishing it. Sometimes success is achieved despite these unreasonable measures, but never because of them. We had just about got to the end of our tether, but fortunately the child was stable enough to defy all our punishments and to proceed on its way of normal development.

However, with one child in every three in towns (the statistics are taken from the first post-war years) the parents' methods of punishment and training were sufficiently wrong to impede this smooth and natural maturing process of the mind and nerves. Basically this failure is due to a wrong assessment of punishment in the training of small children and to the fact that one underrates the child's own natural instincts toward cleanliness, when they are slow to develop. "Punishment," "orderliness" and "naughtiness" are conceptions which make sense only to adults and older children. While it is a question of mind and nerves learning to master complicated body functions, there can never be any naughtiness involved. There can only be the wrong kind of learning. To revert to our former example, it is as if the unconsciously working muscles of the cyclist were to learn how to fall off instead of how to keep their balance.

In just the same way bed-wetting at night is a question of unconscious functions. None of us can say why the kidney excretes small quantities only of water at night and why we are sometimes wakened in spite of this by the urge to urinate. It is really absurd to think that you can conceivably interfere with this unconscious work of learning on the part of the muscles by inflicting punishment. When a boy wants to learn to ride a bicycle, you hold the saddle and handlebars until he has learned to keep his balance. Anyway the punishment comes too late—generally speaking, the next morning. Just think how far ahead a two-year-old child can see emotionally. When it wants something, it must have it at once. Otherwise it thinks it will never get it. Anything refused or denied it for a moment constitutes a final rejection in the child's eyes. It is something which is forbidden. It does not yet know what postponement means. To understand the meaning of "waiting" and "tomorrow" demands considerable work of growing and learning. It takes years, and some people never learn it. But for a two-year-old the interval between its nightly sleep and bed-wetting and waking up the next morning is too great for punishment to have the slightest point. It is, however, sufficient to have the opposite effect, i.e. it makes the child learn the wrong way.

The more one disturbs a child at night and worries it with warnings in the evening, the less soundly it sleeps, the less the reduction in activity of the kidney at night, and therefore the more it wets its bed. That is the logical conclusion of punishment and earnest admonishment.

The way to a child's soul is far for adults. We cannot return to their world of innocence. We can only study it and try to understand it and show the necessary appreciation and trust of this miraculous work of physical and mental development, which follows its own natural laws. Only then is maternal love a powerful engine which helps everything on to a quicker maturity and to full health.

Study the development chart; avoid the too early and futile punishments, which transforms the child's diaper into a barometer of the mother's changing emotions, thereby spoiling her life. Avoid being over-concerned and fussy. Use your intelligence to detect signs of the child's willingness and ability to do things as it develops. That is the right moment. It is scarcely possible to teach others just when that is. One simply has to rely on one's instinct as a mother and must not be led astray by the boasts of other women about the early "cleanliness" of their children.

The ambition of a mother must never be "early," but rather "well-functioning" and "healthy." And one thing above all: each child is an individual with its own laws and speed of development. Compare your children with the chart. They will generally have reached the various stages sooner than indicated on the chart. Those on the chart are dictated by the law of "usually," and not by your own child, whatever it may be like.

13.   Pains and Complaints

WHAT IS PAIN?

"It hurts" is something easily said and everybody knows what it means. However, if one looks into the matter more closely or tries to find out the real meaning of pain in the medical sense, one comes up against a surprising fact. Hardly any investigation has been made into this every-day symptom. There is no watertight theory for pain. There is still no complete answer to the question: Why does it actually hurt?

Now we all know, of course, that pain stimuli reach the brain by definite nerve routes and set off the various kinds of unpleasant sensations which we define as pain. Of course we know the rate at which a pain signal chases over the nerve route from the big toe to the brain. We even know different forms of electric waves which chase over the telephone wires of the nerve routes of our body and which we know to be pain signals. But nevertheless pain cannot be measured. All that we can learn about the intensity of pain felt by another person is couched in such vague expressions as: "It hurts a bit," "It hurts a great deal," or "It is unbearably painful."

But we do not know whether the same pain stimulus, for example, would be felt by one person as "It hurts very much," and by another as "It hurts a little." That is to say, we do not know why different people react to the same pain signal with varying degrees of sensitivity.

But why should there be greater differences in this particular aspect of the work of our nerves than with the other sensory phenomena in healthy people? Let us think, for example, of the human eye's sensitivity to light. It is true there are illnesses which weaken the power of vision, but most people have almost equally sensitive eyes. The same probably applies to the actual sensitivity of our nerves to pain.

ON BEARING PAIN

But somehow this information fails to satisfy us. Every day one comes up against people who appear to endure great pain without a murmur, while others cry at the slightest thing. If we look more closely at the expressions we choose when describing this condition, we suddenly see that we regard the intensity of pain as an object of comparison—something which is common to all people. For we say, "The robust person 'endures' pain better than another." In other words, "He bothers less about the 'disturbance' to his mental equilibrium which the pain causes." And there we have it in a nut-shell. It is the mental attitude of the individual which is the crucial point. We cannot all bear the same pain with the same fortitude, even though we all experience the same degree of pain.

But the question which perplexes us most concerns the

point of pain. Why, in heaven's name, do we have such a thing as pain? It is a very trying and unnecessary part of life and spoils our enjoyment of living. Why can't we do without pain? Yes, why indeed? Now, with pain from the skin the answer is obvious. For example, we would not notice if we had cut ourselves, and the cut would go much deeper without a sudden pain to warn and shock us. There are nervous diseases in which individual limbs go dead and can no longer feel pain. Such unfortunate people continually suffer little injuries, especially burns, on the affected limbs. In this respect our irritating companion through life—pain—is a protective warning signal. We might have the audacity to say, "That is all very well, but why does it go on hurting after we have been warned?" Because, unfortunately, we have to go on being warned.

After one has been injured, the body's repair processes are set in motion, i.e. a damaged tissue, a cut or a tear is stuck together again. Now that of course could not be done very well if the affected part were not constantly rested, i.e. if the injured hand were moved the whole time. If the pain ceased after cutting oneself, one would forget all about one's injury the next minute and by movement would constantly upset the healing process.

THE USEFULNESS OF PAIN

So all these are useful pains. Perhaps they need not always be so severe, but we willingly concede that point—we must have an automatic warning of some sort. But what about the pain which occurs in other illnesses? Well, one can first of all say that pain in an illness compels us to rest and that resting in bed is still a very effective, even though primitive, natural method of cure.

Let us imagine a case of arthritis. The pain forces the affected limb to rest. But what about a stomach pain? What is the use of pain in a sick gall-bladder? One might reply, "These pains serve to send a person to the doctor and so save him from worse dangers." But things cannot be interpreted as simply as that. The natural laws which control all living creatures are not as straightforward as that, especially since there are other serious illnesses in which pain is absent. One might think the system of warning in the simple case of external injuries had outplayed itself in many internal illnesses and therefore become pointless. There are illnesses which cause severe pain but where mere resting of the body does not alone bring recovery. That which for a cut finger constitutes a clever and purposeful process of adaptation to the dangers of the outside world, is in internal illnesses of value only as a guide for the doctor in charge of the case. To the patient himself it is just a troublesome evil. It would appear that such internal illnesses (unlike the dangers of external injury) played no part in the development of living creatures. No provision for them was made in nature's plan of construction. Living creatures, including man, have aimed at health and a high standard of efficiency in their development to adult life. What lay on the other side of this peak on the descending line was not able to exert any decisive influence.

One can perhaps vindicate the pain of illnesses by explaining that pain is not only an unpleasant conscious sensation, which can hinder our work, thought, and certain of our movements; every pain stimulus also sets off countless other automatic nerve stimuli. So in addition to what we consciously feel and actively and voluntarily do against pain, other important processes take place in our body at the same time. These nerve impulses, which are set off by the pain stimulus, below the level of consciousness, alter certain organ functions. The distribution of blood is altered; the intestinal movements are different; the excretion of urine, i.e. the activity of the kidneys, is changed. Innumerable changes automatically take place in our body when we consciously suffer pain. However, with our present-day knowledge it is impossible to say whether these amount to the defense against illness or if these changes in the organ functions of the body are part of our body's efforts to bring about a cure, such as happens with the destruction of invading bacteria. In other words, are pains in themselves healing stimuli? We do not know, and we must leave future generations of research workers to answer this question.

The harmless words "It hurts" still conceal unsolved mysteries of nature.

HEADACHE

The brain substance itself is not responsible for pain stimuli. Headaches generally originate from the nerves in the walls of the blood-vessels which run through the brain. Especially painful is the expansion of these vessel walls which occurs with increased blood-pressure, and so it happens that headaches are found to be a symptom of countless general body disorders and illnesses. But headaches can also be an illness on their own, as, for instance, migraine, which was described on page 259. Many other kinds of headache are, like migraine, caused by mental processes and experiences and consist of pains very similar in quality to the "central" headaches of mental origin. This allergic type of headache occurs in fevers, infectious diseases, inflammation of the nasal sinuses, and actual allergic illnesses.

Headaches occur as a symptom in disorders of the stomach and intestine—including acute stomach upsets and constipation—in kidney diseases, high blood-pressure, gall-bladder and liver complaints, and in tumors of the brain and poisoning.

A special and severe type of headache is called facial neuralgia (trigeminal neuralgia). The trigeminal nerve (so called because it has three branches) conducts the facial skin's sensitivity to touch and pain to the brain. It can become diseased in a similar way to the sciatic nerve (see page 264) and the long-lasting pain which results (incidentally completely useless pain) can become so unbearable that the patient can be helped only by destroying the nerve fibers.

Another frequent cause of headaches is a disorder of vision which has not been properly corrected by spectacles. It may be a very small discrepancy between the distance of the eyes and that of the centers of the two glasses, or such like. For this reason anyone who has suffered from headaches for a long time should have his eyes examined by an oculist. Glasses can often cure headaches which have persisted for a long time.

One should never regard headaches as something which cannot be avoided. In many cases they are an accompanying symptom of other illnesses, which can be diagnosed, even if the doctor's first examination is unsuccessful. Headaches can seriously upset one's health, but they sometimes help the doctor to discover a more deep-seated complaint. Therefore one should try to cure them with the same tenacity as in any other illness. The actual type of headache gives very little clue as to what any underlying illness is. If, however, it seems to be "one-sided," this should be reported to the doctor, as it suggests migraine. The way the pain starts is also important, and whether it disappears gradually or suddenly.

We are all occasionally compelled to cope with a headache without medical help. Some people swear by coffee. But only some kinds of headache are relieved by caffeine, which is present in tea and coffee. One has to find out for oneself. It is especially effective in migraine-like and allergic headaches. The basic substance of most familiar headache powders and headache tablets is aspirin and similar substances.

TOOTHACHE

Toothache is an indefatigable reminder that one should go to the dentist. If the tooth ache becomes worse on eating sweet or salt food or with cold or hot drinks, it is a sign that the origin is superficial (coming from a hole in the enamel which causes irritation in the nerve in the middle of the tooth). But, if the pain becomes worse with pressure (chewing), it is highly probable that the root is affected. There is danger of suppuration in the region of the top of the root and an abscess may result. Should the inflammation of the area around the root be more severe, a feeling of soreness occurs in the throat on the same side. The lymph glands in the neck may swell and become painful.

Toothache should always be treated by a dentist as soon as possible.

Toothache can occur also in healthy teeth. These pains are of a neuralgic nature and people who are subject to sciatica and rheumatism may get them. These pains usually affect a whole row of teeth without the sufferer being able to indicate one particular tooth as the root of the pain. Similarly—i.e. by way of the nerves—toothache in the lower jaw can sometimes be felt in the corresponding tooth in the upper jaw. A tiny air pocket under a filling also can cause a toothache.

Careful rinsing of the mouth with warm liquid soothes superficial toothache (sensitivity to sweet things). With deep toothache, a simple remedy is to steep one's gum in pure brandy or put a few drops of oil of cloves into the cavity. Aspirin tablets will help relieve pain, but they must be swallowed with water to be effective. Holding an aspirin tablet next to an aching tooth will irritate the gum.

SORE THROAT

There are two kinds of sore throat. First a general inflammation of the throat, which in a mild form is felt as an irritation or tickle. It generally accompanies an ordinary cold or chill (see chapter on Infectious Diseases, page 143). Valuable household remedies are hot lemon drinks (with or without sugar), hot milk sweetened with honey, or gargling with salt. Penicillin is completely useless, since bacteria do not play a part in this type.

The second form of sore throat is accompanied by swallowing difficulties and a choking feeling. This is due to inflamed and swollen tonsils (tonsillitis). The responsible bacteria (streptococci) are destroyed by the usual chemotherapeutic drugs. Fruit and vegetable juice enriched with vitamin C is a suitable diet, since the difficulty in swallowing necessitates a liquid diet. Tonsillitis also occurs in measles and scarlet fever. Diphtheria also affects the tonsils. For symptoms and diagnosis, see chapter on Infectious Diseases, page 160.

Pains in the throat may occasionally be caused by inflammation of the thyroid gland, which has no connection with the hormone disorders which are more common with the thyroid.

THROAT COMPLAINTS

Hoarseness without pain requires an examination by an ear, nose and throat specialist.

Swellings in the region of the throat are usually due to disease of the lymph glands. The trouble may be tuberculosis, or may be a disease of the lymphatic system, such as leukemia (see page 192).

An enlarged thyroid gland causes a swelling which is both visible and palpable. This is generally symmetrical on both sides of the front and lower part of the neck, but may be more pronounced on one side. Little lumps which can be felt in the thyroid are usually harmless, but should nevertheless be shown to the doctor as they may be cancerous. The rounder and smoother the lump, the less likely it is to be malignant. Swellings of the thyroid (goiter) can press on the breathing passages. Large swellings usually denote under-functioning of the gland, whereas the swellings are generally only of moderate size when the gland is over-functioning.

The sudden feeling of having a lump in one's throat is almost exclusively due to mental-nervous causes. The cause of the sensation is faulty position of the inner throat muscles caused by nerves. Nervous disorders of the heart (see page 255) often result in similar complaints.

The throat muscles are partly under voluntary control and partly under involuntary influences and so mental-nervous disorders are very common there.

HEART PAIN

Pain and discomfort around the area of the heart (precordial pain) may be regarded as a comforting sign that the heart muscle itself and the heart valves are still intact. They occur predominantly with nervous functional disorders of the heart and mostly when one is resting. They get better when one moves about or works (details on page 255). A simple remedy is to hold one's breath for some time and then breathe slowly; distracting activities are also useful.

A chest pain accompanied by breathlessness which is not quickly relieved by rest may be due to occlusion of a coronary artery. Summon a doctor and lie down.

Pains which radiate from the heart into the left (sometimes the right) arm (especially the inside of the upper arm) indicate constriction of the coronary vessels (causes, page 253). You can best help yourself by resting for a few minutes until the pain has gone. The doctor, who should at any rate be consulted with such attacks, has effective drugs which make the coronary vessels dilate, but these can be obtained only on a prescription.

PAIN IN THE CHEST

A rough feeling deep inside, which causes a slight stabbing pain when breathing, occurs with an inflammation of the lower breathing passages (bronchitis). It is a continuation of the sore throat further inward. Treatment as for chills and colds (see chapter on Infectious Diseases, page 143).

One-sided stabbing pain in the chest occurs with pneumonia. This is accompanied by a raised temperature. Pleurisy also causes very sharp pain and there may be no rise in temperature with this. Breathing becomes painful. The pain is usually in the lower half of the chest. Ordinary aspirin, etc., generally somewhat improves the condition. Of course medical treatment is necessary in pneumonia and pleurisy.

Deep, boring pains which occur at the level of one's shoulder-blades in the back are usually muscular pains, due either to rheumatism or strain. A "slipped disc" (in the neck) may also manifest itself in this way.

Rheumatic pains in the rib muscles are not unknown. They can usually be relieved by rubbing in liniment, just as with pains in the back.

One-sided pain along one or more ribs may be due to neuralgia or may indicate the start of shingles (see chapter on Infectious Diseases, page 148).

Pain which spreads from the right side of the chest to the shoulder can be caused by an inflamed gall-bladder and stones in the gall-bladder. This is the typical symptom of gall-bladder pains. Kidney pains may also be "referred" in a similar way to the lower part of the back of the chest.

ABDOMINAL PAIN

Stomach-ache is probably the most common form. We have all experienced it as a mild cramp in the left upper half and middle of the abdomen after unwise eating. (See "The upset stomach," page 114). This can also occur with stomach ulcers or chronic inflammation of the stomach mucous membrane. The pain is worse if one presses. You can tell whether the duodenum is inflamed or whether there are duodenal ulcers by feeling for a sensitive spot. This is somewhat above the navel, near the bottom of the breastbone. Ulcers also are indicated by a gnawing pain in that area about 45 to 60 minutes after a meal, or pain in the night that is relieved by food.

GALL-BLADDER PAIN

This occurs in the right upper part of the abdomen, generally directly beneath the ribs. ("Gall-bladder and gallstones," see page 72.) Heat is helpful (hot-water bottles).

APPENDIX PAIN

This occurs in the right lower part of the abdomen. (See picture and paragraph, "The cecum and the appendix," page 74.) Pressure makes it worse. Do not take any food and call your doctor.

ABDOMINAL CRAMP

This is a cramp-like tension in individual sections of the intestine, especially the colon. The pain moves about. Heat helps.

PERITONITIS AND INTESTINAL OBSTRUCTION

These cause such severe pains and other complaints that one goes to the doctor without any more ado.

PELVIC PAIN

These are usually on one side and in women are often the result of inflammation of an ovary or Fallopian tube. These disorders usually are accompanied by a discharge. In addition there is pain in the small of the back and increased menstrual pain. These illnesses need proper treatment and possibly surgery.

BLADDER PAIN

This generally takes the form of a sharp pain directly behind the pubic bone. It is almost always accompanied by the desire to pass water. Bladder "chills" are generally purely due to irritation, and bacteria are not involved. But there are, of course, cases of bacterial inflammation of the bladder. The doctor must then decide what treatment to give and chemotherapy must be used. Bacterial inflammation of the bladder, if not treated in time, can be dangerous as the infection may spread up the ureter and affect the kidney.

Then another form of pain is added to the bladder pain. Pains from the kidney and ureter are felt on the affected side in the middle of the abdomen and from there shoot downwards towards the pubic bone. These are cramp-like, stabbing pains, which generally increase in waves and die down again. This is a serious sign and medical examination is imperative. (See also "Colic of the Kidneys," page 393).

PAINS IN THE SMALL OF THE BACK

There are three causes for these and it is very difficult for the sufferer to distinguish between them. Firstly they may be due to kidney disease. Then they are usually felt somewhat above the actual small of the back. Kidney pains are usually on one side and can also be recognized by the fact that the pain increases if one taps gently with one's fist on one side of the spine above the loins. The pains are generally dull, but they may become sharp if there is severe inflammation. The second form of pain in the small of the back arises as a result of arthritis of the vertebral column and the sacral joints. A "slipped disc" is very common (see page 13). Feeling between the vertebrae then usually locates a painful spot. However, the center of the pains may well be in the muscles adjacent to the vertebral column, which have gone into spasm. These changes in the vertebrae may cause pressure on the nerves coming out of the vertebral column. This causes considerable pain, which often radiates along the sciatic nerve into the leg.

These pains in the small of the back may, in individual cases, be relieved sometimes by lying, sometimes by standing, and sometimes by sitting. They are in any case nearly always affected by changes in the position of the body. At all events they require medical advice as it is difficult to differentiate between them. It is senseless to set about a damaged intervertebral disc or a nerve pain due to pressure, by massage, which is good for muscular or rheumatic pains.

The third common cause of pain in the small of the back is especially to be found in women. Malposition, inflammation and injuries to the pelvic organs, especially the womb, very frequently cause pains in the small of the back. These are generally on both sides or in the middle and can only be vaguely localized. That is to say, the sufferer cannot properly indicate the place where the pain really is and where it is worst. For this reason constant pain of this kind should induce a woman to be thoroughly examined by a gynecologist. She can often be cured by suitable methods of treatment. The pains should certainly not be allowed to drag on, since, like any constant pain, they detract from one's enjoyment of life and impair one's vitality and efficiency.

Mention must also be made of a fourth frequent cause of

pain in the small of the back: bad footwear; flat feet; wearing high-heeled shoes for too long, and even corns, which can lead to a cramped foot position—all these can cause pain in the small of the back. The foot muscles form part of a unit which goes right up to the back muscles. Thus it can happen that, passed up from below, faulty positions of the muscles and joints in the small of the back occur, which cause pain. Naturally it is useless to massage oneself. These pains usually get better if one lies down. All pains in the small of the back which cannot be properly accounted for should be examined by orthopedic specialists. So simple a remedy as wearing well-fitting shoes has been known to cure people who have suffered for years from pain in the small of the back.

LUMBAGO

This is a sudden tightening of the muscles in the small of the back. It hurts exceedingly and usually occurs in people who tend to get rheumatism. An unconscious nerve stimulus is usually responsible for this painful occurrence. You can help in such cases by massage, which, however, is very painful. Heat, too, helps to loosen the tension. Anyone who has this often would be well advised to be examined by an orthopedic specialist.

COLIC

Colic was originally called intestinal cramp—derived from the Greek word *kolon*. But nowadays it is used for all particularly violent abdominal cramps. There is an intestinal colic which occurs for instance with severe inflammation of the intestine (dysentery), but also from kinking of the intestine.

Violent cramp-like pains from the gall-bladder are another example of colic. This occurs particularly when small gallstones reach the narrow excretory duct in the bile. This sets up particularly violent cramp movements of the gall-bladder, which in favorable cases squeeze the wedged stone out through the narrow duct into the intestine. With gall-bladder colic the whole of the right upper abdomen is in terrible pain, which radiates upwards in the direction of the right shoulder. The first thing one can do to help oneself is to put hot compresses on the right upper abdomen. The doctor summoned to the case heals the pain with atropine, which helps to combat all kinds of cramp of the digestive organs.

Colic of the Kidneys

This occurs in the area of distribution of kidney and ureter pain (see page 390). This, too, is almost always caused by stones. One can help oneself in the same way as with colic of the gall-bladder. The doctor must always be summoned.

Colic of the Bladder

As for colic of the kidneys.

One speaks also of stomach colic, which may occur with acute and particularly severe inflammation.

In the broadest sense, colic means cramp-like pain, which emanates from internal organs and the severity of which exceeds the limit of endurance.

PAINS IN THE LIMBS AND NERVES

The most understandable and sensible of all pains is the one which we suffer from external injury such as a cut and the inflammation which may ensue. This is the pain which urges us to take care and thus facilitates our cure.

There are three important and common sources of pain in the limbs. Firstly, rheumatism of the muscles and joints and similar painful conditions, which lead to stiffness (see pages 180 and 260).

Secondly, neuritis is not rare, as we know from the description of sciatica (see page 264). Neuritis also occurs in the arms. A special kind is pain in the finger-tips, which occurs in the night toward morning (so-called acroparesthesia), which not only causes pain, but also other unpleasant tingling sensations.

A third kind of pain in the limbs comes from the blood-vessels and the sensitive pain nerves in their walls. It is not easy for the layman to distinguish these pains from those of neuritis. They, too, sometimes become particularly unbearable at night. Vessel cramp pains in the legs (see page 264) usually get better if one lets one's legs hang down so that the weight of the blood increases the blood-pressure and forces it to flow through better. Pain from narrowed arteries gets worse with muscular work, unlike nerve pains. In typical cases they occur as cramp in the calves when walking and vanish again after a short rest. The pain is due to lack of blood-supply to the tissue. Calf cramps at night in otherwise healthy limbs are something similar to lumbago (see page 392).

Inflammation of the sheath covering a tendon causes considerable pain, which occurs especially when the affected joint is moved.

FOOT COMPLAINTS AND PAINS

The foot is an ingenious arch, which maintains its curve by muscular pull and firm tissue ligaments between the bones. This arch must bear the entire weight of the body, and its muscles must balance out this weight. Now we all know that in some people the arch gives way under the pressure of the burden. That is first and foremost a failure on the part of the muscles. It is wrong to blame the bones. Muscular failure and weakness arise most likely as the result of lack of practice and strain. Therefore foot complaints are not due so much to excessive wear and tear as, on the contrary, to lack of use. We cannot escape the fact that constant wearing of shoes with hard, unyielding soles plays an important part in alienating our foot muscles from their true purpose.

Sensible Footwear

There are two precautionary measures which you can adopt. You must give your feet enough space in your shoes, i.e. you must select models which allow the toes enough room in front as well as at the side. Then the toe and foot muscles can come into play while walking, thereby maintaining their strength. This is also helped by soft, flexible soles, which counteract the flat pavement of our streets. It is not always easy to choose shoes from the standard models that are really broad enough in front. Projecting soles often give a deceptive impression of breadth. However, there have been many improvements in this respect and we should never be forced by fashion into pointed shoes.

Foot Training

The second precautionary measure is of course active exercise, which, as is well known, is the first essential for any form of muscle training. Running about barefoot is an exercise which anyone can carry out at home. Moccasins or similar footwear with thin, soft soles are an ideal form of house shoe, since they automatically involve foot training. An excellent method of foot training is to run barefoot on uneven ground out of doors in the country. This needs, however, somewhat "hardened" soles, but once they have become accustomed to it every step brings into play all foot muscles which are not otherwise used. One need not emphasize the value of athletics and long-distance running for acquiring an elegant gait and healthy foot muscles. One has to learn to walk from the hips, with a springy, rolling step.

But there is yet another special kind of foot gymnastics, which can be carried out regularly at home without difficulty. You can do picking-up exercises with the toes, e.g. lifting up a stocking with the foot; catching hold of a pencil between the big toe and second toe and then lifting up the pencil between each pair of toes of both feet in turn. It is particularly valuable to grasp a spread-out hand towel or small bedside mat with one's toes and crush it under the arch of the foot, keeping the heels on the ground. You should sit down to do this. Try it every evening for ten minutes for two weeks. It is worth while. You feel a different person and go on doing so afterwards.

Artificial Supports

If, however, neglect has already affected the feet and the arch has suffered damage, one cannot hope for any relief from such active exercises for a long time, if at all. There is nothing for it but to resort to artificial supports, and these must be well fitted. Otherwise they are useless and place an even greater burden on the foot and cause still worse complaints. (The pain which occurs in the first week while the feet are getting accustomed to the supports, which happens even when the supports fit well, should not be confused with those caused by faulty supports.) Orthopedic specialists are best qualified to judge this and recommend supports. One must consult one of these to be cured of foot troubles. Weakness of the arch does not only manifest itself in pains in the foot. A typical symptom is pain and a feeling of tiredness in the legs, above all in front next to the shin. As said above, pains in the small of the back may also be symptomatic of bad feet.

Corns

These horny formations occur in places where there is pressure but a lack of fleshy padding between the skin and bone of the foot—for example, on the upper surfaces of the toes, especially the little toe, when shoes are too tight. There are two methods for removing them: first, one should buy sensibly made shoes, and here one must be very particular. It is not the price which matters, but comfort. Secondly, intensive foot training is necessary. The correctly moving and balanced foot with taut muscles wearing well-fitting shoes does not get corns or calluses. Only in this way can the cause of corns be eliminated, but of course the poor sufferer cannot wait so long. He needs a short-term remedy and for this the knife is least suitable. The best measures are baths and corn plasters which soften the corn.

Chilblains

Chilblains and other effects of cold wet weather occur very often in sportsmen, farmers, and others whose work requires long periods of exposure to near-freezing temperatures. The body should be well protected against moisture with rubber boots, raincoat, and other foul-weather gear. Symptoms of the onset of chilblains include itching, tingling, or redness of the skin. It is important that normal circulation be restored quickly to relieve the symptoms.

Perspiring Feet

A very trying symptom, which sometimes also occurs in other foot complaints. It is caused by overactivity of the sweat glands and patients with this problem also may experience excessive sweating of the palms, armpits, and other areas. The unpleasant odor that accompanies the odor is the result of activity of bacteria and yeast cells. Frequent and careful cleaning of the feet, aluminum chloride solutions and potassium permanganate compresses are helpful. Drying powders should be used daily in the shoes.

NAUSEA, VOMITING, FEELING OF DIZZINESS

One is accustomed to think of the first two terms as meaning the same thing. But there is a form of nausea which has nothing to do with the stomach. This nausea occurs with a breakdown of the circulation. It appears to emanate from the heart, and apparently the stimuli which cause it originate in the blood-vessels running from the neck to the chest. This kind of nausea precedes a fainting fit (see page 59). It also occurs when one is in very great pain. It sometimes occurs as a permanent condition in heart disease, especially severe in cases where the mind and nerves play an important part (see page 255). Regulation of blood-pressure depends greatly on a person's mental and nervous state, so that sickness can occur as an ailment in itself, just as one can occasionally feel sick with fear or because of a guilty conscience. For the same reason there is always a certain amount of nausea in the physical symptoms accompanying mental depression. For this reason it is possible that when we habitually use the word "bad" there is a deeper medical sense behind it. If one goes about with guilt feelings, one becomes ill because of one's "badness," even if one refuses to accept responsibility for one's guilt and does not wish to recognize it. Very often one cannot recognize it, since one is unable to grasp the implications in the deeper parts of the mind if one is not helped.

Disorders of the sense of balance cause vomiting by way of a nervous reflex. Therefore dizziness causes nausea. This reflex can start in the inner ear as a result of direct stimuli. This explains sea-sickness and the vomiting seen in some diseases of the inner ear. Why we have to be bothered with this reflex between dizziness and vomiting, no one knows. There is no purpose in it.

The feeling of nausea associated with disgust is more closely connected with the stomach. In fact it often leads to vomiting. This, too, can become a psychosomatic illness of its own, which manifests itself in repeated "nervous vomiting." Many chronic appetite disorders have a similar origin and they can go so far that the patients become completely emaciated. This has been known to happen even in children between the ages of six and ten and with young girls during and after puberty when faulty attitudes and inadequate or misleading information on matters of sex prevail. It is always a question of incomprehensible and therefore persistent feelings of guilt and disgust, which every healthy person can well understand when he thinks of those things that can spoil his appetite. With the patients, things which affect the stomach are permanently with them in their subconscious. If one fails to grasp this connection, one cannot cure the condition with tonics or medicines to stimulate the appetite. You can do a great deal for yourself by having a heart to heart talk with an understanding friend. This, of course, especially applies to young people, whose character and personality have not yet become too fixed and hard to change.

Nausea also accompanies inflammation of the stomach mucous membrane (gastritis) (see page 109). This nausea is a precursor of vomiting, which frequently occurs when stomach ulcers form in the region of the pylorus (exit from the stomach) with chronic inflammation of the mucous membrane of the stomach. When heart failure affects the circulation so that the veins become congested with blood in the lower part of the body and the doctor can feel a swollen liver, the sickness of the heart is combined with sickness of the stomach. The congestion with blood of the abdominal organs, including the mucous membrane of the stomach, causes the appetite to fail. Unfortunately the drug digitalis, which is such a blessing, and which generally has to be used in heart failure, sometimes sets up additional inflammation of the stomach mucous membrane in some people. One notices this very quickly and can easily get round it by administering the drug in other forms which are better tolerated.

Vomiting is a nervous reflex present only in those creatures who eat meat or a mixed diet. Herbivores do not vomit. The reflex consists of a reversal of the direction of movement of the muscles of the stomach and the esophagus. In children this is effortless and without great choking or struggling, while adults often nearly kill themselves as the more conscious part of the nerves impedes and upsets the simple process. The vomiting reflex is one of the body's methods of protecting itself, as many have experienced after excessive consumption of alcohol. By vomiting, alcoholic poisoning is prevented.

But vomiting can, like pain, also take on an independent character and become purposeless. That applies, for example, to the vomiting which occurs in unavoidable kinds of poisoning such as occur with serious kidney disease when the kidney is unable to excrete waste matter. Vomiting which occurs with some women in pregnancy is attributed to internal symptoms of "poisoning" because the mother's body is unable to cope with the metabolism of pregnancy. Retching which persists after the stomach has been emptied of its contents is particularly distressing, although by rights there should be nothing left to bring up. The reverse current forced on by the activity of the muscles can even bring up the contents of the small intestine. Then the vomit contains bile since bile is emptied into the duodenum.

The worst form of vomiting occurs with intestinal obstruction. Then not only the stomach contents but also the contents of the intestines are vomited.

Nausea and vomiting can therefore originate in several ways, i.e. heart, circulation, irritation in the stomach and intestine, or an internal poisoning stimulus. The symptom is therefore found in many illnesses. Naturally there cannot be a uniform remedy effective in all these cases.

As has already been mentioned, dizziness comes from disorders of the sense of balance. The receptor organ for this sensation is in the inner ear. There are numerous nerve links from the eye to the brain-center for this sensation. Thus, not only ear complaints, but also sight defects and diseases of the eye, especially incorrect spectacles, can cause a feeling of dizziness.

The most common form of dizziness, usually only slight, occurs from circulatory disorders. This, the ordinary faint, is apparently due to an insufficient blood supply to the brain. It is not so much the supply of blood as an insufficient blood-pressure. If one lies down, this dizziness passes, as the blood from the heart has then to be pumped in a horizontal direction only and does not have to overcome gravity.

In some circulatory disorders there is temporary dizziness every time one gets up from the horizontal position—in bad cases, even with slight changes of position in bed (postural fainting). This is due to a nervous disorder of the nerve reflexes that regulate the width of the blood-vessels in various parts of the body and so stabilize the blood-pressure. When there is hardening of the arteries (see page 252) this regulation becomes especially difficult.

Dizziness at heights, dizziness experienced when a train rushes towards one while standing on the platform, etc., is a mental symptom, caused by complex feelings of fear.

WEAKNESS AND INERTIA

These are symptoms which can occur in almost any illness. They are feelings which indicate a more or less definite breakdown of the body. They are often the only symptoms to indicate a slowly progressive disease—for example, T.B. or heart trouble. A disorder of this sort which persists for a long time should not be ignored. You should seek a careful medical examination. In older people also this should not be regarded as an inevitable symptom of old age, but one of illness.

INSOMNIA

In rare cases this can be caused by organic disease of the brain—for example, as a result of encephalitis (see page 149). Generally, however, sleep is disturbed for neurotic reasons (see "Nervous-functional disorders" pages 247 and 277), and can take the forms either of difficulty in going to sleep or of restless, disturbed nights. The last type of sleep disorder is also found when one is suffering pain. Be careful with sleeping pills. The more powerful barbiturates can easily become a habit and can even give rise to symptoms similar to those experienced by addicts. Drugs containing antihistamine are less harmful. The amount of sleep necessary varies greatly from person to person between six and nine hours.

STUPOR AND UNCONSCIOUSNESS

Between complete alertness and deep coma many degrees of clouding of consciousness and disorders of the consciousness can be recognized. By stupor is meant a condition of sleepiness from which patients can temporarily be roused by shaking or being shouted at. This kind of clouding of the consciousness is most often observed after poisoning, or in severe feverish infectious diseases, after a stroke and after skull injuries. In each case it is due to injury to the nerve cells of the brain—whether this has been caused directly by poisons, by an insufficient supply of blood-sugar or by insufficient blood supply in the final stages of heart failure. It is a serious sign and a doctor must be summoned. The treatment depends on the actual cause, which a layman cannot find out. It is very dangerous to try and give a stuporous or comatose person a drink as there is a danger that he may choke so that inflammation of the lungs may ensue. Place the patient flat on his back and turn the head to one side. If he is pale, keep the head slightly lower than the feet; if he is flushed, keep the head and shoulders slightly raised. For further details see under accidents and their prevention (page 414).

14. Medicines and the Home Medicine Chest

Medicines are substances which have been tested by scientific methods for treatment of patients. The more careful and comprehensive this testing is, the better and safer they are. Nowadays we know in general a great deal about the drugs we use. We have usually tested how they work and seen what effect they have on animals and individual organs. By and large one can say—the more efficacious the drug, the more exactly we know how, when and in what quantity to use it. Naturally we also know that not all the successes of drug treatment can be attributed to the medicine itself (see "The magic of medicine," page 280). But one thing we know for certain—and that is that present-day medicines are not poisons. Therefore one should not feel any superstitious fear that drugs are poisons. Potassium cyanide is very poisonous. Nevertheless, we all consume minute quantities of it in almonds and other foodstuffs. It is just the same with drugs. It is a question of the amount taken by patients. Choosing the correct quantity (dose) is one of the feats of medical science.

Its Use

The form in which medicine is administered to the body is determined by its characteristics. Of course the most convenient way is taking tablets or a liquid. The disadvantage of taking drugs through the mouth is that one does not know exactly what quantity actually gets absorbed by the body, and there is also the fact that some medicinal substances are destroyed in the stomach.

Injections are the ideal form as one can determine exactly the quantity needed. When a doctor prescribes injections, this has nothing to do with the gravity of the illness being treated, nor has the number of injections anything to do with it. One often hears quite amazing things said, such as "He gave me twenty-two injections" (mysterious shiver down one's spine), or "He has been quite poisoned with the injections." One should show a little sense with such vital things as medical treatment, which one has to undergo from time to time. Certainly there may be a certain amount of "magic of medicine" attached to an injection. Some substances are injected straight into the blood-stream. This, some people feel, is a different thing than when the same substances are absorbed through the intestinal wall into the blood. But one must realize and consider why doctors prescribe injections.

The answer is simple—either because of the characteristics of the drug or because one wants to be sure of getting the exact dose. Medical science is no longer magic or witchcraft, but instead a comprehensive and teachable science, which is capable of far greater and much more apparent miracles than any form of sorcery. But the best part about it is that one can believe in these miracles because they are true. We are over a thousand years ahead of thinking in terms of miracles, and it is after all much easier to believe in undeniable truths. To disbelieve them is impossible if one likes to pride oneself on possessing common sense.

EQUIPPING THE HOME MEDICINE-CHEST

This should be an integral part of every home—that is to say, one should have a clean little cupboard where everything necessary for treating illness and first-aid treatment of minor injuries is tidily kept. Most medicine-chests are too small and for this reason cannot be kept sufficiently tidy so as to enable one to find what one needs quickly.

The cupboard must be systematically equipped and all drugs and medicines should be clearly labelled, so that one knows just what they are for. Otherwise one forgets only too quickly what one thing was good for and it lies about for years, taking up room and finally going bad. It is a bad habit to throw all drugs and remains left over from other treatments into the medicine-chest. Again one forgets their purpose and takes them on the wrong occasion, thereby harming oneself. We want to try to compile a simple list of what is indispensable in the home medicine-chest in the hope that readers will, with the help of this book, be able to use them to their best advantage.

3 large squares of clean muslin
   for dressings and bandages
1 elastic bandage
3 packets sterile gauze
Pure white cotton wool
Adhesive strips, 1 in. and
   2 in. wide
Elastoplast
Clinical thermometer
Rubber gloves
1 pair sharp scissors

For external use

96 per cent alcohol—For cleaning skin and instruments
Liquor cresoli saponatus (Lysol)—For disinfecting when
   washing
Tincture of iodine—For disinfecting wounds
Hydrogen peroxide—Diluted for gargling
Pure Vaseline (petroleum jelly)

Remedies for particular illnesses

Aspirin—Pains, headaches, toothache
Milk of Magnesia—For heartburn, belching (better than
   sodium bicarbonate)

Measures and weights when prescribed

1 wine glass	= 3 oz. liquid
1 cup	= 5 oz. liquid
1 tablespoon	= ½ oz.
1 teaspoon	= ⅛ oz.

Children's doses

For calculating these, use Young's formula, which is:

$$\frac{\text{Adult dose} \times \text{age in years}}{\text{Age in years} + 12}$$

The doctor does not always stick to this hard-and-fast rule
since small children can safely take particularly large doses

of certain medicines, while others agree with them far less
than with grown-ups.

THE WRONG USE OF REMEDIES

For some people the drug store and its wares have a strange
fascination. The medicine man of primitive tribes has his
modern counterpart in the glaring advertisement telling of
some wonderful remedy which we can purchase: with the aid
of a few pills we can slim and be sylph-like again; coughs can
be cured in a flash, or we can regain our youth with the help
of a rejuvenating drug. These are but a few of the things which
this type of advertisement promises us.

Nearly everyone who buys such remedies has a sneaking
qualm that he should really go and ask his doctor's advice before he starts to doctor himself. What often happens is that
the person eventually goes to the doctor to ask his advice
when he has already done himself considerable harm by taking some quite unsuitable remedy. The doctor is, fortunately,
at least able to discover what was in the medicine or pills
which the patient has been taking, as every proprietary drug
must, by law, state its actual contents and the chemical names
for them.

Here is an example of the sort of harm people can do to
themselves in this way: a slimming drug which claims that it
causes a person to lose weight rapidly cannot do so without
being harmful to the person who takes it. If you take a drug
that makes you lose five pounds in weight in a day, you may
be stopping your body from absorbing sodium and so you
run a grave and quite unnecessary risk.

There is really scarcely an ailment which some proprietary
drug does not claim to cure. Some people buy advertised
remedies from unethical firms because, dissatisfied with their
own doctor's treatment, they think that they can do better
themselves. Do remember, though, that the science of drugs,
pharmacology, is a very complicated one: the doctor has had
many years of experience in prescribing drugs, while you are
just dabbling in the game. It is very unlikely that you can
dabble successfully, and more than likely that you will get
yourself into very deep water and be grateful in the end when
your doctor is kind enough to fish you out.

If the doctor has prescribed you a remedy, see that it is
labelled clearly and that you understand how to use it. If there

is some left over when your course of treatment is finished, it is often best to throw it away. Left lying about, the label may wear off and you may forget the use of this particular drug and use it in quite the wrong way, or it may grow stale and unfit for use. Some remedies become more concentrated as they get old because the water in the preparation evaporates. This is often true of corn remedies, and they become so strong that, if some of the preparation falls by mistake on the ordinary skin instead of the corn, the patient may get a burn.

There will always be people who hoard remedies at home, and if you feel that you are one of those people who can never get out of this bad habit, at least keep your bottles and boxes in an orderly way. See that they are clearly labelled, that the amount to be taken is stated, and never use any of the hoarded remedies unless you know that they are still fresh, that you are certain about the required dose, and that you clearly understand the drug's use.

15.   Home Remedies and Simple Nursing

Sterilization of instruments. After ordinary washing put them in a pan of boiling water with half a dessertspoonful of soda to 1 pint and boil for five to ten minutes.

DEALING WITH UTENSILS WHICH MAY BE INFECTED. After use never grasp with bare fingers when carrying—use rubber gloves or wrap in a cloth. Boil gloves afterwards.

SOILED CLOTHES (BANDAGES, ETC.). Do not touch with bare fingers. If this cannot be avoided, scrub one's hands carefully immediately afterwards. With injured or cracked fingers use rubber gloves.

CLEANING RUBBER UTENSILS. Rinse thoroughly with plenty of cold water and rinse again with warm soapy water. After this, rinse again carefully with cold water as soap is bad for rubber. When drying see that there are no creases. Wash rubber gloves before removing, first with cold water, then with warm water and soap. Rinse, turn inside out and wash the inside. After drying, turn again, inflate them and sprinkle talcum powder inside.

MAKING BEDS WITH A PATIENT IN. The patient is rolled to one side (Fig. 57). The old bottom sheet is rolled up as far as the middle. The new sheet is placed folded alongside. The outer edge is tucked in and the inner edge also rolled together in the middle. The patient is put on the other side and the process of removing and replacing the sheet is completed.

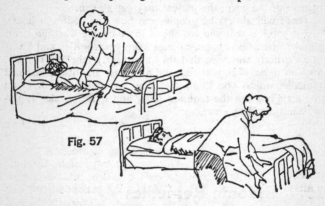

Fig. 57

PROTECTING THE PATIENT FROM DRAFTS is shown in Figure 58.

SUPPORTING THE PATIENT WHEN CHANGING POSITION. Help the patient to draw up his knees. Put one hand under the neck across to the shoulder and the other hand under the hips and pull toward one (Fig. 59).

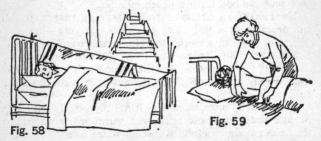

Fig. 58

Fig. 59

LIGHTING IN THE SICK-ROOM. Must be indirect. At night a small lamp placed under the bed often proves satisfactory.

THE FLOOR OF THE SICK-ROOM. Always wipe damp and use

Lysol or something similar in the case of infectious diseases.

SIMPLE AIDS FOR SITTING COMFORTABLY IN BED. Foot support from deckchair. Chair turned round. Simple board (Fig. 60).

Always place a pillow under the knees and if necessary under the hands and have a box to prop against the feet.

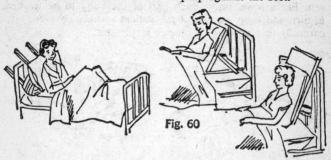

Fig. 60

HELPING THE PATIENT FROM A BED INTO A CHAIR. Dressing-gown and shoes should be put on as far as possible while the patient is lying down. Help to get the patient into an upright position and get the legs out. Then let the patient sit like that for a few minutes (danger of fainting). Grasp the patient under the armpits with the hands (Fig. 61) and help him to stand up. Lead him to the chair (walking backwards yourself), and then sit the patient down. Blankets or rugs to keep the patient warm while sitting are put round the legs from the back to the front so that the ends overlap a long way in front.

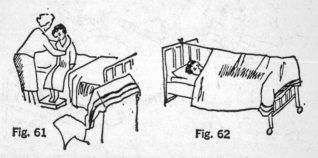

Fig. 61   Fig. 62

Bed cradle (Fig. 62) for preventing uncomfortable pressure from the blankets.

Another comfortable bed seat is shown in Figure 64.

PROTECTING THE FEET FROM THE PRESSURE OF THE BED-CLOTHES. A firm cardboard carton with a hole in one side. Two folded and tied pillows (Fig. 63).

WASHING IN BED. Note position of the wash cloth (Fig. 65). Loose ends must not hang down or the bed clothes will get wet. Put a towel under each part of the body to be washed in turn and keep the rest of the patient warmly covered. Dry carefully and powder all creases in the skin.

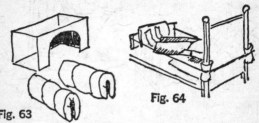

Fig. 63

Fig. 64

FIXED KNEE BOLSTER. A pillow rolled up in a sheet. The ends are twisted together (like a taffy wrapping) and fixed to the bedstead (Fig. 66). The pillows are placed in a slanting direction.

RING TO PREVENT BED-SORES. A five-inch diameter soft rubber tube is stuffed with cotton wool and bent to form a ring (Fig. 68). The ends are fixed by winding a bandage round them. Another covering of muslin or flannel.

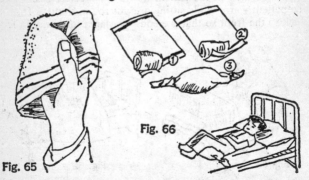

Fig. 65

Fig. 66

BED-TABLES. These can be improvised, e.g. from the projecting folding end of a sewing machine, or, better still, an ironing board placed across the arms of two chairs (Fig. 67).

DEALING WITH RESTLESS PATIENTS. Fold a sheet across the

chest and tuck in firmly under the mattress on both sides (Fig. 70).

The edge of the mattress farthest from the wall should be raised by pillows (Fig. 69). (The patient can then only roll toward the wall.)

Figure 71, on page 410, shows another security device for the exposed side of the bed.

IMPROVISED BED-PANS FOR BEDRIDDEN PATIENTS. Twist a very thick roll of newspaper together, rolling one end of some string together with the paper. Bend the roll to form a ring and bind the ends together. Then take many more layers of paper, cover them with oilcloth, lay them under the ring and roll the edges round it (Fig. 72).

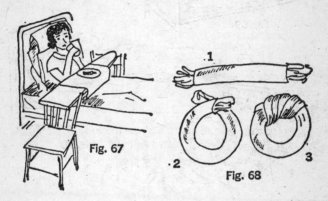

Fig. 67

.1
.2 3
Fig. 68

TAKING THE PATIENT'S PULSE. Place the first three fingers on the wrist pulse. Any emotional excitement or physical exertion falsifies the result. Count for a whole minute.

Normal pulse-rates:

At birth	130-160
Infants	110-130
From 1-7 years	80-120
Older children	80-90
Women	70-80
Men	60-70

TAKING THE PATIENT'S TEMPERATURE. Preferably in the mouth. The thermometer is kept under the tongue for at least one minute. The lips must be closed. Make sure no hot drink has been recently given.

In tiny children and dazed or restless patients the temperature should not be taken in the mouth.

Taking the patient's temperature under the armpit. Wipe the armpit with a dry soft cloth or cotton-wool swab. Dampness causes temperature mistakes. Place the tip of the thermometer in the middle of the armpit with the stem sticking out in front. The patient should hold the shoulder with the other hand in order to prevent movement which would cause temperature mistakes. Leave it there for ten minutes.

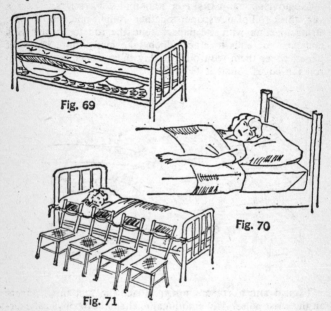

Fig. 69

Fig. 70

Fig. 71

Taking the patient's temperature in the rectum. Adults lie on one side with the knees bent. Infants are held lying on their backs and with their legs up, and the thermometer is inserted about one inch inside the rectum (Fig. 73). It is kept there for two minutes.

Normal temperatures:

Armpit	97.9	degrees
Mouth	98.6	degrees
Rectum	99.3	degrees

Every time the patient's temperature is taken at home it should be written down and the time of day stated, as one's memory is only too liable to let one down.

Cleaning the thermometer. This is done with a cotton-wool

swab moistened with water (not hot!) and soap. Pull it through in a turning movement from above to below.

GIVING THE PATIENT AN ENEMA. The patient should lie on one side, or, another method, on knees and elbows (Fig. 74) on a table covered with oilcloth. In bed a rubber sheet should be used underneath, with newspapers and a large towel. The

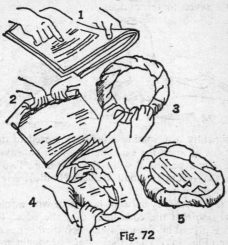

Fig. 72

nozzle of the syringe is rubbed with a lubricant (oil). Let some of the enema fluid run into a basin until the temperature is right (it should not feel too hot nor too cold on one's hand), then close the tap on the apparatus (or hold the container low) and insert. For adults the amount is two pints, for children about one pint according to size. When finished draw the nozzle out slowly and carefully. The fluid should be retained for at least five minutes.

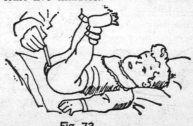

Fig. 73

OBSERVING THE PATIENT'S STOOLS (to tell the doctor). (1)

The number of times the patient's bowels are opened. Degree of firmness. (2) Contents, such as blood, pus or mucus. The color is very important.

OBSERVING THE PATIENT'S URINE (to tell the doctor). Color (dark, light, clear, or cloudy).

Most adults urinate five times in twenty-four hours, every time about seven to ten ounces.

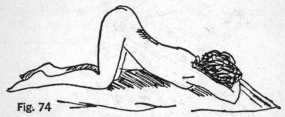

Fig. 74

Any difficulty in urinating must be reported to the doctor.

Specimens of urine for examination should always be taken from the urine passed first in the morning. Two to three ounces are sufficient (a small medicine bottle). Always write the name and date on it.

HOT COMPRESSES. A basin of hot water with a folded towel laid over it so that the ends hang over the edge. The actual compress is placed on the middle, which then hangs down into the water (Fig. 75). Then the water is brought to the boil, the compress is taken out with the hand towel and is wrung out while wrapped up in this (Fig. 76). Carefully wring out and then take the compress out with the tips of one's fingers, shake in order to get rid of surplus steam, then place carefully on the area of skin to be treated.

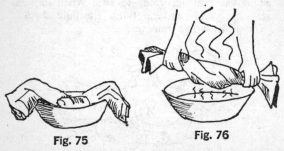

Fig. 75   Fig. 76

STEAM INHALATIONS. With a large carton (or firm paper bag), cover a pitcher of boiling water, containing a few drops of camphorated oil, and cut a square hole for the nose. Then the steam is inhaled as shown in Figure 77.

HOT-WATER BOTTLE. The correct temperature of the water is 110–150 degrees. Do not pour the water directly from the kettle, but from a pitcher, in which the temperature has been measured with a bath thermometer. Never place directly on the skin, always wrap a towel around.

Rubber hot-water bottles are, after use and having been dried, closed while inflated. In this way they last longer.

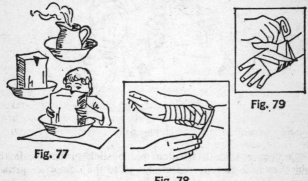

Fig. 77

Fig. 78

Fig. 79

BANDAGES. Two basic types of bandages are the roller bandage, commonly used to hold a sterile gauze dressing in place, and the triangular bandage, made from a large square of cloth. When using a roller bandage on a limb, work upwards in a spiral fashion (Fig. 78), keeping bandage flat against skin.

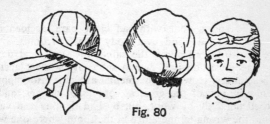

Fig. 80

Figure-of-Eight bandage. (Hand, leaving out the thumb.) See Figure 79. Can be used correspondingly for any joints. *Head bandage with triangular bandage* is shown in Figure 80. *Arm sling with triangular bandage,* Figure 81.

REMOVING A FOREIGN BODY FROM UNDER THE UPPER EYELID.
Gently pull the upper lid down and have the patient look
up. If you see the object, gently try to move it with the tip of
a clean handkerchief or a moist cotton swab. If you can not
see the object with the lid pulled down, turn the upper lid

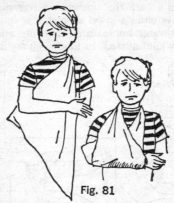

Fig. 81

back over a smooth wooden match stick or pencil. If the
object cannot be removed easily, go to the doctor as quickly
as possible.

16. Accidents and their Prevention

Everybody knows that with sufficient care accidents can
largely be averted. And everybody knows, from the place
where he works, all about the safety measures and devices,
often ingeniously devised, which safeguard against accidents
with machinery. However, the mental aspect is also important.
Tiredness is one of the greatest sources of danger, and this
is caused not only by work, but by bad lighting and ventilation and the wrong temperature in the room where one works.
Lighting. Direct sunlight is harmful while working. With artificial light there should be no dazzle or glare. However, the
light should not come in evenly from all sides as clear vision
is impeded by the lack of shadow.

TENDENCY TO ACCIDENTS

However, the human element in accidents goes much deeper than the mere external effects of over-tiredness, etc. There are people who are more prone to accidents than others. These are not lacking in presence of mind—they usually react particularly quickly. If one must describe a distinguishing characteristic for these people, one can at the most say that they are very impulsive and often act before they think. In addition to this impetuosity there is usually some form of rebellion against any kind of authority, so that even their own reason sometimes constitutes this sort of authority. But in practice the tendency towards accidents in a person can only be recognized by the fact that he or she has more little or big accidents than other people. This is apparent at an early age, so that one should bear this in mind when choosing a profession for the person concerned. Adolescents who have had a lot of accidents in their youth (regardless of whether or not they were to blame) should be discouraged from taking up dangerous occupations. In particular everything should be done to prevent them from becoming chauffeurs or truck drivers.

FIRST AID

WOUNDS. First stop the bleeding by applying pressure directly to the wound or at the nearest key pressure point. Minor wounds can be washed with soap and water and painted with

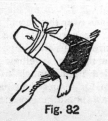

Fig. 82

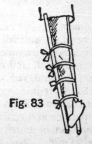

Fig. 83

a mild antiseptic. Larger wounds should be covered with a sterile dressing until a doctor arrives.

Superficial wounds (abrasions). Clean the wound with soap and water after bleeding is stopped. Abrasions are easily infected because dirt and germs are ground into the wound. If the abrasion is small, cover it with an adhesive bandage.

Injured limbs. When bandaging, these should be held up as the bleeding then becomes less on account of the fall of blood-pressure in the blood-vessels. Wounds near joints are always dangerous and require medical attention within six hours.

Arterial bleeding (the blood spurts out of the wound in jets). First measure:—Stop the flow of blood as quickly as possible by applying pressure directly to the wound or by pressing the main artery of the affected limb at a point between the wound and the heart; press the artery tightly against an adjacent bone. It may be helpful to bend the joint above the wound (Fig. 82).

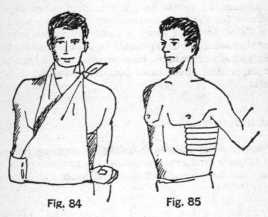

Fig. 84   Fig. 85

Next measure:—a very tight bandage over the wound. Only in severe cases should a tourniquet be applied to the limb (belt, braces, inner tube of bicycle tire). This should be done as high as possible and never too near the knee or elbow joints (danger of paralysis). This is pulled tight enough to stop the bleeding. It must not be kept on for longer than half an hour at the most. Then the tourniquet should be loosened for a few minutes and replaced if needed.

BURNS. Small burns should be covered with a cold wet bandage. Do not open burn blisters. No oil and no ointment.

With larger burns no bandage should be used. But protect the burn area from infection with clean sheets or freshly laundered towels. Keep the patient's head lower than his feet. Give him sweetened liquids to drink if he is able to swallow.

BURNING CLOTHES. Wrap the injured person tightly in rugs or blankets, throw him on the floor and roll him over.

STINGS AND BITES. Apply an ice pack to curtail spread of poison in tissues. Take antihistamines. Notify the doctor if symptoms become worse.

BLEEDING FROM LUNG OR STOMACH. The patient must lie absolutely quiet in shock position (head lower than the feet). Summon a doctor as quickly as possible. Do not give the victim anything to drink, but moisten his mouth with water.

EYE INJURIES. Bathe the eye thoroughly with fresh clean water, unless it is apparent that the eye has been penetrated by a foreign object. Bandage both eyes—always the uninjured one as well, as this prevents unnecessary eye movements. Take the victim to the nearest hospital or doctor's office as quickly as possible.

HEAD INJURIES. In every case, even if there is no visible external wound, lay the patient down flat at once. He must be kept quiet, all movements must be avoided, and he must be carried off carefully in a recumbent position.

ABDOMINAL INJURIES. Do not allow anything to eat or drink. Keep patient flat on his back, head lower than his feet. Transport him to the nearest hospital immediately.

FRACTURES. Keep the patient quiet and still. If there are external injuries the wound should first be covered with a bandage, then the injured limb should be fixed to splints—padded sticks or boards may also be used. The joints near the fracture must be bandaged to the splint in such a way that they cannot move (Fig. 83). Use broad bandages so that the edges do not cause pressure over the fracture site.

DISLOCATIONS AND SPRAINS. The dislocated limb must be handled gently. It is the doctor's job to put it back in position. (Sprains differ from dislocations in that although the joint swells painfully, there is no deformity.) Apply cool compresses.

BROKEN COLLAR-BONE (sport injury). Put the arm in a triangular bandage (see Figure 84).

BROKEN RIBS. Long strips of adhesive tape across the place where the pain is. Take care when sticking them on. There is a danger of internal injuries from the jagged rib ends. For the sake of safety the patient should be removed in a recumbent position. Lay him on the injured side in order not to impede his breathing with the healthy side (see Figure 85).

SPINAL INJURIES. The patient should be laid flat on something firm (board door removed from its hinges, or something similar). Mattresses are too soft.

ELECTRIC SHOCK. First of all, switch off the current. If the current cannot be turned off, do not touch the injured person until you are properly insulated and can safely remove him from the circuit. A long dry piece of wood or a dry length of rope sometimes can be used to separate the victim from the source of electricity. Rubber aprons, rubber shoes, window panes or china may provide insulation in an emergency. Do not touch either the circuit or the injured person without adopting considerable safety precautions. Otherwise one endanger's one's own life. In works where there are high-tension cables there are special instructions.

If the patient is unconscious, apply artificial respiration at once before taking him elsewhere. On recovering consciousness let him have plenty to drink.

BEING STRUCK BY LIGHTNING. Treat as for electric shock. If unconscious, apply artificial respiration immediately.

ACCIDENTS DUE TO HEAT-STROKE OR SUNBURN. Open the clothing. Lay in a shady place. Raise the patient's head and sprinkle him with cool water. If breathing stops, apply artificial respiration. Give cool water but no stimulants.

DROWNING ACCIDENTS. First remove sand, mud, or other obstructions (including chewing gum or dentures), from victim's breathing passages by wiping the inside of the mouth and throat with your fingers or with a cloth wrapped around the fingers. Begin artificial respiration immediately.

FAINTING (see page 59). If breathing stops, apply artificial respiration. If there is vomiting, turn the head to one side.

ACCIDENTS DUE TO EXPOSURE. Frozen limbs, nose and ears. If the frost was intense and the effects great, take the utmost care in touching the patient. Warm the patient in a warm bath or warm room but do not expose him to great heat. Give hot drinks. If the frozen parts of the body are still red or blue and swollen, the danger is not as great as if they are white. Medical treatment as soon as possible is absolutely essential.

TOTAL EXPOSURE (e.g. falling into snowdrift) with a low body temperature. Do not rub with ice or snow. It is best to warm the patient in a warm bath or warm room. If possible give the patient spoonfuls of a warm drink.

EXPOSURE AS A RESULT OF FALLING ASLEEP IN THE OPEN. This is possible, especially when intoxicated, if the temperature is below freezing. Vital body functions decrease. The patient must be rewarmed immediately.

FALLING THROUGH ICE. Do not run directly to the spot. Push ladders, boards, sticks or similar things along first in order to distribute the weight. The best thing is to form a chain of several people lying flat, each one holding firmly on to the feet of the man lying in front of him.

SPLASHING WITH CORROSIVE LIQUIDS. Rinse immediately with plenty of water. Remove clothes. If possible, rinse with dilute vinegar or lemon juice, after alkali splashes, and with soapy water if the splash was acid.

DRINKING CORROSIVE LIQUIDS. See page 128.

FOOT BLISTERS. Only large ones should be pricked. Use a sterile (boiled) needle after having cleaned the skin by painting it with iodine. Do not cut off skin. Use a clean bandage.

SWELLING OF A JOINT. Cool compresses. Keep the patient quiet.

FITS. Lay the patient on something soft. A soft gag (cloth) between the teeth. Do not use force to try and suppress the twitching.

Artificial Respiration

Because even people trained in first aid do not have the necessary experience, or the essential equipment, to distinguish whether or not lack of breathing is a result of disease or accident, some form of artificial respiration should be started at the earliest possible moment. The American Red Cross has determined that the mouth-to-mouth (or mouth-to-nose) tech-

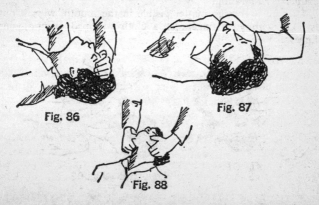

Fig. 86

Fig. 87

Fig. 88

niques of artificial respiration are the most practical for emergency ventilation of an individual of any age who has stopped breathing—especially in the absence of equipment or of help from a second person—regardless of the cause of cessation of breathing.

Any procedure that will obtain and maintain an open air passageway from the lungs to the mouth and provide for an alternate increase and decrease in the size of the chest, internally or externally, will move air in and out of a nonbreathing person. The mouth-to-mouth (or mouth-to-nose) technique has the advantage of providing pressure to inflate the victim's lungs immediately. It also enables the rescuer to obtain more accurate information on the volume, pressure, and timing of efforts needed to inflate the victim's lungs than are afforded by other methods.

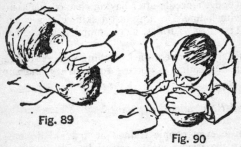

Fig. 89

Fig. 90

When a person is unconscious and not breathing, the base of the tongue tends to press against and block the upper air passageway. The procedures described below should provide for an open air passageway when a lone rescuer must perform artificial respiration.

If there is foreign matter visible in the mouth, wipe it out quickly with your fingers or a cloth wrapped around your fingers.

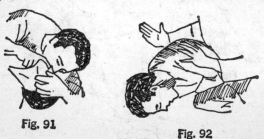

Fig. 91

Fig. 92

1. Tilt the head back so the chin is pointing upward (Fig. 86). Pull or push the jaw into a jutting-out position (Fig. 87 and Fig. 88).

These maneuvers should relieve obstruction of the airway by moving the base of the tongue away from the back of the throat.

2. Open your mouth wide and place it tightly over the victim's mouth. At the same time pinch the victim's nostrils shut (Fig. 89) or close the nostrils with your cheek (Fig. 90). Or close the victim's mouth and place your mouth over the nose (Fig. 91). Blow into the victim's mouth or nose. (Air may be blown through the victim's teeth, even though they may be clenched.)

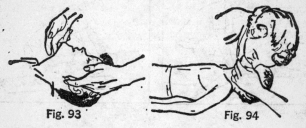

Fig. 93   Fig. 94

The first blowing efforts should determine whether or not obstruction exists.

3. Remove your mouth, turn your head to the side, and listen for the return rush of air that indicates air exchange. Repeat the blowing effort.

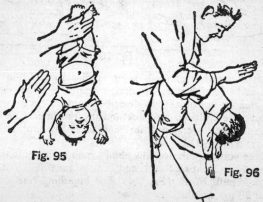

Fig. 95   Fig. 96

For an adult, blow vigorously at the rate of about 12 breaths per minute. For a child, take relatively shallow breaths appropriate for the child's size, at the rate of about 20 per minute.

4. If you are not getting air exchange, recheck the head and jaw position (Fig. 86 or Fig. 87 or Fig. 88). If you still do not get air exchange, quickly turn the victim on his side and administer several sharp blows between the shoulder blades in the hope of dislodging foreign matter (Fig. 92).

Those who do not wish to come in contact with the person may hold a cloth over the victim's mouth or nose and breathe through it. The cloth does not greatly affect the exchange of air.

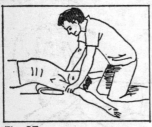

Fig. 97

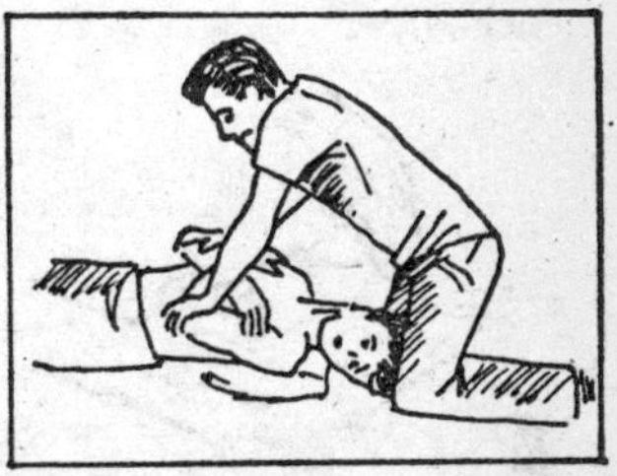

Fig. 98

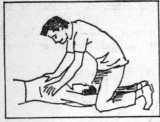

Fig. 99

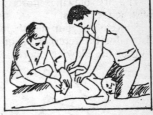

Fig. 100

Mouth-to-mouth technique as it applies to children embodies only a few changes. If foreign matter is visible in the mouth, clean it out quickly as described previously.

1. Place the child on his back and use the fingers of both hands to lift the lower jaw from beneath and behind, so that it juts out (Fig. 93).

2. Place your mouth over the child's mouth *and* nose, making a relatively leakproof seal, and breathe into the child, using shallow puffs of air (Fig. 94). The breathing rate should be about 20 per minute.

If you meet resistance in your blowing efforts, recheck the position of the jaw. If the air passages are still blocked, the child should be suspended momentarily by the ankles (Fig. 95) or inverted over one arm (Fig. 96) and given two or three sharp pats between the shoulder blades, in the hope of dislodging obstructing matter.

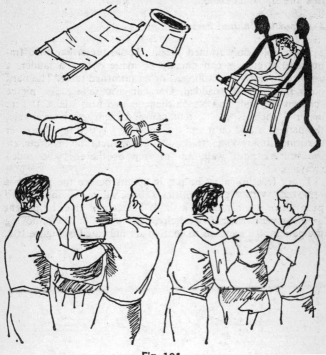

Fig. 101

The easiest manual method of artificial respiration is as follows:

Turn the head to one side. Put a roll of clothing or something similar under the shoulderblades. Kneel behind the patient's head, grasp his arms and carry out the movements as shown in Figures 97–100. After stretching the arms, there must be an interval of two seconds before the next time. When squeezing the chest one must not press too hard (especially with children) as there is a danger of causing internal injury. Repeat the movements ten to fifteen times per minute as regularly as possible. You must go on for at least two hours, unless a doctor decides that there is no hope.

If the patient's arms or shoulders are injured the artificial respiration is carried out by squeezing and releasing the lower ribs and upper abdomen.

Transporting Injured Persons

If possible, only trained people should undertake this. Improvised stretchers can quickly be made out of a ladder, a door removed from its hinges, or an upturned table. The hard parts must be well padded. One can also take sacks, pierce them at the ends and attach them to two firm sticks. If firm material such as sheets, tent canvas or carpets is available, the patient is laid on it and the ends are knotted together over a strong stick. When transporting a patient on a stretcher, the bearers must walk out of step or there is too much swaying.

Every fracture must be put in splints before the patient is removed. With slighter injuries (above all, when the injured person can use his arms) a single helper can give the patient a "piggyback" ride. If two helpers are available for removing the patient, the methods to be used are indicated in Figure 101.

INDEX